Specialty
Contact Lenses:
A Fitter's Guide

Specialty Contact Lenses:

A Fitter's Guide

Carol A. Schwartz, O.D., M.B.A., F.A.A.O.
Associate Professor
Optometric Center at Fullerton
Southern California College of Optometry
Fullerton, California

W.B. SAUNDERS COMPANY
A Division of Harcourt Brace & Company
Philadelphia London Toronto Montreal Sydney Tokyo

W.B. SAUNDERS COMPANY
A Division of Harcourt Brace & Company

The Curtis Center
Independence Square West
Philadelphia, Pennsylvania 19106

Library of Congress Cataloging-in-Publication Data

Schwartz, Carol A.
    Specialty contact lenses: a fitter's guide/Carol A. Schwartz.
—1st ed.

    p. cm.

    ISBN 0–7216–4747–2

    1. Contact lenses.   I. Title.

RE977.C6S38   1996   617.7′523—dc20   95–17561

Specialty Contact Lenses: A Fitter's Guide   ISBN 0–7216–4747–2

Printed in the United States of America.

Last digit is the print number: 9   8   7   6   5   4   3   2   1

To my husband, Robert Standish Billups,
with love
And to the contributors and friends
who made this book possible

Preface

This book is *not* like any other contact lens text on the market. It is not, nor was it ever intended to be, a scholarly tome. Rather, *Specialty Contact Lenses: A Fitter's Guide* is designed to be a quick reference for busy practitioners. We approached authorities in the contact lens field and asked them to imagine the following scenario:

> Your best friend is a vision therapy specialist whose partner does all the contact lens fitting for the practice. The partner is on vacation. A patient presents who requires a specialty contact lens. The fitting cannot be deferred until the partner's return nor can the patient be referred elsewhere. Your friend calls you (the expert) to guide the process of designing a type of unfamiliar lens. This is not the time for theory or a lecture on optics. Your best advice is needed to get your friend's patient fitted *quickly*.

The book that resulted is a compilation of their best advice; a book for practitioners rather than students. It is intended as a ready reference on unusual designs for those who already know how to fit standard contact lenses. There is much useful information in the appendices as well. In addition to basic spherical lens fitting, there are excellent discussions on lens care, modification, and complications. Legal aspects of contact lens fitting are also discussed.

Not everyone is lucky enough to have a friend who is a recognized expert in contact lens fitting. Through this book, it is possible to have the resources of those who are experts. We hope you enjoy it and that it proves to be of benefit to both you and your patients.

CAROL A. SCHWARTZ

Contents

Contributors

KEITH AMES, O.D.
Private Practice
Chillicothe, Ohio
Aspheric Rigid Gas Permeable Lenses

WILLIAM (JOE) BENJAMIN, O.D., Ph.D.
Professor, University of Alabama at Birmingham, School of
Optometry, Birmingham, Alabama
Bitoric Rigid Gas Permeable Lenses

EDWARD S. BENNETT, O.D., M.S.Ed.
Associate Professor and Chief, Contact Lens Service,
University of Missouri-St. Louis, School of Optometry, St.
Louis, Missouri
Back Toric Rigid Gas Permeable Lenses

TIMOTHY B. EDRINGTON, O.D.
Professor, Optometric Center of Fullerton, Southern
California College of Optometry, Fullerton, California
Contact Lens Management of Keratoconus

ARTHUR B. EPSTEIN, O.D.
Director, Contact Lens Service, North Shore University
Hospital, New York University Medical School, Manhasset,
New York
*Post-penetrating Keratoplasty Lens Fitting, Contact Lens
Complications*

NEIL B. GAILMARD, O.D.
Clinical Assistant Professor, Illinois College of Optometry,
Chicago, Illinois; Optometrist, Gailmard Eye Center,
Munster, Indiana
Frequent Replacement and Disposable Lenses

SUSAN M. GAILMARD, O.D.
Optometrist, Gailmard Eye Center, Munster, Indiana
Frequent Replacement and Disposable Lenses

GARY G. GUNDERSON, O.D., M.S.
Associate Professor of Optometry, Illinois College of
Optometry, Chicago, Illinois
Cosmetic Lenses: Special Purposes, X-Chrome Lenses

DAVID W. HANSEN, O.D., F.A.A.O.
Private Practice
Des Moines, Iowa
Presbyopia: Rigid Gas Permeable Bifocal Lenses

VINITA ALLEE HENRY, O.D.
Clinical Associate Professor, University of Missouri-St.
Louis, School of Optometry, St. Louis, Missouri
Extended Wear: Rigid Gas Permeable Lenses

NEIL R. HODUR, O.D.
Chicago, Illinois
Contact Lens Modifications

JANICE M. JURKUS, O.D., M.B.A.
Associate Professor, Illinois College of Optometry, Chicago,
Illinois
Toric Soft Lenses, Presbyopia: Soft Bifocal Contact Lenses

DAVID P. LIBASSI, O.D.
State University of New York, New York, New York
Lens Care and Dispensing

HARUE J. MARSDEN, O.D., M.S.
Assistant Professor, Southern California College of
Optometry, Fullerton, California
Orthokeratology

CHARLES ROBERTS, O.D., F.A.A.O.
Private Practice
San Juan Capistrano, California
Front Toric Rigid Gas Permeable Lenses

CRISTINA M. SCHNIDER, O.D., M.Sc.
Associate Professor and Director, Contact Lens Education
and Research, Pacific University, College of Optometry,
Forest Grove, Oregon
Extended Wear Soft Lenses

BARRY WEINER, O.D.
Private Practice
Ancillary Faculty, Wilmer Clinic, Johns Hopkins Hospital,
Baltimore, Maryland
Post-surgical Fitting: Refractive

MARIAN C. WELLING, J.D., B.S., A.S.
Faculty, University of Missouri-St. Louis, School of
Optometry, St. Louis, Missouri; Attorney, Legal Services of
Eastern Missouri, St. Louis, Missouri
*Questions and Answers About Legal Issues in a Contact
Lens Practice*

KARLA ZADNIK, O.D., Ph.D.
Senior Optometrist, University of California at Berkeley,
School of Optometry; Associate Clinical Professor,
Department of Ophthalmology, University of California,
Davis, School of Medicine, Davis, California
Pediatric Lenses

EDWARD ZIKOSKI, O.D.
Pennsylvania College of Optometry, Preceptor Program,
Philadelphia, Pennsylvania; Staff Optometrist, Saint
Lawrence Rehabilitation Center, Lawrenceville, New Jersey
Aphakia

CHAPTER 1

Back Toric Rigid Gas Permeable Lenses

Edward S. Bennett

The correction of high corneal astigmatic error, often defined as 2.50 D or greater, is best managed by either a back-surface toric or a bitoric rigid gas permeable (RGP) lens. Although fitting the highly astigmatic patient can appear to present a challenge to the practitioner, the fitting of any toric posterior rigid lens design is, in fact, little different than fitting a spherical design. This chapter addresses fitting back-surface toric RGP lenses. Much of this design information also applies to bitoric lenses. Other contact lens alternatives for the highly astigmatic patient include soft toric lenses and both spherical and aspheric RGP lenses.

NON-POSTERIOR SURFACE RGP TORIC OPTIONS

Soft Toric Lenses

Soft toric lenses should not be considered for the majority of highly astigmatic patients but should be considered in cases in which patients are highly motivated toward soft lens wear and exhibit no evidence of corneal distortion. The probability for consistent, high-quality vision correction with a soft toric lens decreases as the refractive cylindrical error increases, because rotation of as little as a few degrees can significantly affect vision performance.

Spherical RGP Lenses

Traditionally, the application of a spherical rigid lens in a highly astigmatic patient was deemed desirable, especially if good centration was achieved, simply because of the reduced expense and the perceived reduction in complexity as compared with posterior toric designs. However, when a spherical lens design is fitted to a highly toric cornea, poor alignment of lens to cornea is present. Typically, a dumbbell-shaped pattern with horizontal bearing and excessive superior and

1

inferior edge clearance exist in high with-the-rule astigmatism, and a bow tie pattern exists in high against-the-rule astigmatism (Fig. 1–1). Clinical reports have indicated that the areas of bearing can result in corneal flattening and possibly distortion over time, whereas the regions of excessive clearance can result in corneal steepening.[1,2] Other potential problems resulting from spherical RGP lens application to a highly astigmatic cornea include lens decentration, flexure-induced compromise in visual acuity, and corneal staining.[3]

Aspheric Designs

An aspheric lens design typically results in a more uniform fluorescein pattern and improved centration than does a spherical design in a highly astigmatic patient. In particular, designs with an elliptical back surface (i.e., progressive and bi-aspheric designs) exhibit good centration in patients with 2 to 3 D of corneal astigmatism. Spherical and aspheric RGP lens designs are indicated in patients with irregular astigmatism or corneal distortion (e.g., from corneal warpage, trauma, keratoconus) in whom posterior toric rigid lenses typically fail to provide (1) adequate visual acuity and (2) little, if any, improvement with aspheric lens designs to minimize subjective symptoms of flare.

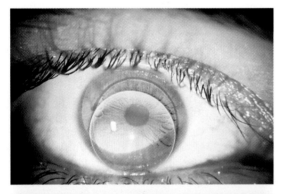

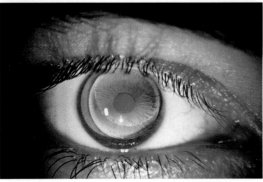

Figure 1–1. A comparison between the dumbbell-shaped fluorescein pattern of a spherical RGP lens on a 3D astigmatic cornea. *Top* can be compared with a back surface toric lens (*bottom*) on this same eye.

BACK-SURFACE TORIC
RGP DESIGN AND FITTING

Back-surface toric lens designs provide better alignment of the posterior lens surface to the cornea (Fig. 1–1B). Therefore, the aforementioned problems of corneal distortion, radical corneal curvature changes, corneal desiccation, and flexure are minimized and often eliminated. Good centration is also often achieved.

Base Curve Selection

There are numerous philosophies on how to determine the base curve radii for a back-surface toric lens. I recommend the design originated by Remba[4] (Table 1–1), although almost any toric base-curve philosophy will be successful. When determining the base curve radii, the tear-layer power will result in a change in power. To determine these values, the following formula from Sarver[5] is used:

$$F_s = F_f + K_f - K_s, \text{ where:}$$

F_s = the back vertex power of the contact lens in the steeper principal meridian (in air)

F_f = the back vertex power of the contact lens in the flatter principal meridian (in air)

K_s = the base curve radius of the contact lens in the steeper principal meridian

K_f = the base curve radius of the contact lens in the flatter principal meridian

The determinations of base curve radii are demonstrated in Example 1–1.

Table 1–1. Remba Back-Surface Toric Design

Corneal Astigmatism	Flat Meridian	Steep Meridian	Keratometry	Tear Lens Correction	Final Base Curve Radii
2 D	Fit 0.25 D flat	Fit 0.25 D flat	42.00 @ 180; 45.00 @ 090	+ 0.50	
3 D	Fit 0.25 D flat	Fit 0.50 D flat		+ 0.25 =	41.75 @ 180; 44.50 @ 090
4 D	Fit 0.25 D flat	Fit 0.75 D flat			
5 D	Fit 0.50 D flat	Fit 0.75 D flat			

Adapted from Remba MJ, Contact lenses and the astigmatic cornea. Contacto 1967;11(2):3843.

EXAMPLE 1–1

Spectacle prescription: $-0.50 \ -3.00 \times 180$
Keratometry: 42.00 @ 180; 45.00 @ 090

According to the philosophy given in Table 1–1, the following base curve radii would be selected:

41.75/44.50, or via Sarver:

$K_f = 42.00 + (-)0.25 = 41.75$ D

$K_s = 45.00 + (-)0.50 = 44.50$ D

$F_f = -0.50 + 0.25 = -0.25$ D

$F_s = -0.25 + (41.75 - 44.50) = -3.00$ D

Final order (empirical): back-surface toric
Base curve radii: 41.75/44.50 D (8.08/7.58 mm)
Power: -0.25 D

Typically, with back-surface toric lenses, only the power of the lens in the flatter corneal meridian is ordered. The power in the steeper meridian is more minus than predicted in Example 1–1 because of an induced cylinder (discussed later) resulting from the back-surface toricity of the lens.

Induced Cylinder

The primary reason back-surface toric lenses are used in favor of a bitoric design in a minority of patients with high corneal astigmatism is the inability to achieve optimal visual acuity because of the problem of induced cylinder. Essentially, a back-surface toric rigid contact lens in situ induces a cylinder in the optical system designed to correct ametropia. The minus cylinder is the result of the difference between the refractive index of the contact lens (n = 1.47 to 1.49 in most RGP lens materials; 1.49 is used here) and the refractive index of the tear lens (n = 1.336). The exact amount is -0.456 times the back-surface toricity. The minus cylinder axis lies along the flatter principal meridian of the toric back surface of the contact lens. This induced cylinder rarely corrects and sometimes compounds the residual astigmatism.

The following contact lens conversion factors are important when determining the changes in power induced by a toric back-surface contact lens:

1. From back-surface lens toricity, as measured with the radiuscope, to contact lens cylinder power in air, measured with the lensometer, multiply by 1.452 (or approximately 1.5).

2. From back-surface lens toricity, measured with the radiuscope, to the contact lens cylinder power measured in fluid (on the eye or induced), multiply by 0.456 (or approximately 0.5).

3. From contact lens cylinder power in air, measured with the lensometer, to the contact lens cylinder power in fluid (on the eye or induced), multiply by 0.314 (or approximately 0.33 or one third).

4. From the contact lens cylinder power in fluid (on the eye or induced), to the contact lens cylinder power in air, measured with the lensometer, multiply by 3.19 (or approximately 3).

This concept can be simplified to a 1:2:3 principle (Fig. 1–2).[6] This principle represents a fractional component by which, if one component is known, the other two can easily be determined. If "2" equals the amount of base curve toricity verified with the radiuscope, "1" equals 1

Per Example 1
Keratometry = 42.00 @ 180
Refraction = −0.50 −3.00 × 180

        (no change at corneal plane)
BCR design (per Remba): 41.75/44.50
                or −2.75 × 180

1

1. Induced cylinder (residual cylinder on eye)
2. Equals 1/2 of back surface (radiuscope) cylinder or
   1/2 × −2.75 = approx. −1.25 × 180

2

1. Back surface (radiuscopic) cylinder
2. Equals −2.75 × 180

3

1. Cylinder power in air (via lensometer)
2. Equals 3/2 times radiuscopic cylinder and
   3/1 times induced cylinder or
   3/2 × −2.75 = approx. −4.00 × 180
   3/1 ×   1.25 = approx. −4.00 × 180

Figure 1–2. The 1:2:3 principle. (*BCR*, base curve radii).

divided by 2, or one half the base curve toricity; "3" equals both three times the "1" value or 1.5 times the base curve toricity. If the base curve toricity equals 2.75 D, the induced cylinder with lens wear is one half of this value or 1.25 D (rounded down from 1.37 D); the value verified with a lensometer is 4.00 D (rounded down from 4.12 D), or 1.5 times the radiuscope value.

In Example 1–1, the amount of cylinder verified with the lensometer is equal to 1.5 times the radiuscopic cylinder, or approximately -4.00×180. Therefore, the steep meridian of this lens would read -4.25 D (i.e., flat meridian $+ -4.00$), and the induced cylinder, which is confirmed by over-refracting the patient, is equal to "3" $-$ "2," or $-4.00 - -2.75 = -1.25 \times 180$. If a plus correcting cylinder of the same amount and axis is applied to the front surface, in this case $+1.25 \times 180$, a spherical power effect bitoric lens is created. This lens can rotate on the eye without affecting vision (see Chap. 4). This is a key factor in deciding between a back surface toric or a bitoric lens, because a bitoric design with the induced cylinder corrected on the front surface will verify with a similar cylinder for both the radiuscope and the lensometer, unless a significant amount of residual astigmatism is also being corrected on the lens surface. In most cases, a back-surface toric lens results in some uncorrected cylinder accompanied by a compromise in vision. The amount of induced cylinder can be reduced simply by decreasing the amount of base curve toricity. However, this is also contrary to the reason why a back surface toric is used—to provide an alignment fitting relationship.

Indications and Contraindications

Primary Indication. One primary indication for a back-surface toric rigid lens design is when the corneal toricity is against-the-rule, and the residual astigmatism is approximately 0.5 times the amount of back-surface toricity of the lens as measured with the radiuscope.[5] In this case, the induced cylinder corrects the residual. This is demonstrated in Example 1–2.

EXAMPLE 1–2

Spectacle prescription: $-0.25 \ -1.75 \times 090$
Keratometry: 41.50 @ 090; 44.75 @ 090
Base curve radii (Remba): 41.25 @ 090; 44.25 @ 090
Induced cylinder: $0.5 \times$ radiuscopic   cylinder = $(0.5 \times -3.00) \times$ 090 = -1.50×090
Residual cylinder: $-1.75 \times 090 - (-)3.25 \times 090 = +1.50 \times 090$

Contraindications. A back-surface toric lens is contraindicated when significant induced astigmatism is created, as described previously. It is also contraindicated in patients with irregular astigmatism, particularly when corneal distortion is present. In these cases, the lens design typically results in compromised vision caused by the optical differences between the lens and an irregular cornea. Likewise, an alignment lens-to-cornea fitting relationship is rarely achieved in these cases.

Other Considerations in Fitting

Lens Material. It is important to use a lens material that is manufacturer-friendly so that it is not difficult for an accurate, high-quality back toric design to be obtained. Often, but not always, depending on the laboratory and the specific material, this is a low-Dk material (i.e., less than 50). However, polymethyl methacrylate (PMMA) and very low-Dk lens materials (i.e., less than 20) are not recommended because they have the potential to induce corneal hypoxia.

Center Thickness. Typically, the center thickness is equal to that recommended by the manufacturer for the more-plus meridian of a spherical lens. If the back toric lens powers are −1.00/−4.00 D for a 30-Dk fluorosilicone acrylate lens material, and the recommended center thickness for a −1.00 D spherical lens of the same material is 0.18 mm, this should be the value ordered for the back-surface toric lens. A representative center-thickness table for low-Dk lens materials is given in Table 1–2.

Overall Diameter. A similar diameter is used with a spherical lens design. Typically, this ranges from 8.8 to 9.8 mm.

Peripheral Curves. Back-surface toric lenses can be designed with

Table 1–2. Center-Thickness Values

Power (D)	Center Thickness (mm)
− 6.00	0.13
− 5.00	0.13
− 4.00	0.14
− 3.00	0.15
− 2.00	0.16
− 1.00	0.18
plano	0.20
+ 1.00	0.22
+ 2.00	0.24
+ 3.00	0.26
+ 4.00	0.28
+ 5.00	0.30
+ 6.00	0.32

Adapted from Remba MJ. Contact lenses and the astigmatic cornea. Contacto 1967;11(2):3843.

spherical or toric peripheral curve radii. Typically, in lower amounts of base curve toricity (i.e., less than 4 D), spherical peripheral curves are used. One method of designing spherical peripheral curve radii is to simply add 1 mm to the average base curve radius value for the secondary curve radius; an additional 2 mm is added for the peripheral curve radius.[3] This is shown in Example 1–3. The refractive information is provided in Example 1–2.

EXAMPLE 1–3

Base curve radii: 41.25/44.25
Base curve radii average (BCR avg): 42.75 (7.89 mm)
Secondary curve radius: BCR avg + 1 mm = ~7.90 + 1 = 8.90 mm

Final lens order:

Material: FP30
Base curve radii: 8.18/7.63
Secondary curve radius: 8.90
Peripheral curve radius: 10.90
Power*: plano
Overall diameter: 9.2
Center thickness: .21 mm
Design: back toric

*The plano power was derived via Remba's base curve radii selection. With 3 D of corneal astigmatism, the flat meridian is designed 0.25 D flat; with a refractive error of −0.25 D present in that meridian, the final lens power is −0.25 + 0.25 = plano.

If the amount of base curve toricity is high, the application of toric secondary curve and peripheral curve radii should be considered. One method for designing these curves is the following:

Toric Secondary Curve Radii. Add 1 mm to the base curve radii. If the base curve radii = 41.00 D (8.23 mm)/46.00 D (7.34 mm), the secondary curve radius = ~8.2 + 1 mm, or 9.2 mm/~7.3 + 1 mm = 8.3 mm.

Toric Peripheral Curve Radii. Add an additional 2 mm to the toric secondary curve radii. Using the previous example, the toric secondary curve radii would equal 9.2 + 2.0 = 11.2 mm/8.3 + 2.0 = 10.3 mm.

Verification

The creation of a back-surface toric or bitoric lens design that exhibits both good optical quality and accurate base curve radii and powers is the sign of a good laboratory. To verify the base curve radii of any posterior surface toric rigid lens, the radiuscopic lens mount is rotated until one mire image comes into focus; that value is recorded. The focusing knob then is turned until the image that is 90 degrees away comes into focus; this value is recorded. Essentially, any back-surface toric rigid lens will have the same radiuscopic appearance as a warped lens. Verifying the power using a lensometer is straightforward. In cases in which no residual astigmatism is present (i.e., refractive cylinder equals corneal cylinder), the air power cylinder should equal approximately 1.6 times the radiuscopic cylinder.

SUMMARY

Back-surface toric rigid contact lenses are indicated in patients with moderate to high corneal astigmatism. Not only is good centration often achieved, but the alignment lens-to-cornea fitting relationship minimizes both radical corneal curvature changes and the possibility of induced corneal distortion. However, back-surface toric rigid lenses induce an astigmatism that often can result in compromised vision.

REFERENCES

1. Wilson SE, Lin DTG, Klyce SD, et al. Topographic changes in contact lens-induced corneal warpage. Ophthalmology 1990;97:734.
2. Wilson SE, Lin DTC, Klyce SD, et al. RGP decentration: a risk factor for corneal warpage. CLAO J 1990;16(3):177.
3. Bennett ES, Blaze P, Remba MJ. Correction of astigmatism. In Bennett ES, Henry VA (eds): *Clinical Manual of Contact Lenses.* Philadelphia, JB Lippincott, 1994;322.
4. Remba MJ. Contact lenses and the astigmatic cornea. Contacto 1967;11(2):3843.
5. Sarver MD, Mandell RB. Toric lenses. In Mandell RB (ed). *Contact Lens Practice.* 4th ed. Springfield, IL, Charles C Thomas, 1988;284.
6. Neefe CW. Prescribing torics: easy as 1:2:3. Contact Lens Forum 1981;6(3):59.

Front Toric Rigid
Gas Permeable Lenses

CHARLES ROBERTS

A prism ballast front toric lens is useful for fitting patients who present with significant refractive astigmatism and little, if any, corneal cylinder. Typically, the refractive cylinder in these patients is ≥ 2.00 D; the corneal cylinder is one half or less of that amount. A spherical lens fitted on such an eye leaves a significant amount of the astigmatism uncorrected, and the visual result would likely be unsatisfactory.

A prism-ballasted contact lens is fitted in the same manner as a spherical base curve contact lens, because that is what a prism ballasted contact lens is: a spherical base curve contact lens that incorporates a cylindrical correction on the anterior surface and utilizes a prism to stabilize the lens on the cornea. This contact lens typically has a prism with a power of 1.00 to 1.50 PD ground base down (Fig. 2–1); the resulting weight differential between the top and bottom edges holds the lens in place. If during a conventional spherical rigid lens fitting, it is found that corneal toricity is 2.00 D or less, and the patient exhibits a significant amount of cylinder in the over-refraction, which improves acuity, this design will be useful.

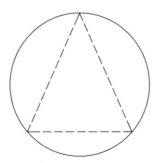

Figure 2–1. A prism is incorporated into a contact lens, making it a prism ballast contact lens.

It is the prism ballast and how the base–apex line is placed in relation to the axis of the cylinder that allows the successful fitting of front surface toric contact lenses. The purpose of the prism ballast is to orient the contact lens on the cornea so the refractive cylinder axis is congruent with a specific meridian. This is the only purpose of adding prism ballast to the contact lens, although it may aid somewhat in centering a high-riding contact lens. By adding a base-down prism, a weight is created in the lower part of the contact lens. In most cases, the contact lens rotates approximately 20 degrees toward the nasal side of the cornea (Fig. 2–2). The base–apex line of the right contact lens rotates in a counterclockwise direction, so that the apex of the prism comes to rest at 110 degrees. The base–apex line of the left contact lens rotates in a clockwise direction, so that the apex of the prism is positioned at 70 degrees (Fig. 2–3).

The nasal rotation of the contact lens is due to the action of the lower eyelid. On blinking, the lower lid makes a spasmodic horizontal movement toward the nose. The base of the prism, which is thick and proximal to the lower lid margin, is pushed upward and to the nasal side. This lid action exerts pressure on the contact lens until the movement ceases, after which the lens can fall back to the normal resting position (Fig. 2–4).

Because of various factors such as the eyelid configuration, the location of the eyelid, the eyelid tightness, and the forcefulness of the blink, the base–apex line of the contact lens may not completely return to the 6-o'clock position. The lens can remain nasally displaced from 15

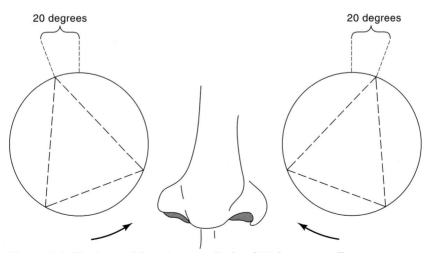

20 degrees   20 degrees

Figure 2–2. The bases of the prisms are displaced 20 degrees nasally.

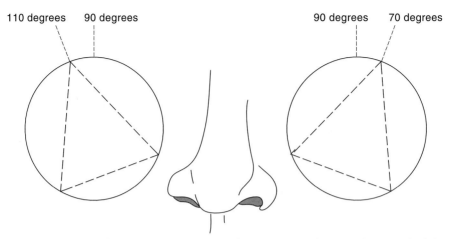

Figure 2–3. The right contact lens base–apex line is positioned at 110 degrees. The left contact lens base–apex line is positioned at 70 degrees.

to 20 degrees. To compensate for this displacement, the lens is often fabricated so that the base of the prism is displaced 10 to 15 degrees nasally from the vertical meridian. The purpose of this displacement is to rotate the contact lens so that it resists the forces exerted by the eyelids and recovers its orientation more quickly after the blink. The base–apex line of the prism ballast contact lens is marked by the

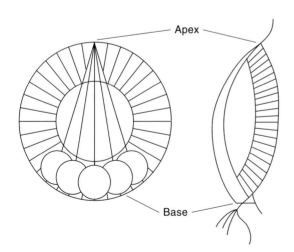

Figure 2–4. The pendulum effect.

manufacturer with depression dots or ultraviolet ink for easy identification. One dot identifies the apex, whereas another dot identifies the base of the prism (Fig. 2–5).

To measure the orientation of a prism ballast contact lens, a line is drawn across the diameter of an ophthalmic trial lens using a wax crayon or white ink visible in dim illumination or under ultraviolet light. This trial lens is inserted into a trial frame, which the patient wears over the diagnostic contact lens (Fig. 2–6). By reducing room illumination and using a Burton lamp or other ultraviolet light source, the placement of the base–apex line of the prism ballast diagnostic contact lens in relation to the diameter line is superimposed on the base–apex line of the prism ballast contact lens to determine rotation movement (RM) (Fig. 2–7). The position of the base–apex line is determined by observing the placement of the ophthalmic trial lens on the compass of the trial frame (Fig. 2–8). The trial frame is removed, and over-refraction is performed.

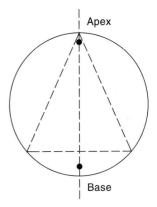

Figure 2–5. Large dots identify the ends of the base–apex line.

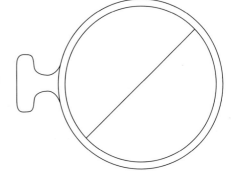

Figure 2–6. A scribed line identifies the diameter line of an ophthalmic trial lens.

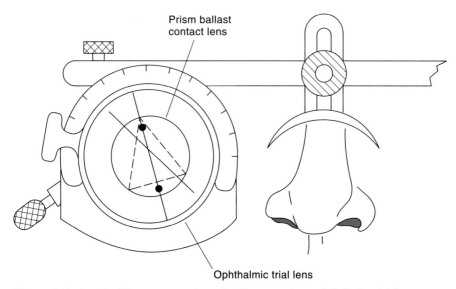

Figure 2–7. A scribed line appears along the diameter of an ophthalmic trial lens.

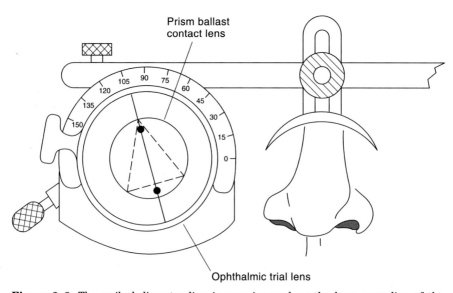

Figure 2–8. The scribed diameter line is superimposed on the base–apex line of the contact lens. The scribed diameter line is positioned at 105 degrees.

ORDERING THE LENS

In all probability, the contact lens fitter rarely has the specific diagnostic prism ballast contact lens required. When this is the case, a spherical base curve, non–prism ballast contact is placed on the eye, and over-refraction is performed over the diagnostic contact lens.

The total power of the prism ballast contact lens (RX_{cl}) is the sum of the power of the diagnostic contact lens (RX_{dx}) and the over-refraction (OR).

$$RX_{cl} = RX_{dx} + OR$$

The amount of rotation of the prism ballast contact lens, or RM, is the algebraic difference between the 90-degree vertical meridian and the point of rest of the base–apex line (BAL). The customary procedure is to maintain the base–apex line at the 90-degree meridian. The prescription axis is adjusted for the amount of nasal rotation, or RM. The adjusted cylinder axis (ACA) is the sum of the cylinder axis (A) and the rotational movement (RM).

$$ACA = A + RM$$

There is no absolute rule concerning the amount of prism required, but less than 1.00 PD will not provide a sufficient weight differential to maintain orientation against the rotational force of the eyelids. A high amount of prism power may result in a thick, heavy contact and is likely to cause discomfort. More prism power is required for plus-powered than minus-powered contact lenses because plus-powered lenses have thinner edges. For the same reason, more ballast may be required in small-diameter, minus-powered lenses. For plus-powered contact lenses with diameters of 9.0 to 9.4 mm and with a sphere power from plano to +4.00 D, the amount of prism power required to stabilize the contact lens is 1.00 to 1.25 PD. For minus-powered prism ballast contact lenses in the same range, 1.25 to 1.50 PD is required for stabilization. When the power is greater than ±4.00 D, the prism should be increased to 1.50 to 1.75 PD.

Table 2–1. Prism Ballast Power Selection

Contact Lens Power	Prism Ballast Power	Contact Lens Power	Prism Ballast Power
plano	1.25	plano	1.00
−1.00	1.25	+1.00	1.00
−2.00	1.25	+2.00	1.00
−3.00	1.50	+3.00	1.25
−4.00	1.50	+4.00	1.25

Adding prism ballast to a contact lens with 8.8 mm total diameter results in less mass than adding it to a contact lens with 10.5 mm total diameter (Fig. 2–9). Both contact lenses have the same amount of prism ballast, but they will not move in the same manner. If all other contact parameters are the same, the larger contact lens will drop more quickly and forcibly onto the lower eyelid after the blink. Remember, prism ballast is prescribed only to orient a contact lens on the cornea and not to correct a high-riding lens. Prism ballast also can be combined with multifocal contact lens designs to reduce rotation and provide additional stability.

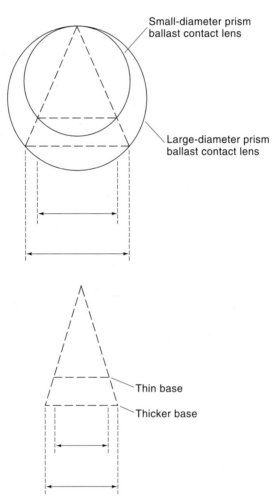

Figure 2–9. A large-diameter prism ballast contact lens will have a larger base and therefore a larger mass than a smaller-diameter lens. As a result, these lenses will move on the eye in different ways, even though they have the same amount of prism ballast.

There is some concern among contact lens practitioners that prism ballast should not be used monocularly. These fitters believe that both contact lenses must have identical prism so the apparent displacement of the visual field is the same for both eyes. Generally, this is not the case. If a monocular front toric patient complains of eye strain, headache, or asthenopia, however, a spherical prism ballast lens can be ordered for the other eye.

If the contact lens has too much weight, it will ride low on the cornea, possibly on the lower lid, and will not move up during the blink. In this case, the tear pump will not be initiated, thereby preventing the exchange of the tear pool from under the contact lens. This may compromise the cornea and cause edema or discomfort. If the prism ballast contact lens does not move, it is advisable to use a flatter-than-K fitting relationship to obtain better movement. Alternatively, a peripheral curve that is flatter or wider than what might otherwise be considered ideal can be used to increase movement.

The edge of the contact lens should be tapered from the front (anterior) surface to the back (posterior) surface to avoid inferior peripheral staining. If tapering does not eliminate peripheral staining, it may be overcome by using a larger-diameter lens.

Truncation may help to prevent the contact lens from rotating beyond its intended position and to provide additional stability. The contact lens should lift slightly with the blink and then settle so that the truncation aligns with the lower eyelid margin. The truncation is most effective if the position of the lower eyelid is normal (i.e., at the limbal area) or slightly high (i.e., above the limbal area). If the lower eyelid is too low (i.e., below the limbal area), the contact lens will not be maintained on the visual axis.

If truncation is used, the bottom of the truncation must be well polished and the edges rounded to minimize the possibility of discom-

Table 2-2. Base Curve Selection

Corneal Toricity (Δk)	Flat Corneal Meridian (K_F)
0	Fit flat by 0.50 D
0.25	Fit flat by 0.25 D
0.50	Fit on flat K
0.75	Fit steep by 0.25 D
1.00	Fit steep by 0.33 D
1.25	Fit steep by 0.42 D
1.50	Fit steep by 0.50 D
1.75	Fit steep by 0.58 D
2.00	Fit steep by 0.67 D

If the corneal toricity is equal to or greater than 2.25 D, then the contact lens of choice is a toric base curve contact lens.

fort. When using a truncated prism ballast contact lens, the vertical diameter should extend about 1.0 mm beyond the superior pupil. The range of the vertical measurement is from 8.6 to 9.2 mm; 9.0 mm is average. The horizontal measurement is 9.0 to 9.6 mm; 9.4 mm is average. The horizontal diameter is 0.4 mm greater than the vertical diameter.

The center thickness of a prism ballast contact lens (CT_{bal}) is the center thickness required to achieve a 0.12-mm apex edge thickness of an uncut contact lens, plus one half of the prism ballast base thickness. The center thickness values are obtained by consulting a center thickness table. Generally, the laboratory computes this value. Fitters who wish to compute center thickness can use the following formula: The formula for the thickness of the prism base is

$$t_b = (p)\,(d) \div 49$$

Where t_b is the thickness of the base of the prism in millimeters, p is the power of the prism in diopters, and d is the contact lens diameter in millimeters.

$$CT_{bal} = (CT) + (t_b/2)$$

Additional edge thickness tends to hold the superior eyelid away from the cornea on the blink and allows the cornea to dry, resulting in peripheral corneal staining.

Table 2–3. Approximate Standard Center Thickness for Plus and Minus Lenses*

	Lens Diameter				
Refractive Power	7.5 to 8.0 mm	8.1 to 8.5 mm	8.6 to 9.0 mm	9.1 to 9.5 mm	9.6 to 10.00 mm
−1.00 to −1.87 D	0.16 mm	0.17 mm	0.18 mm	0.20 mm	0.22 mm
−2.00 to −2.87 D	0.15 mm	0.16 mm	0.17 mm	0.18 mm	0.19 mm
−3.00 to −3.87 D	0.14 mm	0.15 mm	0.16 mm	0.16 mm	0.17 mm
−4.00 to −4.87 D	0.13 mm	0.14 mm	0.15 mm	0.15 mm	0.16 mm
−5.00 to −5.87 D	0.13 mm	0.13 mm	0.14 mm	0.14 mm	0.15 mm
−6.00 to −6.87 D	0.12 mm	0.12 mm	0.13 mm	0.13 mm	0.14 mm
−7.00 and over	0.11 mm	0.11 mm	0.12 mm	0.12 mm	0.13 mm
+1.00 to +1.87 D	0.19 mm	0.20 mm	0.22 mm	0.23 mm	0.25 mm
+2.00 to +2.87 D	0.21 mm	0.22 mm	0.24 mm	0.26 mm	0.28 mm
+3.00 to +3.87 D	0.22 mm	0.24 mm	0.26 mm	0.28 mm	0.31 mm

* If computed center thickness for a standard-thickness minus-powered lens is less than 0.13 mm, an anterior lenticular construction with a 0.13-mm center thickness can be considered. The anterior optic zone is 0.5 mm larger than the posterior optic zone. If ultrathin lenses are desired, 0.03 mm is subtracted from the value in the table.

The total diameter of front toric lenses is typically 8.8 to 9.2 mm; 9.0 mm is average. If the lens is to be truncated, a vertical measurement of 8.8 to 9.2 mm and a horizontal measurement of 9.2 to 9.6 mm (i.e., a truncation height of 0.4 mm) are normal. The optical zone diameter is 7.2 to 7.6 mm; the average is 7.4 mm.

EXAMPLE 2-1

The following example illustrates the steps required to design a prism ballast front surface toric contact lens.

- The patient's right eye has keratometry values of 45.00 @ 90 and 44.00 @ 180.
- The spectacle prescription is −3.50 −3.00 × 180.
- The power of the diagnostic contact lens is −2.00 with a base curve of 44.00 (7.67 mm), 1.25 PD base down.

The diagnostic contact lens is placed on the right eye and time is given for it to stabilize. A trial frame with a marked ophthalmic trial lens is placed over the diagnostic contact lens. The diameter line of the trial lens is aligned over the base–apex line of the diagnostic contact lens, and its placement is observed on the trial frame reticule.

The placement of the diameter line (i.e., BAL) of the ophthalmic trial lens is found to be 100 degrees.

RM = 90 degrees − BAL
RM = 90 degrees − 100 degrees
RM = 10 degrees

The trial frame is removed, and OR is performed. The result of the OR is:

OR = −1.50 −2.50 × 180

The power of the contact lens is the power of the diagnostic contact lens added to the power of the OR.

$RX_{cl} = RX_{dx} + OR$
$RX_{dx} = -2.00$
$+ \text{ OR } -1.50 \ -2.50 \times 180$
$\overline{RX_{cl} \quad -3.50 \ -2.50 \times 180}$

The cylinder axis must be adjusted to reflect the nasal rotation (i.e., RM) of the diagnostic contact lens.

ACA = A + RM
ACA = 180 degrees + −10 degrees
ACA = 170 degrees

One half of the base thickness of the prism (t) of the prism ballast lens is calculated:

$t = (P)(TD) \div 49$
$t = (1.00)(9.0) \div 49$
$t = 9.00 \div 49$
$t = 0.184$ mm

One half of the thickness of the base of the prism is added to the center thickness of a conventional contact lens. The CT of a conventional contact lens with a power of -3.50 is 0.15 mm.

$CT_{bal} = CT + (t/2)$
$CT_{bal} = 0.15 + (0.184/2)$
$CT_{bal} = 0.15 + 0.09$
$CT_{bal} = 0.24$ mm

The contact lens will have the following parameters:

Power: $-3.50 \ -2.50 \times 170$
TD = total diameter: 9.0 mm
OZ = optical zone: 7.4 mm
BC = base curve: 7.67 mm (44.00 D)
SCR/W = secondary curve radius/width: 8.47 mm/.4
PCR/W = peripheral curve radius/width: 11.50 mm/.4
CT: 0.24 mm

BIBLIOGRAPHY

Bennett AG: *Optics of Contact Lenses.* Association of Dispensing Opticians, 1969.
Bennett ES, Grohe RM: *Rigid Gas Permeable Contact Lenses.* Professional Press Books, 1986.
Bier N, Lowther G: *Contact Lens Correction.* Butterworth, 1979.
Creighton PC: *Contact Lenses Fabrication Table.* John R. Creighton, 1964.
Dabezies OH: *Contact Lenses: The CLAO Guide to Basic Science and Clinical Practice.* Little, Brown & Company, 1984.
Filderman IP, White P: Contact Lens Practice and Patient Management, Chilton.
Hanan PR, Morgan JF, Dabezies OH: *Nomenclature, Lens Design, and Fitting Parameters, Contact Lenses.* Little, Brown & Company, 1984.
Mandell RB: *Contact Lens Practice.* Charles C Thomas, 1974.
Roberts CM: *Optics of Contact Lenses.* 1988.
Stein HA, Slatt BJ: *Fitting Guide for Hard and Soft Contact Lenses.* CV Mosby, 1977.

CHAPTER 3

Bitoric Rigid Gas Permeable Lenses

WILLIAM (JOE) BENJAMIN

Considerable mystique has surrounded the prescription of bitoric rigid lenses; yet the basic principles that surround the fitting of spherical rigid lenses to slightly toric corneas (i.e., <2.00 D of corneal toricity) are merely applied to both primary meridians of back toric lenses in the fitting of corneas having greater toricity (i.e., ≥2.00 D of corneal toricity). More emphasis should be placed on the adherence to these basic principles in the case of back-surface toric lenses, because there is less room for error than with spherical lenses. The manufacture of back-surface toric lenses is more difficult and exacting; inaccuracies in the prescription are compounded by heightened financial and other consequences. Meticulous verification of back-surface toric lenses is a necessary requirement for successful prescription. Even so, the required greater level of attention to detail can supply a sense of accomplishment to the practitioner who becomes successful with patients for which optical correction is best undertaken with back-surface toric rigid gas permeable (RGP) corneal lenses.

Back-surface toric lenses are prescribed in cases with high corneal toricity when a spherical RGP lens will not ride appropriately on the toric corneal surface. Most corneas and especially highly toric corneas are with-the-rule, being steeper vertically than horizontally; the initial discussion is concerned with fitting with-the-rule corneas. Management of against-the-rule and oblique corneas is discussed later in this chapter.

The same guidelines apply to back toric lenses that apply to spherical rigid lenses in a lid-attachment fit. The ideal is a lens that is as close to central alignment (on K) as possible, and the lens must be large enough to facilitate lid attachment. The stated goal of an overall alignment fit is difficult to achieve with a significantly toric cornea.[1] As when fitting a spherical lens to a slightly toric cornea, fit the flat corneal meridian on K or a little steeper than K, and fit the steep corneal meridian somewhat flatter than K. The static base curve–corneal surface fitting relation should ideally be one of alignment or slight central clearance (i.e., slightly steep) in the flattest meridian.

21

The static base curve–cornea relation should be flatter than K in the steepest corneal meridian by an amount that allows some rocking of the lens during the blink to promote tear fluid exchange underneath the RGP lens.[2] The overall flat nature of the static fit permits lid attachment of the lenses for those patients whose upper eyelids are able to control the vertical centration of the lenses. Care should be taken so as to avoid an overly flat fit in the vertical meridian, because this creates excessive dynamic rocking, discomfort, and inadequate vertical lens centration because of aggressive lid attachment. If the vertical meridian is fitted too steeply, dynamic lid attachment is generally less effective, and tear fluid flushing is limited.

In general, therefore, prescribe back toric lenses to fit about two thirds to three fourths of the corneal toricity and slightly steeper than K in the flatter horizontal meridian. It is necessary that at least 2.00 D of corneal toricity be present so that the toric back surface can match the cornea to align the optical power meridians in the correct axis and to justify the additional effort and cost of back toric RGP lenses over spherical RGP lenses in terms of enhanced vision and comfort. The static fluorescein pattern of such a lens will have slight central clearance horizontally (slight fluorescence) and will have two zones of slight touch (minimum fluorescence) on the cornea in the horizontal periphery of the optic zone. There will be some tear fluid pooling (significant fluorescence) underneath the static lens superiorly and especially inferiorly in the mid-periphery and periphery of the optic zone (Fig. 3–1). It is important to ensure that the horizontal pattern has slight central clearance if so desired. In the presence of significant tear fluid pooling above and below, the relative lack of

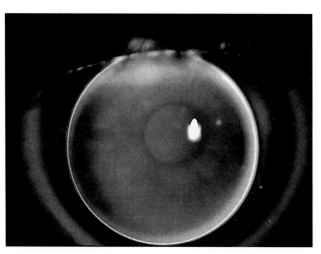

Figure 3–1. A static lid-attachment fit on a with-the-rule cornea showing slight central clearance horizontally and pooling above and below in the steep vertical meridian.

fluorescence horizontally may induce the practitioner to falsely recognize the horizontal pattern as being in alignment or even slightly flat. In some cases, the practitioner may actually want the horizontal pattern to be in alignment or slightly flat across the entire optic zone to obtain greater lid attachment.

As in the case of a spherical RGP lens, dynamic lens centration of a back-surface toric lens is brought about by steepening the overall base curve–cornea relation when an interpalpebral fit is required. In these instances, the full corneal toricity may be prescribed in the posterior surface of a lens having a small optic zone and overall diameter so as to effect vertical lens centration over the apex of the cornea. Prescription of the full corneal cylinder on a with-the-rule cornea will allow the eyelid to slide more easily over the upper lens edge to enhance comfort, reduce vertical movement of the lens on the blink, and to avoid pushing the lens inferiorly on the cornea.

The necessity for an interpalpebral fit incurs the costs of incomplete tear flushing during the blink and less comfort due to blinking over the exposed upper edge of the contact lens. Prescription of full corneal toricity requires more minus power in the steep meridian, thus reducing the supply of oxygen through the higher-minus periphery to the cornea. Fortunately, the oxygen capabilities of RGP materials have greatly increased over the last 10 years,[3] such that incorporation of refractive power should have a less adverse impact on corneal physiology than in the past.[4,5] These newer materials allow the cornea to be more forgiving when optimum tear fluid exchange is not attained.

DIAGNOSTIC SESSION

The first order of business when prescribing a bitoric RGP lens is to hold a diagnostic session to arrive at the back-surface design necessary for optimal lens performance. It is of even more importance in comparison to the fitting of spherical RGP lenses that the evaluation be performed with diagnostic RGP lenses on the eye so that your best educated guess of the proper lens geometry can be ascertained. The cornea is steepest centrally and usually flattens peripherally, but the degree of flattening varies from meridian to meridian and from eye to eye.

The amount and axis of corneal toricity change from the center to the periphery of the cornea. There is no guarantee, for instance, that a cornea having 3.00 D of with-the-rule astigmatism according to keratometry will be 3.00 D in the periphery, or even with-the-rule, for that matter. The central cornea is an irregular surface, although regularity is assumed for purposes of optical correction, and the degree of irregularity increases into the periphery. Therefore, the amount of back-surface toricity that an eye requires must be determined by assessment of the static and dynamic fluorescein patterns of at least one diagnostic rigid contact lens. It is very important that the parameters of the diagnostic lens be accurately verified before proceeding with the diagnostic session.

If You Have Only a Spherical RGP Fitting Set

With a set of spherical lenses, you would select a diagnostic lens in the same way that you would select a diagnostic lens for a spherical RGP lens fitting. The base curve (BC) should be approximately equal, in diopters, to the flat K reading plus 20% of the corneal toricity. The overall diameter (OAD) and optic zone diameter (OZD) of the diagnostic lens should be large enough to attach to the upper lid. A lens with an OAD of 9.5 mm and an OZD of 8.1 mm would probably be appropriate. A smaller lens having an OAD of 9.0 mm and an OZD of 7.8 mm is appropriate in some cases, depending on the corneal diameter, pupil diameter, and upper lid anatomy. If fitting interpalpebrally, use a steeper base curve 9.0-mm diameter lens. Ideally, the refractive power of the diagnostic lens should approximate that of the final prescription. If the diagnostic lens is of significantly different power than that which will be worn by the patient, adjust the lens design according to how you believe incorporation of the final lens power will affect the performance of the final lens.

The basic idea is to place on the eye a representative spherical lens that is close to the appropriate diameter and base curve of the spherical lens you might prescribe if toric lenses were not available. The next step is to assess the static base curve–cornea fitting relation in the flat (horizontal) and steep (vertical) meridians to estimate how much flatter or steeper these two meridians must be fitted. The fitting relation of the horizontal (flattest) meridian is usually not difficult to judge, because the base curve of the lens is not far from the horizontal corneal curvature. Because the diagnostic lens has been chosen to be 20% of the corneal toricity steeper than the flat K, the fitter generally needs to flatten the horizontal base curve for the final back toric lens by a small amount (approximately 0.50 D), depending on the amount of corneal toricity. The diagnostic fit in the vertical (steepest) meridian will be significantly flat; therefore, the base curve selection for the final back toric lens will be much steeper than that of the diagnostic lens. In general, the fitter should steepen this curve by a dioptric value of about 50% of the corneal toricity.

Your best educated guess regarding the degree to which you will steepen this meridian according to the spherical lens fit that you have evaluated will be the factor that has the least accuracy concerning the back-surface design of the final lens. You should check the static and dynamic fluorescein patterns of the final lens when it is first placed on the patient's eye. This is especially true for the steep meridian, to see if you will want to further steepen, or even flatten, the base curves of the back toric prescription the next time you order a lens for that eye.

Do a spherocylindrical over-refraction before taking the spherical diagnostic lens off the eye. In cases of highly toric corneas, the cylinder within the spectacle refraction is substantially the result of corneal astigmatism, and only a minor astigmatic contribution comes from internal (residual) astigmatism. In many instances, you will find that the over-refraction yields only a small cylindrical component.

The cylindrical correction in the over-refraction should be equal to the internal (residual) astigmatism of the eye, but this concept is confused by the fact that so-called rigid spherical gas permeable trial lenses actually flex on toric corneas. The optics of rigid lens flexure has been presented in detail elsewhere, but in practical terms, flexure lessens the correction of corneal astigmatism by decreasing the minus power of the lacrimal lens in the steep meridian.[6] This effect creates an amount of against-the-rule refractive correction on with-the-rule corneas equal to the amount of flexure. As correction for internal astigmatism is generally 0.50 to 0.75 D against-the-rule, the result of flexure can be to underestimate the amount of against-the-rule cylinder showing through an "inflexible" spherical RGP trial lens. If the cylinder in the over-refraction does not match the predicted residual astigmatism, perform over-keratometry to see how much flexure is occurring. Because the back toric lenses to be ordered will match corneal toricity more closely, they will not flex as much as spherical trial lenses on the eye. Bitoric lenses usually do not flex much. The front surfaces of back-surface toric lenses are toric in nearly all instances; hence, the term bitoric. The implication is that over-keratometry cannot practically be used to verify the degree of on-eye bitoric lens flexure.

You may need to alter the overall diameter, the optic zone diameter, or both of the final contact lens prescription according to fit and centration of the diagnostic lens. To a large extent, selection of these parameters is influenced by the corneal diameter, pupil diameter, and eyelid anatomy. You normally will be able to do a good job of determining the toric base curves and powers of the final lens with a spherical RGP diagnostic lens if the corneal toricity is less than 4.00 D. Sometimes, you will have to order a second lens when you update your evaluation of the lens fit and over-refraction after the original lens is dispensed. If the corneal toricity is greater than 4.00 D, you will likely have to treat your original order as a diagnostic lens or fit from a set of bitoric trial lenses (discussed later). The theoretical maximum back-surface toricity able to be manufactured is about 10.00 D. Lenses below 6.00 D of toricity can be easily produced. Above 6.00 D, the laboratory may have difficulties. About 12 to 15 D of corneal toricity is all that can be corrected with RGP contact lenses, unless the toricity is concentrated centrally so that in the periphery, the lenses ride on portions of the cornea that are less toric.

Spherical Power Effect Bitoric Trial Lenses

Connoisseurs of back toric RGP lenses generally own one or two fitting sets of special spherical power effect (SPE) bitoric lenses. The front surfaces of these lenses are made to produce the same optical effect on the eye as does an inflexible spherical lens.[6] A refraction over a SPE bitoric lens yields the same result as does an over-refraction over an inflexible spherical lens having the same overall parameters as the flat meridian of the bitoric. SPE trial sets have back-surface toricities of 2.00, 3.00, or 4.00 D, and they make great trial lenses because it is possible to obtain an accurate over-refraction without worrying about how the lens rotates on the eye. When an SPE bitoric lens rotates on the eye, there is no in-eye cylinder power to rotate with it. A more accurate estimate of how to alter the base curves in the vertical and horizontal meridians to achieve the final lens performance desired can be obtained from the fluorescein pattern in comparison to a spherical trial lens. SPE bitoric lenses can easily be identified because the back-surface toricity in diopters is equal to the refractive cylinder of the lens measured in air with the lensometer.

When using SPE trial lenses for a lid-attachment fit, select a diagnostic lens that has two thirds or three fourths of the corneal toricity and a base curve in the flat meridian that is in alignment with or slightly steeper than that of the cornea. For an interpalpebral fit, select a lens that matches or is slightly steeper than the central K readings. Select a lens from the fitting set that is as close as possible to the predicted best fit. Because the SPE lens fits better than a spherical lens on a highly toric cornea, and because the SPE lens fits in a manner more representative of the final lens to be ordered, your estimate of how much flatter or steeper the two major meridians must be fitted to obtain the best final lens performance will be more accurate. This will be of even greater importance in fitting corneas with toricity greater than 4.00 D. Before taking the lens off the cornea, perform a spherocylindrical over-refraction. The SPE bitoric lens will be more comfortable than a spherical lens; as a result, the refraction over a SPE lens should be more accurate because of reduced reflex tearing. As with spherical trial lenses, the sphero-cylindrical refraction over an SPE bitoric lens in many instances yields only a small cylindrical component equivalent to the internal (i.e., residual) astigmatism of the eye.

Selecting the Peripheral Curves

Much has been said about the benefits of rigid lenses with a spherical base curve and toric peripheral curves versus rigid lenses with toric base curves and a spherical peripheral curve versus rigid lenses with toric central and peripheral surfaces. From a practical point of view, it is a rare cornea that is best fitted with spherical optic zone but requires a toric back peripheral zone. Such a cornea would have little toricity centrally and a lot of toricity peripherally. Likewise, it is a rare cornea that is best fitted with a toric central back surface but without a toric back peripheral zone. Such a cornea would be very toric centrally but have only minor toricity peripherally. All other highly toric corneas require a toric back optic zone and a toric back peripheral zone for best fit.

Follow the same empirically derived guidelines for toric peripheral curves as for spherical peripheral curves, maintaining the same difference between radii of curvature of the two primary meridians in the periphery as in the optic zone. In this way, the junctions between the optic zone, secondary curve, and peripheral curve are concentric and circular. Back surfaces are tri-curve designs in each primary meridian having an axial edge lift of 0.08 to 0.10 mm. If a computer program is not available, the axial edge lift may be approximated in each meridian by producing the secondary and peripheral curves according to Table 3–1.

If, when you assess the diagnostic spherical or SPE lens on the cornea, you see that the peripheral edge clearance is less or more than might be expected for the average cornea, either flatten (i.e., increase axial edge lift and clearance) or steepen (i.e., decrease axial edge lift and clearance) the peripheral curves of the final lens accordingly. Upon dispensing of the initial bitoric prescription, you may further assess the result of your peripheral curve selection and appropriately modify the prescription the next time you order a lens or lenses for the patient. An order form showing the data for two lenses prescribed in Example 3–1 (right eye) and Example 3–2 (left eye) is included in Figure 3–2.

Table 3–1. Approximating Axial Edge Lift

Lens Diameter (OAD/OZD, in mm)	Secondary Curve Radius	Peripheral Curve Radius/Width
9.5/8.1	1.0 mm flatter than BC	2.0 mm flatter than BC/0.2 mm
9.0/7.8	1.5 mm flatter than BC	2.5 mm flatter than BC/0.2 mm
8.5/7.5	2.0 mm flatter than BC	3.0 mm flatter than BC/0.2 mm

BC = base curve; OAD = overall diameter; OZD = optic zone diameter.

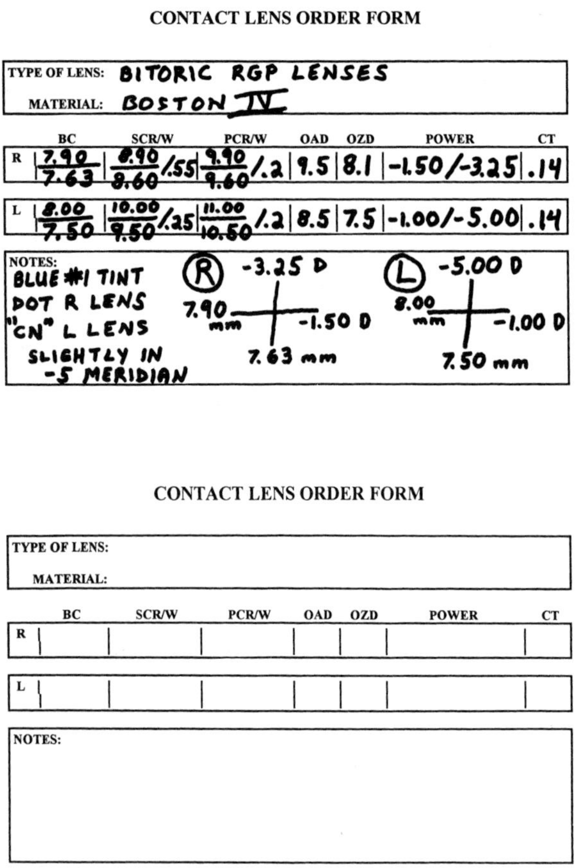

CONTACT LENS ORDER FORM

TYPE OF LENS: **BITORIC RGP LENSES**						
MATERIAL: **BOSTON IV**						
BC	SCR/W	PCR/W	OAD	OZD	POWER	CT
R	**7.90** **7.63**	**8.90** **8.60** /.55	**9.90** **9.60** /.2	**9.5**	**8.1**	**-1.50/-3.25**	**.14**
L	**8.00** **7.50**	**10.00** **9.50** /.25	**11.00** **10.50** /.2	**8.5**	**7.5**	**-1.00/-5.00**	**.14**

NOTES:
BLUE #1 TINT
DOT R LENS
"CN" L LENS
SLIGHTLY IN
-5 MERIDIAN

Figure 3–2. A contact lens order form filled out for the lenses prescribed in Example 1 (right eye) and Example 2 (left eye). The meridional refractive powers and radii of curvature have been spelled out below, in case the laboratory encounters some confusion concerning the parameters listed in the boxes above. The prescription in the left eye calls for a slight CN bevel to be applied to the periphery of the most-minus meridian.

CONTACT LENS ORDER FORM

TYPE OF LENS:						
MATERIAL:						
BC	SCR/W	PCR/W	OAD	OZD	POWER	CT
R						
L						

NOTES:

ORDERING THE FINAL REFRACTIVE POWERS

Bitoric rigid lenses obey all of the optical principles that apply to spherical rigid lenses. All that is necessary is that you pay a little more attention to refractive power in each primary meridian. Figure 3–3 is a version of a Rigid Bitoric Form 1040, which can be used to predict the refractive power of the final lens. You should already know the keratometry measurements of the eye being fitted, the pertinent parameters of the diagnostic contact lens, the central back-surface parameters of the contact lens to be ordered, and the spectacle refraction of the eye referred to the corneal plane so that the basic information section of the form can be filled out. Next, make two estimates of the final contact lens power (Final CLP) in both meridians. The first estimate is based on the spherocylindrical over-refraction (OR) performed over the diagnostic contact lens power (Diag. CLP) and the

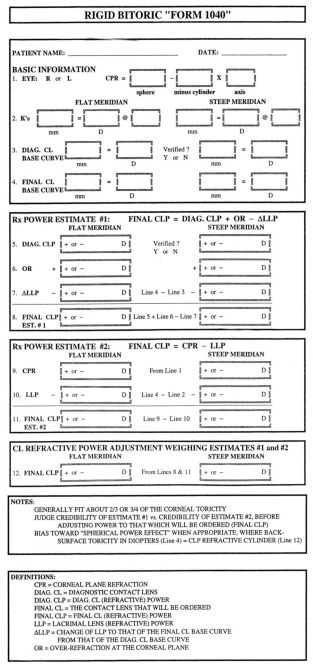

Figure 3–3. A worksheet for derivation of the refractive correction for rigid contact lenses, to be used especially in cases of back-surface toricity (bitoric rigid gas permeable lenses).

change in the power of the lacrimal lens in the final base curve compared to the base curve of the diagnostic lens (ΔLLP). Remember that a base curve change of 0.05 mm is roughly equivalent to a power change of 0.25 D. The second estimate is based on the spectacle refraction referred to the corneal plane (i.e., the corneal plane refraction, or CPR) and the lacrimal lens power (LLP) of the final lens as computed from the K readings and final base curves. The last evaluation of refractive power is a comparison of the first and second estimates, and prescription of the final CLP is based on your evaluation of the credibility of these two estimates.

EXAMPLE 3–1:

Spherical Power Effect. Look at Example 3–1 shown in Figure 3–4 with the basic information as listed in the upper section of the document. The corneal cylinder is equal to the refractive cylinder; therefore, we expect no internal (residual) cylinder to show up in a refraction over the diagnostic lens, which is a − 3.00 D spherical RGP lens with a base curve of 7.90 mm. An over-refraction of − 0.50 − 1.00 × 090 is obtained. The toric base curves selected on the basis of the diagnostic lens fit are 7.90 and 7.63 mm.

Proceed to compute the first and second final CLP estimates from the data accumulated and according to the established equations shown on the Rigid Bitoric Form 1040. Perhaps you identify the fact that some flexure of the spherical diagnostic lens accounts for the discrepancy between the two final power estimates in the vertical meridian, and measure over-keratometry readings to see if flexure does indeed exist. The over-K readings do indicate that the spherical diagnostic lens is flexing by 1.00 D. This would not be expected for a final back toric lens that would be more closely aligned with the toric central corneal curvature. Thus, the final CLP was selected to be closer to the second estimate in the hope that the back toric RGP lens will not flex nearly as much as the diagnostic lens.

Note that the final contact lens ordered in Example 3–1 is very nearly a bitoric lens having the SPE on the eye. The final lens power is only 0.25 D away from being equal to the back-surface toricity in diopters. When this lens rotates on the eye, only 0.25 D of cylinder rotates with the lens—a negligible amount that is unnoticed by the patient.

EXAMPLE 3–2:

Cylindrical Power Effect. Look at Example 3–2 shown in Figure 3–5 with the basic information as listed in the upper section of the document. The corneal cylinder is not equal to the refractive cylinder; therefore, we expect some internal (residual) cylinder to show up in a

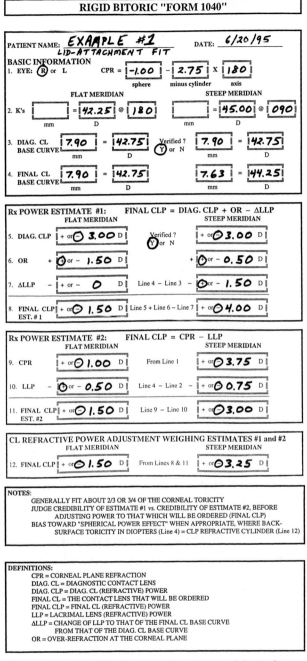

Figure 3–4. The worksheet as filled out for Example 1, a lid-attachment fitting on the right eye of a 2.75 D with-the-rule toric cornea. Between two thirds and three fourths of the corneal toricity has been prescribed in the back surface of the contact lens.

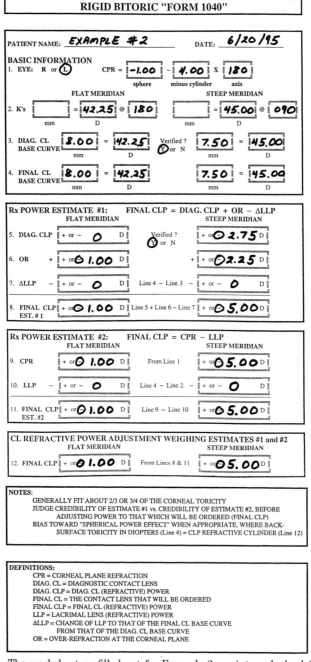

Figure 3-5. The worksheet as filled out for Example 2, an interpalpebral fitting on the left eye of a 2.75 D with-the-rule toric cornea. The full corneal toricity has been prescribed in the back surface of the contact lens.

refraction over the diagnostic lens, which is an SPE bitoric with power of plano/− 2.75 D and base curves of 8.00 and 7.50 mm. An over-refraction of − 1.00 − 1.25 × 090 is obtained. The toric base curves selected for the final prescription on the basis of the static and dynamic fluorescein patterns of the diagnostic lens are 8.00 and 7.50 mm for an interpalpebral fit in which the base curves match the central corneal curvatures.

Proceed to compute the first and second final CLP estimates from the data accumulated and according to the established equations shown on the Rigid Bitoric Form 1040. In this case, an uncommon instance occurred: both estimates came out the same! The final CLP is − 1.00 D with − 4.00 D of cylinder in the steep meridian.

Note that the final contact lens ordered in this example is a back toric lens with a CPE on the eye. The final lens power is 1.25 D away from being equal to back-surface toricity in diopters. When this lens rotates on the eye, 1.25 D of the cylinder will rotate with the lens, a significant amount that could be noticed by the patient. More attention must be paid to lenses that have 1.00 D or more effective cylindrical power, so that stable lens rotation is achieved to obtain the correct axis orientation for the effective cylinder.

Fortunately, corneal astigmatism accounts for the majority of refractive astigmatism in cases in which back toric lenses are needed, so that internal (residual) cylinder rotating with the CPE lens is usually small and relatively insignificant. In cases in which significant effective cylinder power could be prescribed, one technique is to bias the sphero-cylindrical contact lens power in the direction of the SPE and in this manner reduce the amount of effective on-eye cylinder.

It is beyond the scope of this chapter to point out the optical concepts that result in a peculiarity about the final contact lens in Example 3–2; the back surface of this lens corrects for all of the refractive cylinder in this case. Thus, the front surface of the lens must be spherical.[6] The final contact lens is a back toric/front surface sphere, technically not a bitoric lens, although it is nevertheless representative of the CPE. It is often unrecognized that the term back-surface toric, rather than the word bitoric, is a more accurate descriptor of the kind of rigid contact lens discussed in this chapter.

FRONT SURFACE DESIGN: ADJUSTING FOR INCORPORATION OF REFRACTIVE POWER

The final CLPs in Example 3–1 are in the low-minus range and do not greatly influence the fitting and rotation of the final lenses in comparison with the diagnostic lens, which is of similar power. Because the lens is nearly an SPE bitoric, an amount of unexpected lens rotation has little effect on the optical correction of the ametropia. However, when the refractive powers of the final contact lens will be different from those of the diagnostic lens, I generally make some educated guesses as to the manner in which the final lens may fit differently and try to compensate for any adverse effects by adjusting the design of the back toric lens. With respect to vertical lens centration, this compensation process is similar to that employed in prescribing spherical RGP lenses.

There are no great mysteries about the adjustments and compensations for final refractive power in the vertical centration of back toric lenses that are not covered in more detail in other chapters with respect to spherical lenses. In the past, however, manufacturers were not prepared to add a lenticular flange to the front surface of a bitoric RGP lens, although a flange could be produced for the rare case in which a back toric/front surface sphere was necessary (see Example 3–2). Today, on the other hand, lenses with front surface toricity can be manufactured in lenticular designs as a result of improvements in computer control and lathing precision. For a lid-attachment fit, minus lenses that are less minus than about − 2.00 D and especially lenses having plus power will likely require a lenticular construction in which a minus carrier is utilized to obtain greater lid attachment. The more pronounced the minus carrier, the more eyelid attachment is achieved, which vertically centers the lens. The lens also may be fitted slightly flatter than normal to enhance lid attachment.

In the case of an interpalpebral fit, lenticular designs with a plano carrier or minus carrier can be prescribed to decrease the mass and the thickness of lenses having powers greater than + 2.00 D. Lenticularization can help compensate for inferior lens centration as a result of excessive mass of full-cut plus lenses. Because the interpalpebral design may already have been steepened slightly to obtain centration of the diagnostic lens, additional steepening of the fit could result in tear fluid stagnation and poor central corneal physiology. A difference in the design of bitoric lenses compared with spherical lenses is that the fitter must contend with the powers of two primary meridians instead of only a single power for the entire lens. Thus, lenticularization may be required, even though the final refractive power of only one of the meridians may have an adverse impact on the manner in which the lens centers. Lenticularization has the added advantage of thinning the central optic cap, allowing more oxygen to the cornea under the center of the RGP lens, where tear fluid exchange is least efficient.

More often, however, contact lens practitioners encounter the problem of prescribing significantly more minus power than was in the diagnostic lens, so that the upper lid is expected to attach too aggressively to the final lens. Starting at about − 5.00 D, prescribe a CN bevel, which is actually a form of minus lenticular that is easy for the laboratory to manufacture. In Figure 3–2, the order for the left lens calls for a CN bevel. Laboratories, however, will determine the actual parameters of the CN bevel, and the practitioner will have to accept the consequences of not defining the front surface more specifically. I am willing to accept those consequences with lens powers in the − 5.00 to − 7.00 D range, but I become increasingly uneasy with the use of CN bevels as the refractive power rises above this range, especially when dealing with bitoric lenses. Above 8.00 D of minus power, specify the exact front surface design desired in the most-minus meridian, including the front optic zone diameter, junction thickness, and uncut edge thickness.

One caveat is that the specified uncut edge thickness of the lenticularized most-minus meridian must be the same or less than the predicted uncut edge thickness of the least-minus meridian before lenticularization. An example of a back toric lens order with these elements is shown in Figure 3–6 (Example 1, right eye; Example 2, left eye). The uncut edge thickness listed for the lenticularized most-minus meridians are equivalent to the uncut edge thicknesses of the unlenticularized least-minus meridians. If the edge thicknesses were specified to be lower than those of the unlenticularized least-minus meridians, the least-minus meridian would become lenticularized as well.

For the interpalpebral fit, the edges of non-lenticularized high-minus lenses are uncomfortable because they are thick. These lenses tend to move excessively during the blink and can be driven inferiorly on the cornea by the upper eyelid margin. A CN bevel or minus lenticular design can be prescribed to allow the lid to slide more easily over the upper lens edge to enhance comfort, reduce vertical movement of the lens on the blink, and to avoid pushing the lens inferiorly on the cornea. Lenticularization may be required even though the final refractive power of only one of the meridians may have a predictably adverse impact on lens centration or comfort. Minus lenticularization has the added advantage of thinning the periphery of a high-minus lens, allowing greater oxygenation of the cornea under the periphery of the RGP lens, which is of special importance in the meridian of most-minus power.

The edge of an unlenticularized bitoric RGP lens is of varying thickness around its circumference. This presents a greatly different situation than that of a spherical RGP lens. Unfortunately, back toric rigid lenses rotate on the eye in response to eyelid forces invoking the "watermelon seed" effect or the minus carrier effect. Bitoric lens rotation on the eye as a result of the equilibrium between these two

CONTACT LENS ORDER FORM

| TYPE OF LENS: **BITORIC RGP LENSES** |
| MATERIAL: **FLUOROPERM 60** |

	BC	SCR/W	PCR/W	OAD	OZD	POWER	CT
R	$\frac{7.75}{7.20}$	$\frac{9.00}{8.40}$/45	$\frac{10.00}{9.40}$/.2	9.2	7.9	-5.00/-9.00	.15
L	$\frac{7.80}{7.40}$	$\frac{9.00}{8.60}$/45	$\frac{10.00}{9.60}$/.2	9.2	7.9	-4.50/-8.25	.15

NOTES: **BLUE #1 TINT; DOT R LENS**
MINUS LENTICULAR IN MOST⊙MERIDIAN

	JUNCTION THICKNESS	UNCUT EDGE THICKNESS	FRONT OZD
R	.35	.22	8.0
L	.33	.21	8.0

CONTACT LENS ORDER FORM

| TYPE OF LENS: |
| MATERIAL: |

	BC	SCR/W	PCR/W	OAD	OZD	POWER	CT
R							
L							

NOTES:

Figure 3-6. A contact lens order form as filled out for lenses prescribed with a minus lenticular design in the most-minus (i.e., steeper) meridian. In addition to the usual bitoric figures, the exact parameters related to the front surface design are detailed in the notes below. In this case, the uncut edge thicknesses of the lenticularized most-minus meridians are the same as the calculated uncut edge thicknesses of the unlenticularized least-minus meridians.

competing effects can be seemingly inexplicable and may not be adequately predictable during the diagnostic fitting session. Although the optical correction will not be significantly affected by rotation of SPE or near-SPE bitoric lenses for the majority of bitoric RGP lens wearers, as noted in Example 3–1, visual performance will suffer for those patients wearing mis-oriented bitoric lenses with significant on-eye cylindrical power (CPE).

These rotations can be minimized by altering the periphery of the contact lens. Lenticular designs may be employed. However, when the final lens is dispensed to the patient, lid forces often rotate the CPE prescription enough to significantly disturb vision. An in-office modification procedure has been recommended for correction of the rotation of RGP lenses from that initially seen on the eye.[7] I often utilize another method of lessening the visual influence of off-axis effective cylinder: biasing the cylinder power of the final RGP lens in the direction of the spherical power effect (SPE).

HIGHLY AGAINST-THE-RULE AND OBLIQUELY TORIC CORNEAS

The thickest portion of the minus-powered back toric lens edge is situated superiorly, such that the minus carrier effect most often results when the upper eyelid overhangs onto a with-the-rule cornea by 2 mm or more. The lens is usually fitted flat in the vertical meridian, facilitating lid attachment and tear fluid flushing induced by rocking of the lens during the blink. If the refractive power of the lens does not allow lid attachment, there are ways to increase the attachment (discussed previously). If the lens attaches too aggressively there are ways to decrease the degree of lid attachment (discussed previously). However, the situation is somewhat different when prescribing for against-the-rule or oblique corneas.

Prescribing for the Against-the-Rule Cornea

If the base curves of a conventional back toric lens align with the appropriate against-the-rule corneal meridians, the thick portions of the minus lens periphery will be positioned horizontally in the interpalpebral space, and the thin portions of the periphery will be located superiorly and inferiorly. This probably will be excellent for an interpalpebral fit, because the upper eyelid should slide easily over the top edge of the lens with minimal effect on lens centration. In an interpalpebral fit we have prescribed the full corneal toricity, often in a slightly steep manner; therefore, the lens should not significantly decenter right or left of the flat (vertical) corneal meridian. In a lid-attachment fit, which is far more prevalent than the interpalpebral fit, the lid may do one of two things to the conventional minus back toric lens: force the lens inferiorly, as in the watermelon seed effect, such that the opposite of lid attachment occurs, or attach strongly to the nasal or temporal portion of the thicker lens edge and rotate the lens considerably off axis after the blink. The lens will also have a tendency to decenter right or left, away from the flatter vertical corneal meridian.

It is important to alter the fitting philosophy for lid attachment of bitoric lenses in patients with against-the-rule corneas. An alignment fit in the vertical (flat) meridian and prescription of the full corneal toricity in the horizontal (steep) meridian should increase the chances of lateral centration, but the beneficial rocking motion necessary for optimum tear fluid exchange will be lost. The fit is steeper in the vertical meridian than that for the equivalent with-the-rule corneal fit. We will therefore have to concentrate on lid attachment with plus and low-minus lenses by use of the minus carrier in a plus lenticular design. The plus lenticular design should also decrease the variation of peripheral thickness around the edge circumference of the lens, so that the lens is less prone to off-axis rotation and can be oriented primarily by the match between the toric back surface and the cornea.

If the lens is to be of high-minus power, there will not be as much lid attachment to worry about when fitting the against-the-rule cornea, if the least-minus meridian orients vertically. We can decrease off-axis rotation by prescribing a minus lenticular design, emphasizing its use in the horizontal (i.e., more-minus) meridian to decrease lid grasp of the otherwise thick lateral edges. Fortunately, bitoric lenses requiring significant effective cylinder are not as prevalent as those nearly exhibiting the spherical power effect. Therefore, corrections for off-axis lens rotation by prescription of special lens designs and by in-office modification as discussed previously are not often necessary.[7]

Prescribing for the Obliquely Toric Cornea

Assume the base curves of a conventional bitoric lens align with a flat meridian at 045° and a steep meridian at 135° on the obliquely toric right cornea of a patient. The thick portions of the minus lens periphery will be positioned superotemporally and inferonasally, and the thin portions of the periphery will be located superonasally and inferotemporally. In the case of an interpalpebral fit, it is likely that the upper eyelid will slide over the superonasal edge of the lens but not as adequately over the superotemporal edge. As a result, the lens may rotate or decenter inferonasally. The upper lid in a lid-attachment fit may do one of two things to the conventional minus back toric lens. First, the lid could force the thick, superotemporal lens edge inferiorly as in the watermelon seed effect, such that counterclockwise lens rotation occurs. The lens will have a tendency to decenter inferonasally below the flat oblique corneal meridian. Second, the lid could attach strongly to the thick, superotemporal lens edge and rotate the lens clockwise with blinking. The lens will have a tendency to decenter superotemporally above the flat oblique corneal meridian.

It is important, therefore, to alter the fitting philosophy for bitoric lenses in cases of obliquely toric corneas. An alignment fit in the flat meridian and prescription of the full corneal toricity in the steep meridian should increase the chances of lateral and vertical centration. The overall fit will be steeper than that for the equivalent with-the-rule lid-attachment fit, so we will have to concentrate on lid attachment with plus and low-minus lenses by use of the minus carrier in a plus lenticular design. As with against-the-rule corneas, the plus lenticular design should also decrease the variation of peripheral thickness around the edge circumference of the lens, so that the lens is less prone to off-axis rotation and can be oriented primarily by the match between the toric back surface and the cornea. If the lens is to be of high-minus power, decrease rotation by prescribing a minus lenticular design in the meridian of most minus power. Bitoric lenses requiring significant effective cylinder are not as prevalent as those nearly exhibiting the spherical power effect. Therefore, corrections for off-axis lens rotation by prescription of special lens designs and by in-office modification are not often necessary.

Prescription of Bitoric Crossed Cylinder RGP Lenses

Up to this point, we have been assuming that corneal astigmatism, internal (residual) astigmatism, and refractive astigmatism are of the same or similar axis orientation. This is usually a safe assumption, because corneal astigmatism and refractive astigmatism are often within 10 degrees of each other. A crossed alignment within this range would only lead to a small (i.e., <0.50 D of cylinder) discrepancy in calculations for refractive correction in the contact lens prescription.

In most cases of high corneal toricity, corneal cylinder is the largest contributor to refractive cylinder, and the influence of internal astigmatism is minor. Thus, even if the internal astigmatism was aligned at an oblique angle with the corneal cylinder, the visual effect of the internal astigmatism could be small. The cylinder axes of the corneal and refractive cylinders would still be similar. We proceed with the bitoric lens prescription, ignoring the fact that a situation of crossed cylinders exists, knowing that a small amount of uncorrected astigmatism probably will not be visually significant.

As a general rule, contact lens practitioners ignore the effect of crossed cylinders when corneal astigmatic correction and refractive astigmatism are crossed less than 10 degrees. It is a good idea to always compare the corneal and refractive cylinder axes at the beginning of a bitoric contact lens fitting to screen for more pronounced cases of crossed astigmatic components that could influence the prescription of refractive power.

As the magnitude of internal (residual) astigmatism increases, the alignment of the corneal cylinder axis and the internal cylinder axis becomes more critical. This is noted by the practitioner when corneal astigmatic correction and refractive astigmatism differ by more than 10 degrees. To the extent that they differ by more than 10 degrees, internal astigmatism is of greater magnitude relative to corneal astigmatism, or its axis of cylinder more obliquely oriented with that of corneal astigmatism. When the spherical or SPE bitoric diagnostic lens is placed on the cornea, significant residual astigmatism should be revealed in the over-refraction at an axis oblique to that of the corneal cylinder. If you add the corneal astigmatic correction calculated from the K readings and the residual cylinder from the over-refraction in the well-known, although complicated, manner necessary for crossed cylinders, the resultant should equal the refractive cylinder. A good lens design computer program has the capability of determining the results of crossed cylinders.

As in any other CPE bitoric lens fit, the effective on-eye (residual) cylinder must be added to the front surface of the correction for corneal astigmatism, which is essentially equivalent to an SPE bitoric lens. After all, if there was no residual cylinder, the optimum correction would, in fact, be an SPE bitoric lens correcting for only corneal astigmatism. The problem is that the axis of residual cylinder is oblique to the astigmatic axis of the toric front surface of the SPE equivalent. Therefore, the proper front surface of the final CPE prescription must be derived by adding these two crossed cylinder powers together. The primary meridians of the final toric front surface of the CPE lens will not be in alignment with the meridians of the toric back surface; hence, the term crossed cylinder bitoric lens. Provided the practitioner has the ingenuity to formulate a prescription in the form of a bitoric lens having toric front and back surfaces of different axes, modern lathing processes are able to manufacture bitoric crossed cylinder lenses according to the prescription.

SUMMARY

Prescription of bitoric RGP corneal lenses should be done with the knowledge that a second or occasionally even a third lens will be necessary before the eye is optimally fitted. The practitioner must be a little more meticulous about the details of the fitting, be more fastidious about verification of the contact lenses used for diagnosis and prior to dispensing, and make a larger educated guess about final lens powers and parameters in comparison to the equivalent spherical RGP fitting. In addition, if the bitoric lens power should deviate slightly from that desired, the practitioner cannot alter lens power in the office, as with spherical RGP lenses. Edge thicknesses can sometimes induce seemingly inexplicable lens rotations on the eye in response to eyelid forces, rotations that may not be adequately predictable during the diagnostic fitting session. For these reasons, on occasion it reduces the potential for practitioner and patient frustration to order back surface toric lenses on a per-case basis. It is a simple matter to avoid undue expectations by educating the patient in the more difficult bitoric cases: for instance, when against-the-rule or obliquely toric corneas also require significant effective on-eye cylinder (i.e., CPE). One of the toughest prescriptions in the area of contact lens practice is the bitoric crossed cylinder lens, especially if corneal toricity is oblique or against-the-rule.

Fortunately, however, there are several positive factors that work in favor of excellent vision with bitoric RGP lenses. The overwhelming majority of highly toric corneas are with-the-rule. This allows a fitting method that captures the beneficial aspects of lid attachment and allows plenty of tear fluid exchange. In most cases, the bitoric correction approximates the SPE. Thus, lens rotations on the cornea do not usually result in visual decrements. Even in cases in which significant effective cylinder is present to rotate with the lens, as in the CPE, the visual result is usually acceptable until a second lens can be received with adjustments made on the basis of the initial lens fit. The magnitude of internal (residual) astigmatism is usually minor in comparison to refractive astigmatism in cases of highly toric corneas, and it is the residual cylinder that composes the effective cylinder of a CPE lens.

Today, more so than in the past, it is possible to adjust the centration and rotation of back-surface toric lenses with plus lenticular and minus lenticular designs, because lenses with toric front surfaces can now be lenticularized. The oxygen permeabilities of RGP materials have risen so greatly that lens parameters promoting tear fluid exchange are not as critical as they once were, and the deleterious impact of lens design and refractive power on corneal oxygenation have been significantly alleviated. Therefore, the potential for success with bitoric RGP lenses has never been higher. To take advantage of this updated technology, practitioners must be versed in the art and science of rigid lens prescription and simultaneously be eager to take on challenges that entice them to break away from the soft lens mentality.

REFERENCES

1. Silbert JA: Rigid lens correction of astigmatism. In Bennett ES, Weissman BA (eds). *Clinical Contact Lens Practice.* Philadelphia, JB Lippincott, 1991, pp 1–42.
2. Mandell RB: *Contact Lens Practice.* Springfield, IL, Charles C Thomas, 1988, p 284.
3. Benjamin WJ: EOP and Dk/L: The quest for hyper transmissibility. Am Optometric Assoc, 1993; 643:196.
4. Richardson SS, Benjamin WJ: Oxygen profiles and contact lens design. Contact Lens Spect 1993; 8(3):57.
5. Benjamin WJ: RGP material selection strategy and the gel/RGP oxygen "gap." International Contact Lens Clinic 1993; 20(9&10):200.
6. Benjamin WJ: Visual optics of contacts lens wear. In Bennett ES, Weissman BE (eds). *Clinical Contact Lens Practice.* Philadelphia, JB Lippincott, 1991, pp 1–24.
7. Benjamin WJ, Borish IM: Presbyopia and the influence of aging on prescription of contact lenses. In Guillon M, Ruben CM (eds). *Textbook of Contact Lens Practice.* London, Chapman & Hall, 1994, p 830.

CHAPTER 4

Toric Soft Lenses

JANICE M. JURKUS

Soft toric lens fitting is no longer the challenge it once was. Better lens design and parameter availability have made the correction of refractive astigmatism with soft lenses easier than ever. Fitting soft toric lenses, as with any specialty lens, requires a step-wise, logical approach. There are five questions the fitter should ask and answer when prescribing a soft toric lens.

1. Does this patient need a toric correction?
The answer is yes if the patient's refraction has a cylinder power equal to or greater than one fourth (25%) of the spherical power. For example, if a patient has a refraction of $-0.50 - 0.75 \times 180$, he or she would benefit visually from a toric lens design, because the cylinder is the major portion of the correction. On the other hand, a patient with a prescription $-3.50 - 0.75 \times 180$ may have acceptable vision with a spherical equivalent correction, because the amount of astigmatism is only one fifth of the total power.

2. Which type of toric soft contact lens is appropriate for the patient?
Toric soft lenses must provide an acceptable physiologic fit and remain in a stable position, producing little, if any, rotary movement. Soft toric lenses are stabilized with either prism ballast or thin-zone design. In general, the prism ballast design is indicated for with-the-rule astigmats, because the thicker portion of the lens is in the vertical meridian (Fig. 4–1). Thin-zone design lenses, which have the thickest portion in the horizontal meridian, are somewhat more stable for against-the-rule astigmats (Fig. 4–2).

All soft lenses conform to the corneal curvature when on the eye. The less the lens has to bend, the more stable it is. The placement of the cylindrical surface on the front of the lens, or front toric design, is useful for more spherical corneas. Back-surface toric design should be considered for use on more highly cylindrical corneas. Larger-diameter lenses make use of the scleral surface for increased stabilization; therefore, they may also be useful for the more toric cornea. These guidelines are not strict dictums. The lens fit and rotational character-

Table 4–1. Soft Toric Lenses

Marking	Brand	Stabilization	Toric Surface
5, 6, 7 o'clock	B & L Optima Toric	Prism	Front
	PBH Hydrocurve 3	Prism	Back
	PBH CSI Clarity toric	Prism	Back
5:30, 6, 6:30 o'clock	Hydron Ultra T	Prism	Front
3, 6, 9 o'clock	Ciba Spectrum Toric	Prism	Back
6 o'clock	Coast Hydrosoft Toric	Prism	Back
	PBH Hydrocurve II	Prism	Back
	Sunsoft Eclipse/Toric	Prism	Back
	Kontur 55 Toric	Prism	Back
Bi-directional	WJ Durasoft 3 Optifit Toric thin zone		Back
	WJ Durasoft 2 Optifit Toric thin zone		Back
3, 9 o'clock	Ciba Torisoft	Thin zone	Front

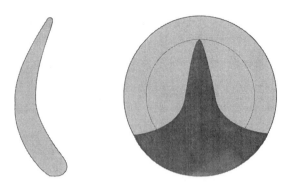

Figure 4–1. In the prism ballast soft lens design, the dark areas are thicker and, therefore, heavier.

Prism Ballast Design

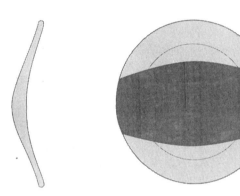

Figure 4–2. In the thin zone toric design, the dark areas are thicker; thinner areas are superior and inferior and slip under the eyelids.

Thin Zone Design

istics can also be influenced by the shape of the eye, the lid configuration, and the lid tension. Today's fitter can use many designs and expect success with a good toric lens fit (Table 4–1).

3. What trial lens parameters should be selected?
Guidelines for lens size and base curve for spherical lens are used for toric lenses as well. Most manufacturers offer a limited number of base curves. If more than one base curve is offered, use the steeper base curve if the central keratometry values are greater than 45.00 D. Use the flatter base curve if the central keratometry values are 41.00 D or less. The midrange base curve is used for average keratometry values. The lens must fully cover the cornea and produce even centration. A common soft toric lens diameter is 14.5 mm.

After base curve and diameter have been selected, trial lens power must be considered. Always begin with cylinder power axis. Select an axis as close to refractive axis as possible. Cylinder power is the next variable to consider. If the exact cylinder power is not available, use the closest *smaller* amount. The sphere power of the trial lens should be within ± 4.00 D of the refractive sphere power. Remember, both sphere and cylinder power must be converted for vertex distance if the power in either is greater than ± 4.00 D.

4. Does the lens fit?

It is best to assess centration a few minutes after lens placement. If the lens decenters to the superortemporal direction or falls to the inferior position with edge lift, the fit is too loose. If the lens does not move with the blink, and conjunctival blanching is observed temporally, the fit is too tight. Make the appropriate lens change. After it has been determined that the lens centers and provides full corneal coverage, it is best to let it equilibrate on the eye before making the final analysis. Most soft toric lenses are made of mid- to high-water-content materials (e.g., ≥45%) and are thicker than spherical designs. The usual equilibration time required for toric lenses is 20 to 30 minutes. The goal is a lens that centers well, moves easily with the blink, fully covers the cornea, and does not rotate more than 20 degrees.

5. What power do I order to make the patient see well?

The final question is most important. To determine the correct power, perform a spherical over-refraction. Remember, the trial lens should have the same cylinder power and axis as the patient's refraction converted for vertex distance, so astigmatism should be fully corrected. If acuity is not within one line of best visual acuity with a spherical over-refraction, check for lens rotation. Lens rotation may be compensated for if it is less than 20 degrees and the lens is stable. Any rotation greater than 20 degrees indicates an inadequate fit, and the base curve, size, or both should be re-evaluated. If the rotation is the "creeping-up" type, the lens is too tight. If the rotation is the "swinging" type, the fit is too loose.

Soft toric lenses are marked at the thickest point on the lens. When on the eye, markings of prism ballast lenses should be at the 6-o'clock, inferior position. Thin-zone designs may be marked at the 3- and 9-o'clock positions, or horizontal position. If the lens torques so the markings are to the observer's left (i.e., clockwise), the number of degrees of rotation should be added to the spectacle axis. If the lens moves so that the markings are shifted to the observer's right (i.e., counterclockwise) the number of degrees is subtracted from the spectacle axis. The mnemonic is LARS (left add, right subtract). Usually, compensation is made if the amount of rotation is between 10 and 20 degrees and stable. There is approximately a one-half line increase in vision for each 10-degree change. For example, a patient with the spectacle correction of $-0.50 - 0.75 \times 180$ is wearing a trial lens with a power of $-2.00 - 0.75 \times 175$. The over-refraction is $+1.50$, but only results in 20/25+ acuity. The lens fits well, but the lens markings are positioned 15 degrees to the fitter's right and are stable there. The power to be ordered is $-0.50 - 0.75 \times 165$ ($180 - 15 = 165$). The lens delivered to the patient should position exactly as did the trial lens; the marks should be stable and seen at the 15-degree counterclockwise position. You would expect visual acuity to be 20/20.

In some instances, the lens does not rotate and fits well, yet the spherical over-refraction does not provide acceptable vision. In such a case, do a sphero-cylindrical over-refraction, checking for resultant cross-cylinder power effect. If such resultant cross-cylinder exists, a composite power must be calculated. One way to determine the power is to telephone the manufacturer's consultant and request that they calculate resultant power. The fitter may also obtain a resultant cross-cylinder computer program.*

The practitioner may also measure resultant cross-cylinder power using an easy technique. Using spectacle trial lenses and frame, set the cylinder power and axis of the trial contact lens in the rear well. In front of that, place the cylinder power of the over-refraction at the correct axis (Fig. 4–3), and measure the two-lens combination with a lensometer (Fig. 4–4). The total spherical power to be ordered is the sum of the sphere values found in the trial contact lens, the over-refraction, and the lensometry measurement. Combine the cylinder power and axis as measured by lensometry with the total sphere power.

For example, a patient is wearing a trial lens power $-3.00 - 1.75 \times 180$. There is no rotation of the lens, but an over-refraction of $+0.50 - 1.00 \times 030$ is necessary to provide good vision. The fitter places a hand-held cylinder lens of -1.75×180 and -1.00×030 in a trial frame and measures the resultant power on the lensometer. The combined power reads $-0.25 - 2.25 \times 010$. The power to be ordered is the sum of all the spheres $[(-3.00) + (+0.50) + (-0.25) = -2.75]$ combined with the cylinder and axis as measured by lensometry (-2.25×010). The power of the lens to be ordered for the patient should be $-2.75 - 2.25 \times 010$. The axis may have to be rounded to the nearest 10 degrees, because many soft toric lenses are only available in 10-degree increments. This lens, when dispensed, should demonstrate the same fitting and rotational characteristics as did the trial lens, but it will also provide good visual correction. A worksheet for this procedure is shown in Box 4–1.

---

* The Sunsoft Corporation (6805 Academy Parkway West, Albuquerque, NM 87109: 800–526–2020) offers a pre-programmed calculator that computes resultant cross-cylinder.

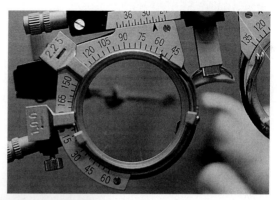

Figure 4–3. Cylinder powers of the trial lens and over-refraction are both placed in a trial frame.

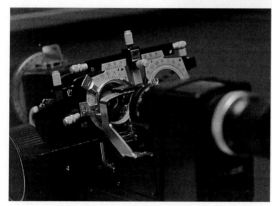

Figure 4–4. The combination of the crossed cylinders is measured by lensometry.

BOX 4–1. RESULTANT CROSS-CYLINDER WORKSHEET

Always work in minus cylinder form.

1. Record trial contact lens power:
   Sphere 1 _____ Cylinder 1 _____ Axis 1 _____.
2. Record sphero-cylindrical over-refraction:
   Sphere 2 _____ Cylinder 2 _____ Axis 2 _____.
3. Place cylinder 1 and cylinder 2 in a trial frame. Measure using lensometer. Record lensometer measurement:
   Sphere 3 _____ Cylinder 3 _____ Axis 3 _____.
4. Add sphere powers:
   sphere 1 _____
   + sphere 2 _____
   + sphere 3 _____
   = Final sphere _____.
5. Power to order:
   Final sphere _____ Cylinder 3 _____ Axis 3 _____.

PROBLEM SOLVING

Problems encountered with soft toric lenses fall into three inter-related categories: vision, comfort, and physiologic response. Fluctuating vision problems are usually the result of a poorly centered, loose lens. In these cases, the fitter may also see the lens rocking back and forth around the stabilization position. Decentration and rocking are improved by using a larger or steeper lens.

Unstable vision that changes with each blink may be the result of poor lens draping caused by a too-tight fit. Tight lenses may also exhibit a continual, creeping rotation of the lens markings. This may be corrected by changing to a lens with a smaller diameter or a flatter base curve.

If the lens appears to fit well but vision is not clear, do an over-refraction and determine resultant power. If the over-refraction does not improve vision, consider using a different type of lens.

The problem of discomfort with a well-fitted toric lens is the result of either excessive thickness or lens drying. The use of artificial tears, different lens water contents or thinner designs may be useful. The newer soft toric lenses appear to be quite comfortable for most patients with normal tear function, so this finding is becoming rare.

Physiologic problems such as edema, staining, and vascularization are treated in exactly the same manner as with spherical soft lenses (see Appendix i). In general, reducing any hypoxic response by increasing oxygen availability to the cornea is the recommended treatment.

EMPIRICAL FITTING

If diagnostic toric soft lenses are not available empirically, design a lens using the guidelines described for trial lens selection, order the lenses under a warranted plan, and consider them the first trial lens. If they do not perform as perfectly as expected, order a second lens after identifying and rectifying the problem.

The correction of astigmatism with soft toric lenses takes only a little more time than the fitting of spherical soft lenses, but the improvement in patient vision and satisfaction is well worth the extra effort.

BIBLIOGRAPHY

Bennett ES, Henry VA: *Clinical Manual of Contact Lenses.* Philadelphia, JB Lippincott, 1994.

Jurkus JM: Contact lens problem solving. Contact Lens Forum. 1990;October:43.

Manufacturer's fitting guides: Each manufacturer produces fitting guides for their soft toric lenses.

Remba MJ, Clompus RJ: Astigmatic soft contact lenses. *Problems in Optometry.* Vol. 2, No. 2. Philadelphia, JB Lippincott, 1990, p 281.

Tyler's Quarterly Soft Contact Lens Parameter Guide: A Quarterly Reference Guide, 5901 H. Street, Little Rock, AR 72205.

CHAPTER 5

Aspheric Rigid Gas Permeable Lenses

KEITH AMES

Aspheric rigid gas permeable (RGP) contact lenses are utilized for two reasons in contact lens practice: to take advantage of the physical fitting characteristics and to take advantage of the optical properties of the aspheric lens surface. Aspheric RGP lenses more precisely align with the aspheric shape of the cornea, thus providing certain fitting advantages. The gradual shift in refractive power as the aspheric surface flattens has been employed to achieve an add effect for presbyopic patients. Although the aspheric shape can be generated on either surface of the lens, it is almost always used on the posterior lens surface, and only this application is discussed in this chapter. A basic understanding of aspheric geometry is all that is necessary to effectively use these lenses in clinical practice.

BOX 5–1. DO THIS FIRST

1. Keratometry
2. Refraction
3. Biomicroscopy
4. Assess lid position
5. Select initial trial lens or lens to be ordered based on manufacturer's fitting guide

---

An aspheric contact lens flattens from the center to the periphery. The degree of flattening can vary and is usually described as the eccentricity or e value. Figure 5–1 shows that eccentricity values can range from less than 1 (an elliptical shape) to more than 1 (a hyperbolic shape). The clinician needs only to understand that the higher the e value, the higher the degree of flattening. Lenses with e values of less than 1 have low-to-moderate flattening and are commonly employed to enhance the physical fitting characteristics of the contact

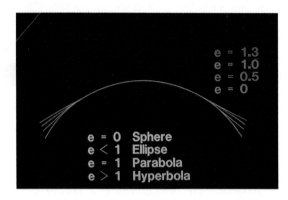

Figure 5-1. Aspheric shapes of varying e values.

lens. Lenses with e values greater than 1 have moderate-to-high flattening and are usually prescribed to achieve an add effect for the presbyopic patient.

The e value or rate of flattening can vary across the surface of the lens. Some designs employ a constant rate of flattening, whereas others have several distinct zones with different rates of flattening. A third type of surface has a continuously changing rate of flattening defined by a specific mathematic formula. The fitting and optical properties of the contact lens are dependent on the width and degree of flattening of the various zones across the posterior surface of the lens. The most commonly used aspheric designs consist of a relatively wide central zone of minimal flattening surrounded by a wider zone of greater flattening.

FITTING PRINCIPLES

Much unnecessary confusion arises over the actual fitting of the various aspheric lens designs. It is enough for practitioners to know that as aspheric zones become wider and flatter, the lens will fit flatter on the eye. Therefore, the contact lens fitter must select a steeper base curve to compensate. Aspheric lenses with low e values designed to enhance fitting characteristics generally require only a slightly steeper base curve compared with an equivalent diameter multi-curve spherical lens to achieve a similar fitting relation. Aspheric lenses with higher e values used in presbyopic correction require correspondingly steeper base curves.

Manufacturers generally do not disclose the proprietary design data necessary to allow practitioners to calculate or predict the base curve adjustment required to compensate for the posterior surface flattening. This is not necessary, because the manufacturer provides fitting guidelines that tell the practitioner what base curve compensation to make.

Comparing the aspheric guidelines with your typical spherical fitting approach will tell much about the geometry of the aspheric design. For example, if an aspheric fitting guide selects a base curve 0.1 mm steeper than the base curve you would have normally selected for a typical spherical lens, you know the aspheric lens has a low-to-moderate degree of flattening. Conversely, aspheric designs that fit 0.2 to 0.3 mm steeper than usual must be flattening at a very high rate.

WHY FIT ASPHERICS
WITH SLIGHT FLATTENING?

Aspheric posterior-surface RGP lenses of low-to-moderate flattening are generally fitted to enhance the physical fitting characteristics of the lens. The cornea is aspheric, and it has been shown that aspheric RGP lenses more closely align with the aspheric surface of the cornea and offer certain fitting advantages.[1-4] To understand how aspheric lenses can improve fitting, it is necessary to understand the limitations of conventional multi-curve spherical lenses. Multi-curve spherical lenses have several inherent disadvantages. The transition zones between peripheral curves are difficult to control. Manufacturing inconsistency is common, and this often leads to distinct, poorly blended junctions, which can decrease comfort and cause visual disturbances such as flare. These problems dictate that multi-curve designs must maintain a large optic zone to keep these transition zones away from the visual axis. However, these large optic zones are spherical and therefore are unable to align with the aspheric geometry of the cornea. The distinct junction between the optic and peripheral zones of the lens usually forms a distinct, narrow bearing zone on the cornea.

Aspheric lenses can eliminate the junctional areas on the posterior surface of the lens, thus allowing for smaller optic zones to be used. This relative lack of junctions can improve patient comfort and reduce visual complaints such as flare and glare. Figures 5–2 and 5–3 show the difference between typical blended, multi-curve spherical lenses and aspheric lenses. Note the lack of a discernable junction area on the aspheric lenses. Using a smaller optic area, the bearing zone that is formed between the lens and cornea is spread over a wide area. Figures 5–4 and 5–5 demonstrate the wider peripheral alignment achieved with an aspheric lens compared with a multi-curve spherical lens.

This wider zone of alignment is largely responsible for the unique and clinically useful fitting characteristics displayed by posterior-surface aspheric RGP lenses. Studies have demonstrated that aspheric lenses are more likely to maintain a centered position on the eye as the central fitting relationship changes.[5,6] Lenses that are fitted excessively flat will not decenter as superiorly, nor will lenses that are fitted

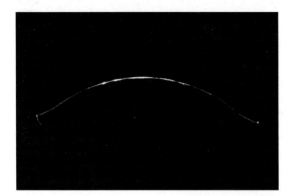

Figure 5-2. Posterior profile of a multi-curve spherical lens.

Figure 5-3. Posterior profile of an aspheric lens.

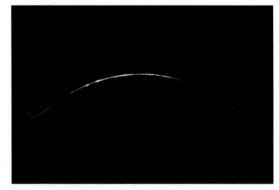

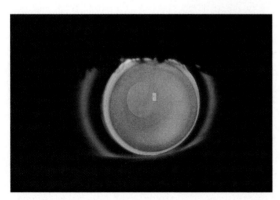

Figure 5-4. Corneal alignment of a multi-curve spherical lens.

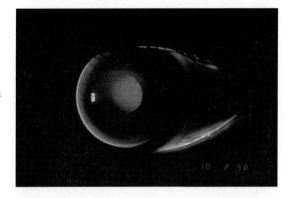

Figure 5–5. Corneal alignment of an aspheric lens.

excessively steep decenter as inferiorly compared with spherical lenses. Additionally, aspheric lenses show less variation in the fluorescein pattern as the central fitting relation changes compared with spherical lenses. Cumulatively, these characteristics show that aspheric lenses are less sensitive to base curve selection than spherical lenses; therefore, the clinician can be less precise in his or her base curve selection and still obtain an acceptable fit. Simply put, aspheric lenses can allow for a greater margin of error in fitting.

WHY FIT ASPHERICS WITH EXTREME FLATTENING?

Aspheric posterior-surface RGP lenses of moderate-to-high flattening are usually fitted to achieve a plus-power add effect for presbyopic patients. The extreme peripheral flattening causes a greater plus-lesser minus-power shift for near correction. These lenses must be fitted much steeper than a typical multi-curve spherical lens because of the flat fitting characteristics related to the high rate of peripheral flattening. Normally, these lenses maintain a centered position on the eye. The bifocal effect achieved is simultaneous, because distance-focused light (i.e., through the lens center) and near-focused light (i.e., through the mid-periphery) are presented to the eye at the same time. The near add effect may be enhanced if the lens translates or moves upward in downgaze during near tasks.

Certain atypical eye conditions warrant an aspheric lens of moderate-to-high flattening for physical fitting purposes. Keratoconus is the most common example. The central region of a keratoconic cornea is extremely steep and is surrounded by a much flatter mid-peripheral area. A contact lens must be fitted with a steep base curve to bridge the central cone but must then flatten at an extremely fast rate to align the much flatter periphery. An aspheric posterior-surface lens is ideally suited to accomplish this. Although the same effect can be achieved with an appropriately designed multi-curve spherical lens, manufacturing of the spherical lens is much more problematic. The multiple curves required to produce this geometry are difficult to reproduce consistently. Interestingly, refractive surgery produces a cornea opposite in character, with a flatter central region and a steeper mid-periphery. Aspheric designs are now being produced with geometries to match (i.e., lenses that steepen in the periphery to assist in the post-surgical refractive correction of these patients).

Although aspheric lenses can benefit most patients, there are specific clinical situations in which aspheric lenses are especially useful in preventing or solving fitting and visual problems. The following case studies demonstrate how the general fitting principles can be applied to assist commonly encountered patients.

CASE STUDY 5–1

Clinical Presentation

K readings: OD 42.00/43.00 @ 85
OS 42.00/43.25 @ 90

Refraction: OD +1.50 −.75 × 170
OS +1.75 −.75 × 180

Contact lens parameters:
Diameter: 9.5 OU
Design/material: Tricurve/Boston RXD
Base curve: 42.50 OU
Power: +1.00 OD
+1.25 OS

Fitting Characteristics

The lenses decenter inferiorly with moderate apical pooling. Lens movement is minimal and moderate, confluent, 3-9 staining is present.

The hyperope whose lenses decenter inferiorly presents a common clinical problem. The center of gravity of the lens causes it to drop, which can lead to desiccation, corneal staining, and discomfort. Practitioners typically try to fit a multi-curve spherical plus lens steeper, but this often leads to greater inferior decentration. If a more centered fit is achieved, the lens often will show a harsh bearing zone in the mid-periphery with minimal movement and poor tear exchange. This patient can be refitted with an aspheric lens, which should maintain a more vertically centered position on the eye. Even with steeper base curve selection, the mid-peripheral flattening of aspheric designs minimize the bearing zone and help promote lens movement and tear exchange. In some cases, especially with higher plus powers, minus carrier lenticulation is required, regardless of lens design, to achieve adequate centration.

CASE STUDY 5–2

Clinical Presentation

K readings: OD 46.00/46.50 @ 90
OS 45.75/46.75 @ 95

Refraction: OD −6.00 − .75 × 180
OS −6.25 −1.00 × 180

Contact lens parameters:
Diameter: 9.5 OU
Design/material: Tricurve/Fluoroperm 30
Base curve: 45.25 OU
Power: −5.00 OD
−5.25 OS

Fitting Characteristics

The lenses position very superiorly, with the upper edge of the lens extending beyond the superior limbus and creating an impression arc stain on the superior conjunctiva. The patient complains of variable vision and glare with bright lights.

The myope whose lenses decenter superiorly is another common clinical problem. The thick edge of a high-minus lens interacts with the lid and is naturally pulled upward. Although this effect is beneficial for many patients, excessive decentration can lead to superior limbal pathology and poor visual performance. This effect is difficult to counteract with standard multi-curve spherical lenses but can often be reduced by fitting an aspheric lens. The propensity for aspheric lenses to maintain a centered position on the eye can be used to the patient's advantage in this situation. The wide, mid-peripheral alignment formed between the lens and cornea maximizes the lens–cornea attraction and minimizes the lens–lid interaction so that lid-induced decentration is reduced.

CASE STUDY 5–3

Clinical Presentation

K readings: OD 43.00/44.50 @ 95 (wide palpebral apertures)
OS 43.00/44.75 @ 180 (no upper lid limbal coverage)

Refraction: OD -3.00 -1.25 $\times$ 180
OS -3.00 -1.75 $\times$ 180

Contact lens parameters:
  Diameter: 9.9 OU
  Design/material: Tricurve/Boston RXD
  Base curve: 42.25 OU
  Power: -2.25 OU

Fitting Characteristics

The lenses position very inferiorly. The lenses are picked up only with a firm and complete blink but drop immediately. The patient complains of lens awareness, and the front surface of the lens shows incomplete wetting. Larger and flatter lenses have been tried, but no improvement in lens positioning has been obtained.

Patients with wide palpebral apertures must usually be fitted with smaller and steeper lenses to achieve acceptable centration. The upper lids of these patients are too high to effectively pull the lens up regardless of how large and flat an RGP lens is selected. Therefore, the lens will drop unless a steeper central fit is achieved so that there is greater attraction between the cornea and lens. Aspheric lenses can be fitted relatively steep centrally and maintain an aligned mid-periphery with adequate edge lift because of the controlled flattening in the periphery of the lens. Aspheric lenses therefore are ideal for intrapalpebral fitting and for this type of patient.

PROBLEM-SOLVING

Problem-solving with an aspheric lens is not unlike that with conventional multi-curve spherical lenses, with a few important exceptions. After the initial diagnostic or prescribed lens is placed on the eye, the fitting performance is evaluated with a biomicroscope. Fluorescein and the blue filter of the biomicroscope are used to assess the positioning of the lens and the lens–cornea relationship. An auxiliary Wratten #12 filter can be placed in front of the optics of the biomicroscope to enhance the fluorescein pattern. This is especially useful with lenses containing ultraviolet-absorbing agents and with aspheric designs, because variations in the tear layer behind aspheric lenses are often very subtle. Ideally, the aspheric lens should be centered or slightly superior on the eye and show a wide area of alignment from center to edge. Minimal bearing in the mid-periphery should be observed, and minimal-to-moderate edge lift should be present. Movement should be smooth and moderate, perhaps slightly less than that typically seen with conventional spherical lenses. If this fitting appearance is not

Table 5-1. Control of Fitting Characteristics

Fitting Appearance	Parameter Adjustment
Excessive apical pooling	Flatten base curve
Mid-peripheral bearing	Flatten base curve
Insufficient edge lift	Increase diameter Flatten base curve
Excessive edge lift	Decrease diameter Steepen base curve
Excessive decentration	Steepen base curve

observed, the diameter and base curve can be adjusted within a given design to enhance fitting and performance.

Parameter variations commonly employed with aspheric lenses are similar in principle to those with spherical lenses with one important exception. Because the rate of flattening with spherical lenses is constant in the periphery, edge clearance will generally decrease as the diameter is increased because of increased sagittal depth. Aspheric lenses, on the other hand, generally show greater peripheral flattening as the diameter increases, so that edge clearance increases as diameter increases. Table 5-1 shows common parameter adjustments to control fitting characteristics.

CONCLUSION

Aspheric lenses should be an important part of any contact lens practice. They can be used to enhance fitting characteristics and to provide an add effect for presbyopic patients. Their effective utilization does not require any special skill or extraordinary knowledge of optics or lens design. Aspheric fitting principles are generally consistent with the fitting principles used by all practitioners to fit conventional multi-curve spherical lenses and can be easily mastered with a minimum of clinical experience.

REFERENCES

1. Kiely PM, Smith G, Carney LG: The mean shape of the human cornea. Optica Acta 1982; 29:1027.
2. Goldberg JB: Clinical advantages of aspheric contact lenses. Optometry Weekly 1974; 65:902.
3. Goldberg JB: Some characteristics of ellipsoidal corneal lenses. Optometry Weekly 1975; 66:1089.
4. Lebow KA: Aspheric and ellipsoidal corneal lenses. J Am Optom Assoc 1976; 47:322.
5. Ames KS, Erickson P: Optimizing aspheric and spheric rigid lens performance. CLAO J 1987; 13:165.
6. Ames KS, Jones F: Spherical vs. aspheric designs: a clinical difference? Contact Lens Forum 1988; 13:19.

CHAPTER 6

Presbyopia: Rigid Gas Permeable Bifocal Lenses

DAVID W. HANSEN

The frustrations of presbyopia led Benjamin Franklin to design and use the first bifocal spectacle lenses. This challenge was presented to the contact lens field by William Feinbloom in 1936, when he filed his first patent application for a bifocal contact lens. These early scleral lenses incorporated the principle of translating alternating images; today, there are many multifocal contact lens designs and materials to enhance their comfort. Faced with the challenges of presbyopia and binocular vision dysfunction, we must incorporate the new technology to meet the needs of our patients. These patients want convenience, comfort, and clarity, and we want the same for them. Where do we begin?

DO THESE FIRST

Needs Versus Wants. A patient's needs or wants are predicated on the theory that all options regarding presbyopia or binocular distur-

---

BOX 6-1. DO THESE FIRST

1. Case history, including:

   - Contact lens history
   - Medical history
   - Occupational and avocational history
   - Needs and motivation

2. Measure:

   - Refraction
   - Position of eyelids
   - Corneal curvature
   - Pupil size

---

bance problems are known. The goal is to explain the new technologic advances in multi-focal contact lenses to the patient.

Medical History. Are there previous systemic problems or contraindications, such as uncontrolled diabetes or hypertension, which may cause acuity fluctuations?

Medication History. Have the patient list the drugs and medications he or she takes regularly, as well as those taken on an as-needed basis. This list should also include over-the-counter medications, which may affect lacrimal production and ocular dryness. Drugs that produce ocular dryness include birth control pills, antihistamines, diuretics, hormone medications, and thyroid medications.

Ocular History. A careful history of previous ocular surgeries, including eyelid surgery, blepharoplasty, strabismus surgery, or other corneal abnormalities, is important. Investigate the treatment of previous corneal foreign bodies or abrasions, whether caused by contact lenses or by the external environment.

Contact Lens History. Has the patient been a contact lens wearer in the past? If so, what kind of lenses were worn? Investigate the previously successful wearing schedule (i.e., years, months, days, and hours per day). Were there complications? If the lenses were comfortable, how was the visual acuity? It is also important to understand previous contact lens history, including reasons for unsuccessful contact lens wear, especially with bifocal or multi-focal contact lenses. Determine whether the patient has had previous experience with monovision lenses. Most successful monovision patients make poor candidates for multi-focal contact lenses. Monovision provides a disparity between the two eyes; therefore, binocularity is sometimes disrupted in the early stages of multi-focal contact lens adaptation.

Motivation. Most patients can adapt to a rigid gas permeable (RGP) contact lens, even if they were former soft lens wearers or have never worn contact lenses. RGP lens options can be presented in a positive way to ease the discomfort of the patient. It must also be determined whether the patient truly wants to wear contact lenses. If the patient is enthused about contact lenses, then acceptance of this modality will be more favorable.

Occupation and Avocation. Careful scrutiny of the patient's occupation and avocation aids in achieving proper design. It is very important to ascertain whether the patient uses computers in his or her daily life. If the patient works with a CRT for at least 30% of his or her day at home and at work, consider a simultaneous or aspheric design. If the patient uses a computer for less than 30% of his or her day, simultaneous design is not mandatory. If leisure activities require mid-range vision, fit the patient with a simultaneous or aspheric design.

Criteria of Design. Determining patient needs greatly reduces design time and/or the length of the diagnostic appointment. Refraction and corneal topography are integral parts of the design function but are worthless unless the patient attains his or her needs. If the patient is a former polymethyl methacrylate (PMMA) or RGP single-vision contact lens wearer with computer needs, fit a simultaneous or aspheric lens. Patients who have not worn contact lenses in the past or have worn soft lenses usually respond favorably to a simultaneous or aspheric design.

Fees. Contact lens fees should be addressed from the beginning. Not only is it our obligation to explain options for the contact lens candidate, but it is our responsibility to explain the higher costs of materials, designs, and professional care needed to fit a multi-focal RGP lens.

SELECTING A DESIGN

Before the diagnostic appointment, determine the two key design factors.

1. The key to design is determining what the patient needs. The patient's primary concern or concerns must be ascertained in the history.

2. Computer usage is the primary criterion for design selection. If the patient uses a computer or has intermediate needs, Figure 6–1 illustrates the steps for selecting a lens design.

OTHER FACTORS TO CONSIDER

Refraction. The key component in selecting a design by refraction is astigmatism.

Eyelids. The external structure of the eye is an integral part of the overall design function. The two eyelids will act independently or in synergy to manipulate the lens. Assessment of lid position is important for improving acuity.

Corneal Measurement. The shape and curvature of the cornea is another factor in the overall success of the lens design. If the patient has a cornea of approximately 40.00 D, use a simultaneous design, such as a Lifestyle Hi-Rider, or a translating design, such as ACC bifocal (Salvatori), Tangent Streak (GT Laboratories) or Fluoroperm ST

BOX 6–2. ASTIGMATISM FLOWCHART
If no residual astigmatism → simultaneous or translating design
If residual astigmatism → translating design

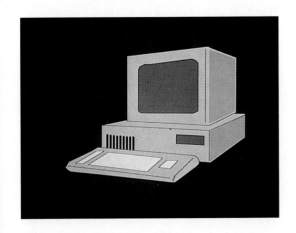

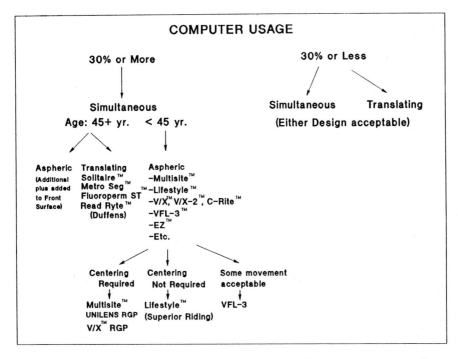

Figure 6–1. Computer usage is a key factor for choosing the appropriate contact lens design for the patient.

(Paragon Vision Sciences). For average corneas (i.e., 41.00–46.00 D), the fitter may use almost any design. For steep corneas (i.e., > 46.00 D), an aspheric center, Bivision, or deCarle design is usually recommended.

Age. Because the amount of the presbyopic component is usually dictated by the age of the patient, it is important to categorize age criteria.

1. If the patient is younger than 45 years of age, I recommend a simultaneous (i.e., aspheric) design. These include Multisite (Salvatori); VFL-3 (Conforma); Lifestyle Hi-Rider (Permeable Technologies); V/X RPG, V/X-2, C-Rite (GBF Laboratories); EZ Bifocal (Concise); and Unilens RGP (Unilens).

2. If the patient is older than 45 years of age, many of the simultaneous or aspheric designs can be used by adding plus power to the front surface or by incorporating a front-surface aspheric curve. If this is not acceptable, consider a translating design.

OTHER THINGS TO DO FIRST

A comprehensive visual examination means many things to many practitioners; but there are certain elements that are needed other than the refraction and health assessment of the eye. We must also determine the binocular function for distance and near vision. There are several key factors involved in integral parts of the comprehensive examination.

Refraction

We usually use the manifest refraction to aid in the prescription determination, but cycloplegic information is also helpful in binocular dysfunction patients.

Keratometry

Keratometry readings, especially those taken by automated keratometry incorporating peripheral assessment, are most helpful for aspheric designs. Keratometry establishes the apex of the cornea, thereby providing additional information to assist in centering the contact lens. For example, if the apex of the cornea is decentered down and in, an aspheric design may not be appropriate, because the patient will see through an intermediate part of the lens. These small frustrations can be alleviated by careful assessment.

External Examination

Cornea. Corneal assessment measurements, especially the visible iris diameter (VID), will help the practitioner determine the design size.

Pupil Size. Mesopic (normal) and scotopic (dim) illumination can rule out certain designs. If the patient has extraordinarily large pupils (i.e., > 5 mm), he or she is usually not a good candidate for an aspheric or simultaneous design. All other patient history criteria may indicate that the patient should be fitted for an aspheric design, but if the pupil size is extremely large, it is not appropriate to start with a "pupil-dependent" design.

Eyelid Assessment. Measure the position of the lids with respect to the cornea. Also assess the tension of the eyelids, and document ptosis or other eyelid abnormalities. Palpebral aperture is a critical evaluation for the overall diameter of the lens. Small palpebral apertures usually require smaller diameter lenses (i.e., 9.2 mm or less) (Fig. 6–2).

Conjunctiva. Conjunctival abnormalities should be documented. Pingueculae can cause convection currents of the lacrimal tear meniscus to be altered, as can pterygia and other conjunctival hypertrophy problems. If the patient has formerly worn PMMA or RGP lenses, dellen or 3–9 corneal dryness changes can affect the conjunctiva near the limbus.

All of the previously described external assessments should be carefully monitored with bio-microscopy using fluorescein and rose bengal stains. It is also important to evert the lids to determine any palpebral conjunctival changes, including dryness, potential allergy hypertrophy blebs, the effects of drugs, or artifacts. Once sodium fluorescein has been instilled, tear break-up time (BUT) should be measured. Patients with dry eyes, especially those who are presbyopic, can be fitted with multi-focal RPG lenses and often are helped by punctal plugs, which produce a lacrimal reservoir to make the contact lens more comfortable (Fig. 6–3).

Figure 6–2. A translating design lens utilizes the lower lid for positioning.

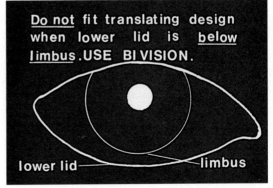

Do not fit translating design when lower lid is below limbus. USE BI VISION.

lower lid — limbus

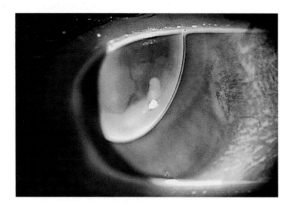

Figure 6–3. Dellen caused by vascular limbal keratitis may be a contraindication for a multifocal contact lens.

THINGS WE NEED TO KNOW

A multi-focal contact lens diagnostic appointment initially helps the practitioner determine the overall success or failure of this modality. The following list guides the fitting process.

1. Selecting the design. Select either a simultaneous or translating lens. It should be obvious which design will work the best from the previous evaluation.

2. Neutralization of diagnostic lenses. The diagnostic contact lenses should be evaluated for accurate parameters. Don't assume anything: make sure the lenses are checked at each appointment for each patient.

3. Applying contact lenses. When applying the contact lens, explain that the diagnostic lens usually is not the correct prescription but that you are determining the fit of the lens.

4. Adaptation. Adaptation for a multi-focal design should take 30 to 45 minutes. Don't be too concerned about the overall length of this visit. The patient must know that you are trying to determine long-term rather than short-term goals. Multi-focal lenses that do not seat properly give the practitioner a false sense of security and many times will cost more money and time in the long run.

5. Visual acuity. After the lenses have settled, visual acuity should be determined, even if the prescription is anticipated to be incorrect.

6. Retinoscopy. Retinoscopy gives an assessment of the overall refraction and position of the contact lenses. The brightness of the reflex helps determine the quality of the optics.

7. Over-refraction. Over-refraction at this point in the diagnostic procedure is done with a Phoroptor to determine the distance prescription.

BOX 6–3. THINGS YOU NEED TO KNOW

1. Computer users do best with simultaneous or aspheric designs
2. Patients with residual astigmatism do best with translating designs
3. Flat or steep corneas are best fitted with aspheric designs
4. Patients with large pupils are best fitted with translating designs
5. Allow at least 30 minutes for adaptation to trial lenses

8. Trial lens with over-refraction. After assessing the over-refraction, a trial lens helps design the near prescription. Using a single-cell trial frame is very convenient. It allows the patient to anticipate the principles of accommodation. We must remember that multi-focal and bifocal contact lenses produce a translating effect for the patient looking from far to near through the intermediate zone.

9. Burton lamp fluorescein assessment. Look for binocular positioning of the contact lenses with the Burton lamp. Watch for movement of the lens on each eye, and assess eyelid interaction. If fitting a translating design, the segment position should be evaluated. If a simultaneous contact lens design is used, the center of the distance area should be positioned directly in alignment with the pupil for best visual acuity.

10. Slit lamp evaluation with fluorescein.

Tear film assessment
Contact lens–cornea relation

- If the contact lens is too flat, steepen the base curve.
- If the contact lens is too steep, flatten the base curve.
- If the contact lens moves temporally, steepen the base curve.
- If the contact lens moves nasally, flatten the base curve.
- If the translating design contact lens rotates nasally, it is too steep; loosen the lens.
- If the translating design rotates temporally, it is too loose; tighten the lens. Most generally, steepening the base curve will help in this circumstance.

Lens–lid relation. Much attention has been given to the superior lid, but it also is important to watch the lower lid for interaction. If the contact lens is under the lower lid, steepen the base curve or reduce the diameter. If the contact lens is tangent to the lower lid, fit a translating contact lens.

MY BEST ADVICE

The ultimate goal in fitting a contact lens is to provide convenience, comfort, and clarity. Vision that includes an easy accommodation from far to near through an intermediate zone without jump provides the best patient convenience.

SIMULTANEOUS DESIGNS

Simultaneous (Aspheric) Designs

If the patient can wear an aspheric or simultaneous lens, start with this design. These lenses require careful centering to produce the simultaneous effect, but flare and glare is always a potential problem. Front-cut adds may be altered by cleaning procedures; therefore, solution compliance is important. Aspheric designs are high-eccentricity posterior aspheric designs, which usually have a spherical front surface. These lenses include Multisite (Salvatori); VFL, VFL-2, and VFL-3 (Conforma); APA, V/X, V/X-2, and C-Rite (GBF Laboratories); Lifestyle Hi-Rider (Permeable Technologies); Unilens RGP (Unilens); and EZ Bifocal (Concise). Although aspheric designs usually require a well-centered lens, they produce good intermediate acuity and are excellent for computer operators. They are comfortable lenses because of the aspheric base curve. The Unilens™ RGP, Multisite™, V/X RGP, and EZ™ Bifocal lenses all require precision centering.

For all the previously described aspheric lenses, fit the initial base curve steeper than the flattest K reading. In cases of corneal astigmatism, increase the steepness of the base curve to achieve a better lens–cornea relation. For example, if a patient has corneal readings of 42.00/45.00 (3.00 D of corneal astigmatism), fit the lens 4.00 D steeper than K: in this example, 46.00 D. This measurement only gives the starting diagnostic base curve parameter. After the lens is placed on the eye, the overall fluorescein pattern, the position of the lens, and the visual acuity help to determine the final lens parameters. The VFL-3 lens is usually fitted 2.00 D steeper than K; the Unilens RGP lens is fitted 1.50 D steeper than K; the Multisite lens is fitted 3.00 to 4.00 D steeper than K; and the V/X RGP lens is fitted approximately 4.00 to 5.00 D steeper than K. The increase in steepness affects the amount of reading prescription that can be generated by the aspheric curve. For those patients in whom centration is more difficult, a VFL-3 lens provides a little flexibility with the intermediate zone, even though centration is suggested (Fig. 6–4).

The Lifestyle Hi-Rider lens is fitted flatter than other designs. Ideally, the Lifestyle Hi-Rider lens is fitted so that the equivalent base curve of the lens is approximately 0.1 mm flatter than the flattest

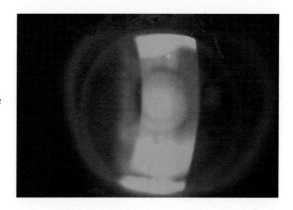

Figure 6–4. Multisite aspheric lens in the central position.

corneal curvature. This fitting relation promotes a slight upward lens decentration. Lens position underneath the superior lid is encouraged. Lifestyle Hi-Rider lenses are available in a 9.0-mm and a 9.5-mm overall diameter lens, and the near add is maximized when the upper edge of the lens rides superior to the limbus. The 9.0-mm lenses are recommended unless the patient has a large corneal diameter or large palpebral aperture (Figs. 6–5 and 6–6).

Simultaneous (Non-aspheric) Design

The deCarle or ACC Bivision (Salvatori) simultaneous lenses are back-surface add designs that reduce flare and glare. They also require a well-centered lens but produce good optics for distance and near vision. There is no intermediate zone; therefore, computer operators may have acuity problems. The ACC Bivision contact lens is a non-prism, annu-

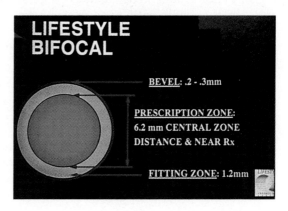

Figure 6–5. Lifestyle Hi-Rider design lens. (Courtesy of Ken Lebow, OD, and Permeable Technologies, Inc.)

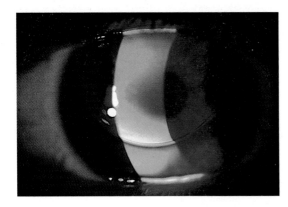

Figure 6–6. Lifestyle Hi-Rider lens in a superior position for proper alignment.

Figure 6–7. Bivision simultaneous bifocal lens demonstrating fluorescein central alignment.

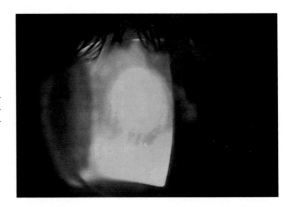

lar design with the distance segment on the geometrical center. Adds are available from + 1.00 to + 3.75 D. This lightweight design fits like a single-vision lens. The distance segment is positioned centrally in front of the pupil with an average 3.4-mm diameter distance zone. Patients with large pupils may present problems; simultaneous non-aspheric lenses are not recommended for these patients (Fig. 6–7).

TRANSLATING DESIGNS

One-Piece Crescent

The One-Piece Crescent lens is a front-surface design with a spherical base curve. The lens should be fitted so that the segment is located below the inferior pupillary rim. The translating design allows for distance and near viewing (Fig. 6–8).

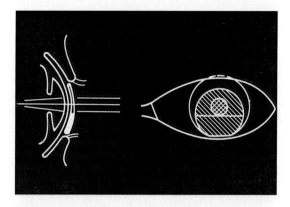

Figure 6–8. Diagrams of translating movement of contact lenses.

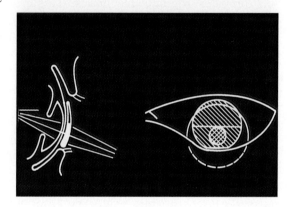

Tangent Streak

The Tangent Streak lens (GT Laboratories) is a unique, one-piece, rigid, "no-jump" design in which the distance and reading curves meet at the geometric center of the lens. This bifocal segment is fitted higher than most translating lenses and is usually positioned 0.3 mm into the pupillary zone. This front-cut design may cause flare and glare at night because of potential rotation of the lens and is thicker than most other bifocal designs because of the tangent cut on the front surface. The lens is fitted on K or slightly flatter than K to allow good translation. The lens should ride with its lower edge near the lower lid for good translation (Fig. 6–9).

Decentered deCarle Translating Design

The ACC translating design (Salvatori) is a decentered deCarle annular concave design. This lens is usually prism ballasted and truncated for better translation. The average distance segment size is 4.0 mm

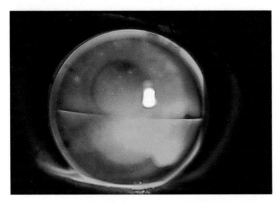

Figure 6-9. Tangent Streak bifocal contact lens in central gaze.

and provides reproducible optics. This translating design is usually used when the lower lid is tangential to the limbus and there is sufficient tonicity of the lids (Fig. 6–10). It also can be used to position a high-riding lens when critical near vision is a major concern. These bifocal designs can be made in add powers of + 1.00 to + 3.75 D in many different gas permeable materials.

Fluoroperm ST Bifocal

The Fluoroperm ST Bifocal (Paragon Vision Sciences) is a high-index, encapsulated, monocentric segment lens that is prism ballasted with the segment placed inferiorly. When the eye is in primary gaze, the near segment is positioned lower than in other segmented designs; normally 0.4 to 0.7 mm below the lower pupillary margin. Prism and mass will help lower the lens on the eye to produce good translation. I recommend following the manufacturer's suggested guidelines (Table 6–1). This lens is usually fitted as a 9.4- by 9.0-mm diameter lens (Figs. 6–11 and 6–12). The Fluoroperm ST translating lens is very thin and comfortable, even for patients who have never worn contact lenses.

Solitaire Bifocal

The Solitaire Bifocal lens (TruForm Optics) produces a prismatic reading lens with a monocentric distance segment cut on the top part of the lens using the same visual axis. The add portion extends around the segment on the upper half of the lens, and the removal of weight in forming this distance segment makes the Solitaire lens inherently bottom-heavy, thus requiring less prism to assist contact lens orientation. The Solitaire lens should not lag. This lens is fitted with the inferior lid near the lower limbus. The patient should not have a low superior lid, which may limit the distance field of view. The Solitaire lens also may not provide enough clearance between the lens and the

Table 6–1. Fluoroperm ST Bifocal Lens Manufacturer's Suggested Guidelines

Parameters

Lens diameter: 7.00–10.50 mm
Base curve: 6.50–9.00 mm
Distance power: + 12.00 to − 20.00 D
Add power: + 0.75 to + 2.00 D
Prism: 1– 4 PD
Prism axis: 0–180 degrees
Center thickness: 0.10–0.70 mm
Segment height: 3.00–5.00 mm

Corneal Toricity	Base Curve
Spherical	0.50 D flatter than K
0.25–1.50 D	K–0.50 D steeper than K
1.50–2.75 D	0.75 D steeper than K
2.75 D	1/3 steeper than K

Distance Power	Prism
+ ≥ 4.00 D	1.25 PD
+ 2.00 to + 4.00 D	1.50 PD
Plano to + 2.00 D	1.75 PD
Plano to − 2.00 D	2.00 PD
− 2.00 to − 4.00 D	2.25 PD
− 4.00 to − 6.00 D	2.50 PD
> − 6.00 D	3.00 PD

Courtesy of Paragon Vision Sciences, Phoenix, Arizona.

superior lid, causing lid capture. This design is highly recommended for patients with an average-to-small pupil size. Patients with small lid apertures usually have more problems with translation of this lens. When selecting the base curve, use Table 6–2.

Solitaire lenses are made of Boston RXD material. Tri-curve designs are usually best, but aspheric designs can be mechanically produced. Two diopters of prism are usually sufficient for translation; however, higher-minus lenses may require more prism. The lenses are usually not truncated if the proper edge shape is manufactured and the lens orients accurately. Lens size should never be larger than 2 mm less than the size of the lid aperture.

Walman OPC One-Piece Crescent Bifocal

The Walman OPC lens is a one-piece crescent translating bifocal lens. The distance power is located in the superior segment and the add power in the inferior segment. This thin lens design provides a trans-

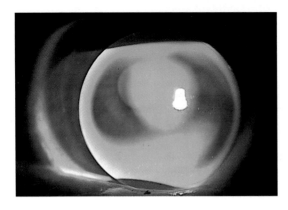

Figure 6–10. ACC translating bifocal lens showing distance segment over pupil.

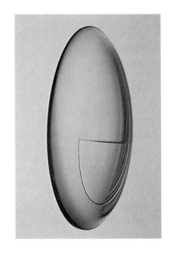

Figure 6–11. Fluoroperm ST translating bifocal lens. (Courtesy of Paragon Vision Sciences.)

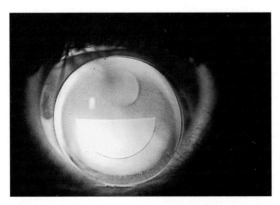

Figure 6–12. Fluoroperm ST bifocal lens fitted properly on the eye. (Courtesy of Bruce Bridgewater, OD, and Paragon Vision Sciences.)

Table 6–2. Parameters for the Solataire Bifocal Lens

Corneal Cylinder	Base Curve
Spherical	0.50 D flatter than K
0.25–0.75 D	0.25 D flatter than K
1.00–1.75 D	K–0.25 D steeper than K
2.00–2.25 D	0.50 D steeper than K

lating bifocal with excellent visual acuity. Because the segment line is not as apparent with the biomicroscopy examination as with other segmented designs, I determine the segment height using an ophthalmoscope. If the segment is too high or too low, compensation should be made by re-designing the segment height. This lens is manufactured with the computerized DAC lens lathe, which ensures more uniform, consistent optics.

Menicon USA, Inc. currently has two designs made of Menicon's SF-P RGP material. The translating bifocal designs are classic— Crescent Seg and Decentered Target. The high Dk material provides excellent oxygen transmission through these translating lens designs. The 9.4 mm standard diameter of the SF-P is available in standard base curves of 6.50 to 9.00 mm in 0.5 mm increments. Powers are + 9.75 to − 25.00 D in 0.25 D increments. The same increments are offered for add powered lenses, which are available in powers of + 1.00 to + 3.00 D. Custom parameters are also available.

TROUBLESHOOTING MULTI-FOCAL CONTACT LENSES

A. Simultaneous (aspheric) designs
　1. Visual acuity
　　a. If near acuity is poor and the contact lens slips under the lower lid, more add power should be designed into the contact lens (i.e., steeper aspheric base curve, or add the plus power to the front surface) (Fig. 6–13).
　　b. If the distance visual acuity is poor and the contact lens is not centering, modify the lens by adding more minus, or residual astigmatism of more than 0.75 D will result.
　　　The key for the aspheric design is to fit the contact lens steep to ensure maximum centering of the contact lens.
　2. Lens position
　　a. If the lens rides high, steepen the base curve, or prism may be used if necessary.

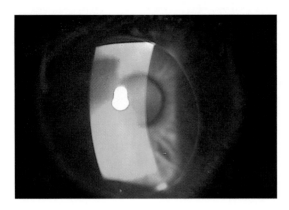

Figure 6–13. The multisite aspheric design lens fitted too flat on the eye causing lagging of lens.

    b. If the lens rides low, use a flatter or larger lens.

    c. Lateral decentration is usually caused by lid configuration or a displaced corneal apex. Therefore, if the lens rides nasally, flatten the base curve. If the lens rides temporally, steepen the base curve.

B. Translating designs

    1. Visual acuity. Compare the over-refractive findings with the expected finding.

    2. Lens position.

        a. Distance segment is too high. If the lens is resting on the lower lid, truncate to lower the distance segment. If the lens is not resting on the lower lid and is being captured by the upper lid, try steepening the lens, increasing the prism, or reducing the diameter (Figs. 6–14 and 6–15).

        b. Distance segment is too low. Decrease the prism, or order a non-truncated diameter.

        c. Rotation of truncation. If the lens rotates nasally, flatten the base curve. If the lens rotates temporally, steepen the base curve (Figs. 6–16 to 6–19).

Troubleshooting the Lifestyle Hi-Rider Lens

Adjustments to the Lifestyle Hi-Rider lens do not require much office time. If the lens is not translating and is producing poor near visual acuity, flatten the base curve 0.1 mm to move the lens upward on the cornea. The Lifestyle Hi-Rider base curve of the lens is specified as the curve of the peripheral fitting zone, called the equivalent base curve (EQBC), rather than the curvature of the central apical radius of the lens, which is the traditional base curve. If the distance vision is blurred with the initial diagnostic lens, use a slightly steeper EQBC to improve the distance vision without adversely affecting the near

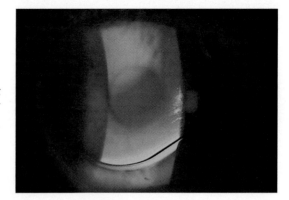

Figure 6–14. ACC translating bifocal lens riding high as a result of lid capture.

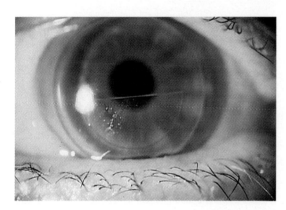

Figure 6–15. Fluoroperm ST translating bifocal lens with segment fitted too high.

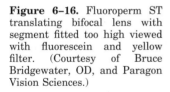

Figure 6–16. Fluoroperm ST translating bifocal lens with segment fitted too high viewed with fluorescein and yellow filter. (Courtesy of Bruce Bridgewater, OD, and Paragon Vision Sciences.)

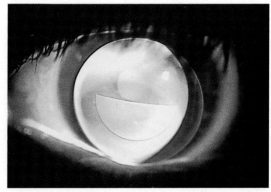

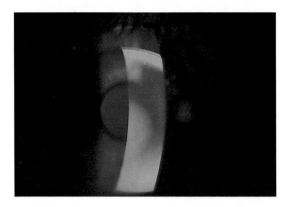

Figure 6-17. ACC translating bifocal lens fitted too low, causing flare and visual disturbance.

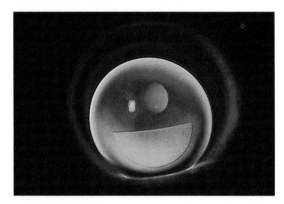

Figure 6-18. Fluoroperm ST bifocal lens with proper segment height and fluorescein pattern. (Courtesy of Bruce Bridgewater, OD, and Paragon Vision Sciences.)

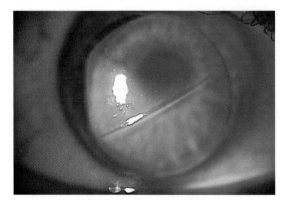

Figure 6-19. Solitaire bifocal lens with nasal rotation, indicating that the lens is too steep.

acuity. Ideally, this lens is fitted with the EQBC of the lens approximately 0.1 mm flatter than the flattest corneal curvature and produces a slight upward decentration of the lens. Adjustments of the lens superiorly and inferiorly in front of the pupil will allow the patient to eventually have maximal vision for distance, intermediate, and near.

SUMMARY

With new technology and computerized lathes, we are now able to expand the ranges for visual acuity on most simultaneous lenses. The aspheric curves can be adjusted to accommodate the prescription for far and near vision. Therefore, the aspheric modality can be considered the primary lens of choice. Those patients with residual astigmatism or wide ranges of near visual demands may be best suited for a translating design.

Computer usage is the key factor when deciding on the initial bifocal design. The second most important criterion is the age of the patient. Most translating designs can provide higher prescriptions and so are better suited to later-stage presbyopes. Emerging presbyopes do well with the VFL-3 or the Lifestyle Hi-Rider lens. Aspheric or thin translating designs are used for most patients who have never worn contact lenses or whose only experience is with hydrogel lenses.

Fitting RGP multi-focal lenses requires a unique knowledge about the patient's demands and needs. However, I encourage you to tackle this very rewarding specialty area. Small adjustments in base curve and diameter will help achieve most of the needs of these patients. Bifocal contact lens designs have expanded greatly with the arrival of new manufacturing technologies and materials. Accurate pre-selection of patients and educating patients with regard to their expectations will enhance your bifocal contact lens practice.

BIBLIOGRAPHY

Arner RS: A simplified design for the Moss-Arner bifocal contact lens. Am J Optom Arch 1965;43:464.

Bennett E: Insights on choosing an RGP multifocal design. Spectrum 1994;Mar:19.

Bennett ES, Becherer PD, Shaw RD, Henry VA: Bifocal contact lenses in the 1990s. Contact Lens Forum, 1990;April:33.

Birnbaum MH: An esophoric shift associated with sustained fixation. Am J Optom Physiol Optics 1985;62:732.

Caffery BI, Josephson JE: Rigid bifocal lens correction. Clin Contact Lens Pract 1993;42:1.

Christenson GN, Korth CJ, Marcolivio J: An investigation of the esophoria shift and its relationship to parameters of the fixation disparity curve. J Behavior Optom 1990;1:179.

deCarle J: The deCarle bifocal contact lens. Contacto 1959;3(1):5.

Fitting Guide Lifestyle Hi-Rider. Virginia Beach, Virginia, Permeable Technologies, 1993.

Fitting Guide V/X bifocal contact lenses. Montreal, Canada, GBF Laboratory, 1992.

Hammon F: Tips—how to fit multifocal contact lenses. Eyecare Business 1994;Feb:52.

Hansen DW: Current concepts of RGP multifocal contact lenses. Pract Optom 1992;3(2):70.

Hansen DW: How to fit the Lifestyle Hi-Rider. Spectrum 1993;Oct:36.

Josephson JE, Caffery BE: Monovision vs. aspheric bifocal contact lenses: a crossover study. J Am Optom Assoc, 1987;58(8):87.

Lebow KA: Presbyopic correction: Lifestyle aspheric bifocal contact lenses. Optom Today 1994:Jan/Feb:21.

Lebow K, Goldberg J: Characteristics of binocular vision found for presbyopic patients wearing single vision contact lenses. J Am Optom Assoc 1975;46:1116.

McGill EC, Erickson P: The effect of monovision lenses on the near-point range of single binocular vision. J Am Optom Assoc, 1991; 62(11):828.

McGill EC, Erickson P: Sighting dominance and monovision distance binocular fusional ranges. J Am Optom Assoc, 1991;62(10):738.

McLendon JH, Burcham JL, Pheiffer CH: Presbyopic patterns and single vision contact lenses II. South J Optom 1968;10:7.

Moss HI: Bifocal contact lenses—a review. Am J Optom Arch 1962;39:653.

The Near Add-Vantage Bifocal Fitting Guide. Sarasota, Florida, Salvatori Ophthalmics, 1990.

Schor C, Narayan V: Graphical analysis of prism adaptation, convergence accommodation, and accommodative convergence. Am J Optom Physiol Optics 1982;59:774.

Sheedy JE, Harris MG, Gan CM: Does the presbyopic visual system adapt to contact lenses? Optom Vision Science 1993;70(6):482.

Stenhouse-Stewart DD: Some observations on a tendency to nearpoint esophoria and possible contributory factors. Br J Ophthalmol 1945;29:37.

Van Meter WS, Gussler JR, Litteral G: Clinical evaluation of three bifocal contact lenses. CLAO J 1990;16(3):203.

CHAPTER 7

Presbyopia: Soft Bifocal Contact Lenses

JANICE M. JURKUS

One of your 44-year-old soft lens–wearing patients finally admits he cannot see well enough to read. He does not want to wear reading glasses over his contact lenses and has heard about soft bifocal contact lenses. He wants to know, "Are soft bifocal contact lenses perfected yet?" The answer is, "Yes, for some people." A careful matching of the patient's needs and expectations with available soft bifocal lens designs will help produce patient satisfaction.

SOFT BIFOCAL LENS TYPES

There are many bifocal soft contact lenses on the market. The majority are of the simultaneous vision design, in which optics for near and distance powers are positioned over the visual axis at the same time, and the patient learns to selectively ignore the rays that are out of focus. The different types of simultaneous vision design lenses are:

1. Simultaneous vision, aspheric back surface
2. Simultaneous vision, aspheric front surface
3. Simultaneous vision, diffractive optics
4. Simultaneous vision, concentric, near center
5. Simultaneous vision, concentric, far center

PATIENT SELECTION

Successful prescribing of bifocal soft contact lenses for the presbyopic patient requires careful patient selection. Three major aspects of the patient's ocular condition must be evaluated for appropriate lens selection:

1. Anterior segment status
2. Refractive error and stage of presbyopia
3. Visual demands and expectations

79

BOX 7-1. DO THESE FIRST

1. Discuss visual demands and expectations
2. Assure health of the anterior segment
3. Test tear film quantity and quality
4. Measure pupil in both dim and bright illumination
5. Trial fit appropriate lens type

Anterior Segment Status

As a patient ages, physiologic changes occur. The eye of a 48-year-old person is different than the eye of a 28-year-old person. The older eye has undergone changes in both quality and quantity of the tear layer. The tear layer must be evaluated to determine whether it can comfortably support a contact lens. Checking the inferior tear prism for excessive debris, performing a test of tear break-up time, and/or performing the phenol red thread test (see Appendix 1) will help diagnose non-pathologic dry eye, which is common in the presbyopic population. Non-pathologic dry eye will influence lens material and water content selection. An often used adage is, "the drier the eye, the harder the lens," the premise being that many practitioners have noticed that patients with dry eyes do better with low-water-content or rigid gas permeable lenses than with high-water-content materials. The consensus of clinical opinion is that high-water-content lenses allow water and tears to evaporate when exposed to the environment, thus robbing the dry eye of fluid, which is already in short supply. For this reason, lower-water-content, thicker lenses should be considered when fitting presbyopic patients.

Normal aging also affects corneal clarity. The presbyopic cornea with endothelial morphologic and functional changes may be more prone to swelling and edema. Epithelial disruption caused by dry eye can increase the staining rate.

Older eyelids usually have reduced lid tension and may not exert as much force to move a soft lens as those of younger patients. One must be careful to note lid closure and blink rate, because lens wetting relies on the completeness of these functions.

Contact lens thickness, water content, and replacement rate should be determined by the anterior segment evaluation. The guidelines used for all soft lens selection hold true for the presbyope.

Refractive Error and Stage of Presbyopia

Presbyopes with myopic corrections in excess of -2.00 D or hyperopic correction in excess of $+1.00$ D have a greater need for correction and are usually more motivated to wear contact lenses than are emmetropic presbyopes. Because soft lens bifocals are available only in spherical powers, vision is best if the amount of refractive astigmatism is less than 0.75 D or 25% of the sphere power.

The major deciding factor on the type of soft lens bifocal to fit is the amount of the patient's presbyopia. The *emerging presbyope* who needs a $+0.50$ to $+0.75$ D add may be best served by "pushing plus" binocularly with single-vision distance lenses. For example, a $+3.00$ D hyperope may get 20/15 acuity at distance but be troubled when doing computer work. This patient may accept slightly reduced distance acuity if near and intermediate vision are more comfortable with a $+3.50$ D distance lens.

The *early presbyope,* who has an add requirement of $+1.00$ to $+1.50$ D, will benefit from a simultaneous vision back-surface aspheric lens. These lenses generally provide comfortable near vision up to $+1.25$ D adds. Another consideration for these patients is monovision lenses.

Mid-range presbyopes, requiring adds of $+1.75$ to $+2.25$ D, often enjoy good acuity with monovision lenses. Other designs that can be considered are simultaneous vision diffractive, simultaneous vision front-surface aspheric, or simultaneous vision concentric lens designs.

The *advanced presbyope* requiring an add of $+2.50$ D or higher is generally not visually successful with bifocal soft lenses. Bifocal soft lenses can be used for modified monovision to provide an increased range of distance, intermediate, and near vision. For example, if a right eye–dominant patient has a correction of OD -3.50 sphere, OS -3.75 sphere, and an add of $+2.50$, simultaneous aspheric lenses (effective add of $+1.25$ D) with powers of -3.50 OD and -2.25 OS will give the effect of approximately $+0.75$ D intermediate correction for the right eye and $+2.50$ D at near for the left eye. More often, the mature presbyope may need reading glasses over contact lenses for near work. Rigid gas permeable designs are also effective for higher add powers.

Visual Demands

The presbyopic contact lens wearer will have to make some vision adjustments. Compromises in range of vision must be considered. If the patient has mainly distance needs with occasional near requirements, simultaneous vision with back aspheric bifocals can be used.

The patient who does computer work and thus has intermediate and near demands can use simultaneous vision aspheric designs, pushing plus to expand the near range. Distance-correcting "driving" glasses can be used to improve far vision. The patient with mainly near, occasional intermediate, and slight distance vision demands can use concentric or simultaneous vision aspheric front-surface designs.

Addressing the patient's visual demands may necessitate the explanation of expectation modification. The mature, presbyopic eye does not see the same as the 20-year-old eye did. The patient should be counseled to expect some compromise in visual acuity.

FITTING BIFOCAL SOFT LENSES

After the type of bifocal soft lens to prescribe has been decided, the fitting procedure is straightforward. All types of soft bifocals must:

1. Provide full corneal coverage
2. Center evenly on the cornea
3. Show perceptible to 1 mm of movement with the blink
4. Provide acceptable acuity at near and far

Simultaneous Vision, Aspheric Back Surface

Lenses in this category are easy to fit. A few of the brand names of aspheric back-surface bifocals are B&L PA1, Occasions, and PBH Hydrocurve II bifocals. The only parameter the fitter determines is the distance power, which should be equal to the patient's spherical equivalent prescription. The base curve, size, and add power are standard and are determined by the manufacturer. These lenses must center

---

BOX 7–2. THINGS YOU SHOULD KNOW

1. The drier the eye, the "harder" the lens should be
2. Patients with insignificant distance corrections are usually not adequately motivated
3. If the add is $\leq +0.75$ D, consider pushing plus at distance
4. For patients with adds from $+1.00 - +1.50$ D, consider simultaneous vision back-surface aspheric designs
5. For patients with adds from $+1.75 - +2.25$ D, consider monovision
6. Patients with adds $> +2.50$ D are generally less successful with soft bifocals

well to provide best acuity. If they do not center on diagnostic fitting, try a different lens design. The usable add power is about + 1.25 D.

Simultaneous Vision, Aspheric Front Surface

The usual front-surface aspheric design, as in the Unilens Aspheric, has a central near zone with a gradual change to the distance power in the mid-periphery. The power of this design is determined by adding one half the add power to the distance spherical equivalent correction. A looser fit is desired; the lens should exhibit approximately 2 mm of movement on upgaze. The standard Unilens offers a choice of 8.7- or 9.0-mm base curve with a 14.0-mm diameter. Add power is slightly greater than that provided by back aspheric designs, about + 1.75 D.

Diffractive Optics, Simultaneous Vision

This unique design uses two different types of optics, refractive and diffractive, to produce the far and near powers. The Ocular Science/ American Hydron Echelon lens is the only lens utilizing this design. The parameter selection is confined to the distance and near power, because the size and base curve are standard. The distance power should equal the patient's spherical equivalent distance prescription. Add powers of + 1.50, + 2.00, and + 2.50 D are available. The separation of the phase plate rings defines add power. Patients may experience ghosting and a three-dimensional effect while wearing these lenses. Visual adaptation may take up to 8 weeks. Vision in dim illumination may be slightly decreased.

Simultaneous Vision, Concentric, Near Center

Simultaneous center-near lenses have a distinct power zone, with the near power located centrally over the pupil. They therefore are pupil size dependent; if the pupil is smaller than the center zone, the patient will lose distance correction. The near zone is usually available in a large (i.e., 3.0–3.5 mm) and small (i.e., 2.3–2.5 mm) diameter. By prescribing the smaller near add zone on the dominant eye and the larger zone on the non-dominant eye, modified monovision can be prescribed. Centration is essential and can be observed by performing distance ophthalmoscopy and noting how much of the pupil is covered by the near power reflex. The near zone will appear as a dark area against the backlit pupil. Some lenses of this type are the Ciba Spectrum Bifocal, Alges Bifocal, and Simulvue.

Simultaneous Vision, Concentric, Far Center

Lenses of the distance center–near surround design, such as Ciba's Bisoft, are also pupil size dependent; therefore, centration is mandatory. The power to be prescribed for distance should equal the spherical equivalent power; adds range from + 1.50 to + 3.00 D in 0.50 D steps. It may be useful to use an add power slightly higher than that of the spectacle refraction, but be aware that patients may experience a ghosting or halo effect in dim illumination. Patients with small pupils may not obtain effective near vision with this design, particularly in bright illumination.

SUMMARY

Regardless of the type of soft lens bifocal prescribed, the fitter must also be aware that lens drying, surface coating, and other complications that occur with single-vision soft lenses also occur with soft bifocals. Awareness and management of both visual and physiologic complications are required.

Prescribing soft lens bifocals is an art. The fitter must identify the patient's visual needs and help create realistic expectations regarding soft bifocal contact lens performance. Matching patient desires with the most appropriate soft contact lens bifocal design can provide adequate vision and satisfied patients.

BIBLIOGRAPHY

Bennett ES, Becherer PD, Shaw RF, Henry VA: Bifocal contact lenses in the 1990's. Contact Lens Forum 1990;Apr: 33–47.
Bennet ES, Henry VA: *Clinical Manual of Contact Lenses*. JB Lippincott, 1994; 362–398.

CHAPTER 8

Presbyopia: Monovision

CAROL A. SCHWARTZ

Monovision is the fastest, easiest, most effective way of fitting multifocal contact lenses. The system consists of fitting each of the eyes to serve a different purpose; typically, one eye is fitted with a single-vision lens correcting distance vision, and the other eye is fitted for near vision. In some cases, a multifocal lens may be used to create a trifocal effect; this is known as modified monovision. Key factors in monovision fitting include patient motivation, patient selection, and problem-solving; fitting of the lenses is identical to that for conventional single-vision contact lenses.

After the patient has been deemed suitable for monovision, the fitting is a simple, straightforward process. When screening monovision candidates, the fitter must take three factors into consideration: visual requirements, lifestyle, and physiologic needs.

VISUAL REQUIREMENTS

Distance refractive error should be fully correctable; small amounts of astigmatism, which might be ignored when fitting single-vision lenses, may be critical to the monovision wearer. If one eye is slightly amblyopic, it should be fitted for near; if near vision through this eye is unacceptable, the patient is probably better suited to bifocal spectacles than contact lenses.

Near requirements are more important diagnostically. Presbyopic correction of less than 1.00 D is generally insufficient to induce the selective suppression necessary for monovision. Hyperopic patients requiring an add of less than 1.00 D often find that soft contact lenses, particularly

---

BOX 8–1. DO THESE FIRST

1. Determine distance correction
2. Determine near add and ranges
3. Determine dominant eye
4. Question patient about working positions, which may influence choice of near eye
5. Demonstrate monovision if diagnostic lenses are available

spin-cast designs, delay the need for near correction. Myopic and emmetropic patients are not as fortunate. In these cases, pushing an add in
excess of actual need (generally 1.25 D) often is successful.

The fitter may wish to approach older presbyopes (i.e., those with near
additions of 2.00 D or more) with caution, because these patients have firmly ingrained visual habits which are often very difficult to break. In
addition, the patient may find the anisometropia induced by monovision
correction unacceptable. For these reasons, success rates for such patients
being fitted with their first monovision correction are generally lower
than those for younger presbyopes. The exception is emmetropic presbyopes who have relied on reading-only spectacles; their visual habits
have been poorly formed, and they are usually as successful entering
monovision as younger patients. Increasing the add of a current monovision patient to more than 2.00 D also generally is trouble-free.

Patients who require intermediate correction may also be fitted with
monovision, although generally in a modified monovision system. Emmetropic and myopic patients whose distance correction approximates
their near add often do well when fitted with one lens.

LIFESTYLE FACTORS

The ideal monovision patient is motivated to avoid wearing glasses,
works at both near and far distances in approximately equal measure,
and has no contraindications for contact lens use. Office workers are
generally ideal candidates, as is anyone frequently in the public eye.

For activities such as long-distance driving or piloting a private
plane, stereopsis is crucial to safety. Patients who routinely engage
in such activities must be counseled not to wear their monovision
correction while doing so, although monovision may be worn on other
occasions. Patients who spend prolonged hours doing near work may
find monovision more comfortable if the dominant eye is fitted for
near; alternatively, they may benefit from a slight spectacle reading
addition and bright room illumination. Patients who must read in
upward or straight-ahead gaze are especially suited to monovision.
Examples of such patients include pharmacists and auto mechanics.

Presbyopic computer users have special visual requirements: they
must be able to read both at intermediate and distance zones in primary gaze, as well as the near zone in downward gaze. Such patients
are ideally suited to monovision and modified monovision. If the patient has a small pupil, the fitter may consider reducing the add
slightly to allow him or her to use one lens for both intermediate and
near work, leaving the contralateral eye fully corrected for distance.
Alternatively, modified monovision should be considered.

All other vocational and avocational contraindications to contact lens
wear apply equally to monovision patients: exposure to fumes and
dust, dry or humidity-controlled environments, or operating hazardous

machinery. Presbyopic patients whose work precludes any sort of contact lens wear will find monovision soft lens correction easier to adapt to than bifocal contact lenses but more difficult than bifocal spectacles.

PHYSICAL FACTORS

Monovision patients must fulfill all general criteria for contact lens wear. Pupil size should also be taken into consideration; those with small pupils (i.e., ≤ 2 mm) enjoy a greater depth of field, in some cases approaching a trifocal effect. In general, patients with small pupils will be happier with monovision when their tasks include intermediate zone needs.

Many patients fitted with monovision experience lenticular changes evidenced by an increase in against-the-rule astigmatism. Although manifest in the refraction, this newly acquired cylinder often does not improve acuity. Unless there is subjective improvement in vision, there is no need to correct these changes; of more benefit to many patients is improved lighting.

Careful assessment of tear volume should be done prior to fitting, because many patients who desire monovision correction suffer from marginal dry eye as a result of hormonal changes associated with the aging process. For these patients, rigid lenses may be preferable. Tear substitutes or punctal occlusion may make any type of contact lens

Table 8-1. Monovision Screening Criteria

	Prognosis		
Factor	*Poor*	*Fair*	*Excellent*
Age (y)	≥ 55	50–55	40–49
Add (D)	≥ 2.00	< 1.00	1.00–1.75
Distance prescription	$\leq \pm 0.75$ D	cyl ≥ 1 D OU	Monocular prescription
Previous mode of correction	None	Spectacles	Contact lenses
Motivation	Low	Moderate	High
Pupil Size (mm)	>3	2–3	<2
Apprehension of I&R	Yes	Slight	None
Occupational needs	Critical N/F only Poor light	Much near	All zones CRT oper.
Avocational needs	Stereocritical	Near intense	General
Column total Weighted total Total score	$\times 1$	$\times 2$	$\times 3$

To quantify potential monovision success, circle the answer that best describes the patient regarding each of the criteria. Add the number of circles in each column and multiply by that column's weighting factor. Add the total weighted score for the three columns to achieve a final grand total that reflects this patient's probable success in monovision. Prognosis: excellent 22–27, good 12–21, poor 9–11.

OU = both eyes; I&R = insertion and removal; N/F = near/far; CRT = cathode ray tube (i.e., computer).

more comfortable for such individuals. Table 8–1 is a monovision screening form that can be used to simplify patient selection.

FITTING TECHNIQUE

The actual fitting of monovision is very simple. After the patient has been screened, the fitting proceeds as normal; however, eye dominancy must be assessed. Tests of eye dominance are described in Box 8–2. None of these tests are 100% accurate; therefore, the fitter may wish to use more than one test. One should also question the patient about occupational or recreational tasks that may require a particular eye to be fitted for near or distance vision. An example would be a typist whose work station cannot be altered; the eye closest to the copy should be fitted for near work.

After eye dominance has been determined, lenses may be fitted as follows: full distance correction in one eye, full near correction in the

---

BOX 8–2. EYE-DOMINANCY TESTS

1. *Hole-in-hand.* Have the patient make a hole with their hands and sight a small distance object by centering it in the hole. While they continue to hold this position, alternately occlude each eye, asking the patient each time if the object remains centered. If the target remains centered, the dominant eye is open; if it moves, the non-dominant eye is open. Carefully watch the patient while they perform this task—they may move their hands toward the dominant eye.
2. *Hole-in-card.* The same test can be performed using a sheet of plain white cardboard in which a 10-mm hole has been cut in the center. Sighting and alternate occlusion is performed as for the hole-in-hand test.
3. *Thumb-sighting.* The patient is asked to stretch their arm to the fullest extent with the thumb extended upward. They are then asked to superimpose their thumb on a small distance target. The eyes are alternately occluded, and dominancy is determined in the same manner as in other tests.
4. *Most plus at near.* If sighting tests are inconclusive, determine which eye can accept more plus at near. This is generally the non-dominant eye.
5. *Balancing brightness.* When performing binocular balancing during the refraction, the patient is asked which target is brighter. The brighter target is being viewed by the dominant eye.

other. Because presbyopic patients often find it difficult to handle lenses, a tinted lens is almost universally used. More often than is typical in general contact lens practice, monovision deals with hyperopic patients; center thickness is therefore of concern. If soft contact lenses are being fitted, a high-water-content material may be necessary to ensure sufficient oxygen supply to the cornea. A Dk of 40 to 60 is recommended in a rigid lens; in addition, the fitter may consider a minus lenticular carrier to avoid low-riding lenses.

Some fitters have recommended dispensing three lenses to each monovision patient, two distance lenses and one reading lens, the premise being that when involved in intensive distance-only activities, the patient will remove the near lens. Although this procedure seems reasonable from the standpoint of maintaining stereopsis at distance, in reality, it generally fails because of inconvenience. Over-glasses to correct the anisometropia also rarely succeed and are generally unpopular with patients. A better procedure is to explain the third-lens concept to the patient as a possibility.

Modified Monovision

Some patients with critical demand in the intermediate zone find they need trifocal contact lenses. They may be accomplished with a technique known as modified monovision, in which one eye is fitted with a multifocal lens. The near eye is typically fitted with a multifocal lens designed to correct for intermediate and near distances. Concentric designs, which contain a central distance zone, are well suited for this purpose. The distance eye remains fitted with a single-vision lens.

PATIENT MANAGEMENT

Perhaps the greatest problem with monovision is that of explaining it to the patient. Unless the patient is familiar with successful monovision wearers, they generally find the technique implausible. One way to motivate patients as well as screen them for monovision success is called the demonstration technique. Before entering into a discussion of monovision, diagnostic lenses in the approximate monovision prescription are placed on the patient, who is then allowed to adapt. After one-half hour, the fitter should be able to determine if monovision is appropriate for this patient, because they have experimented with it on their own. All the fitter need do is explain the technique; the patient has already been convinced it will work and is motivated to continue the fitting.

If no diagnostic lenses are available, the fitter must rely on an oral explanation. Oral explanations are rarely as motivational as demonstrations and tend to be more time-consuming. Several concepts from the psychology of selling may be helpful. First, it is important to list all available options from worst (bifocal spectacles) to best (monovision). Cite a credible person as being successful with the technique; for example, one of the many U.S. presidents who has worn monovision or one of the patient's acquaintances. Last, understate the success rate, and stress the length of time the technique has been in use.

It is typical for presbyopic wearers to take slightly longer to learn insertion and removal. Tinted lenses will help hyperopic patients see the lenses on the eye and in their hand. Monovision patients should be instructed to insert the near lens first and remove it last. It is also wise to prepare a handout explaining the technique, listing common symptoms of adaptation and suggesting that the patient experience night driving in monovision first as a passenger, then attempt driving when he or she has more fully adapted. The patient should also be cautioned to pay extra attention to room illumination in the first weeks of adaptation. Spare pairs of lenses are often very attractive to the monovision patient who quickly becomes dependent on his or her contact lenses.

PROBLEM-SOLVING

Most symptoms of monovision adaptation disappear within 14 days; for this reason, many fitters delay the first checkup whenever possible. A study by Josephson found that 55% of patients adapted to monovision within 1 week, 25% adapted in 2 weeks, and the remaining 20% never adapted. Many of the monovision problems listed in Table 8–2 spontaneously disappear when the patient has fully adapted. Of those that do not resolve within 2 weeks, the majority are caused by fitting the inappropriate eye for near. If any symptom persists after the adapta-

Table 8–2. Problem-Solving Monovision Fittings

Symptom	Probable Cause	Solution
Asthenopia: transient	Adaptative	Wait at least 1 mo for full adaptation (average is 2 wk)
Asthenopia: frequent or prolonged	Power or optics off	Verify and correct
	Uncorrected cylinder	Refit with toric or rigid gas permeable lenses
	Incorrect add power	See Blur, persistent
	Patient not suitable	Refit with another modality
Blur: distance	Optical problem	Verify power and optics
	Uncorrected cylinder in distance eye	Refit distance eye with toric lens
	Not suppressing—add too low	Refit with higher ($\geq +1.25$ D) add

Table 8-2. Problem-Solving Monovision Fittings *Continued*

Symptom	Probable Cause	Solution
Blur: intermediate	Large intermediate demand	Reduce add slightly (0.50 D) Refit with modified monovision; bifocal in near eye If task-specific and not routine, refit with third lens for intermediate use only
Blur: near, constant	Incorrect add power	Over-refract and adjust power
Blur: near, task-specific	Excessive near demand in occupation or hobby	Over-spectacles for task only
Difficulty handling lens	Can't see lens	Refit with tinted lens— remove near lens LAST, insert near lens FIRST
Difficulty with insertion and removal	Old habits	Schedule 2-day session— learn to care for lenses first, wear 4 h, return to learn insertion and removal
Dry eyes	Reduced tear production Lens drying	Increased use of lubricants Refit with thicker, lower-water-content lenses or more wettable rigid gas permeable lenses
Fatigue	Excessive close work	Over-spectacles: plus over distance eye, plano over near eye
Flare	Optical zone too small	Measure pupil in normal and dim illumination, refit with optic zone at least 2 mm larger than scotopic pupil
	Tint reducing light entering pupil	Limit to annular and visibility tinted lenses
Frequent lens loss or damage	Patient not able to see lens well when handling	Refit with tinted lenses
Headache	Young presbyope: accommodating with distance eye	Increase add to 1.25 D; if problem persists, delay monovision until add requirements increase

Table continued on following page

Table 8–2. Problem-Solving Monovision Fittings *Continued*

Symptom	Probable Cause	Solution
Involuntary eye-switching	If transient: visual stress	If during adaptation: do nothing; if due to temporary change in circumstance (e.g., tax time) refrain from monovision use until stress alleviated
	If persistent: eyes fitted incorrectly	Refit distance eye for near and vice versa
Light-headedness	If transient: adaptative symptom	Delay action for 2 wks
	If persistent: possible systemic problem	Refer to internist
Low-riding rigid gas permeable lenses	Lens too heavy	Refit with lenticular, minus carrier, or larger overall diameter design
Night driving difficult	Complains of flare	See "Flare"
	Complains of poor vision or loss of spatial relations	Over-spectacles with minus added to near eye or third lens for prolonged night driving
Non-suppression	Add insufficient to cause suppression in early presbyope	Use at least 1.25 D add to force suppression
Persistent blur or haze	Incorrect lens power	Over-refract and refit
	Edema	Refit with greater Dk lens
	Constant: poor optics	New lens
	Uncorrected cylinder	Refit with toric or rigid gas permeable lenses
	Add too low	Increase add by 0.50 D
	Add >2 D (new wearer)	Patient unsuitable for monovision or cut add by 0.50 D
	Wrong eye for near	Switch eyes
Slight or intermittent blur or haze	Adaptative within 2 wk of fitting	Counsel patient to increase lighting, wait
	Poor fit	See Persistent blur or haze
Vague complaints of discomfort	Wrong eye for near	Switch eyes
	Intermediate demand (especially if myopic, low add)	Refit with modified monovision, bifocal on near eye

tion period, the recommended solutions are listed in Table 8–2 in order of likelihood.

BIBLIOGRAPHY

Back A, et al: The comparative visual performance of monovision and various concentric bifocals. Transcript: British Contact Lens Assn: Annual Clinical Conference, 1987;4:46.

Charman WN: Theoretical aspects of monovision contact lens correction. Contact Lens Monthly 1980;Feb: 19–22.

Farnsworth C: What's so hard about monovision? Rev Optom 1984;Aug: 32–35.

Garland MA: Monovision and related techniques in the management of presbyopia. CLAO J 1987;13(3):179–181.

Harris MG, Classe JG: Clinicolegal considerations of monovision. Optom Assoc 1988;59(6):491–495.

Heath DA, et al: Suppression behavior analyzed as a function of monovision addition of power. Am J Opt Physiol Optics 1986;63(3):198–201.

Josephson JE, Caffery B: Bifocal hydrogel lenses: an overview. J Am Optom Assoc 1986;57(3):190–195.

Josephson JE, Caffrey BE: Monovision vs. aspheric bifocal contact lenses: a crossover study. J Am Optom Assoc 1987;58(8):652–653.

Koetting RA: Monocular fitting: a viable alternative for the presbyope. J Am Optom Assoc 1982;53(2):134–135.

Koetting RA: Monovision contact lens fitting in presbyopia. Optom Extension Program, Nov., 1983, 11–15.

Koetting RA: Stereopsis in presbyopes fitted with single vision contact lenses. J Am Acad Optom Physiol Optics. 1970;Jul:557–561.

Lester RW: The bifocal contact lens today. California Optom Assoc 1959;28(1):22.

London R: Monovision correction for diplopia. J Am Optom Assoc 1987;58(7):568–570.

Loshin DS, et al: Binocular summation with monovision contact lens correction for presbyopia. Int Contact Lens Clin 1982;9(3):162–165.

McGeehon M: Survey: practitioners unhappy with current bifocal lenses. Contact Lens Forum 1988;13(6).

Meier GD: Monovision contact lens fitting and functional vision. Optometric Extension Program 1983;1:3.

Nolan JA, Nolan JJ: Driving with monovision. Optom Monthly 1984;Aug:308–313.

Nolan JA, Nolan JJ: Monovision with glasses. Optom Monthly 1983;Mar:130–133.

Pence NA: Modified trivision: a modified monovision technique specifically for trifocal candidates. Int Contact Lens Clin 1987;14(12):484–488.

Rothman SM: Monovision fitting of contact lenses for presbyopia: review and personal comments. J Optom Vision Development 1985;16:19–21.

Sanchez FJ: Monovision—which eye for near? Contact Lens Forum 1988;13(6).

Schor C, Landsman L, Erickson P: Ocular dominance and the interocular suppression of blur in monovision. Am J Optom Physiol Optics 1987;64(10):723–730.

Sheedy JE, et al: Monovision contact lens wear and occupational task performance. Am J Optom Physiol Optics 1988;65:1.

Weinstock FJ: Techniques and designs of soft bifocal lenses. Contact Lens Forum 1988;13(10):14–18.

Williams CE: An evaluation of the CSI Plus series with emphasis on monovision fitting. Int Contact Lens Clin 1983;10(3).

Wood WW: Monovision does work! Optom Management 1985;Sep:49–56.

CHAPTER 9

Extended Wear Soft Lenses

CRISTINA M. SCHNIDER

Fitting soft lenses for extended wear has become less fashionable in recent years because of concerns about the increased risk of corneal complications, despite advances in our understanding of the underlying mechanisms of these problems. However, extended wear lenses are still a very popular modality with patients considering contact lens wear. With appropriate patient education, fitting, and follow-up, it can still be a useful addition to the various contact lens options in clinical practice.

The most important advice to anyone fitting soft lenses for extended wear is to begin with only the best patients. This requires careful assessment of the entire ocular surface and tear film, in addition to the patient's motivation and hygiene. Slit lamp biomicroscopy should be carefully performed, first with white light, and then with fluorescein and cobalt blue light with a yellow-gold barrier filter for optimal viewing of the fluorescein. White-light observation should begin with the pre-corneal tear film, because this layer is easily disturbed by other procedures. Using diffuse illumination and/or the area of specular re-

---

BOX 9–1. DO THESE FIRST

1. Evaluate tear film to rule out:
   - Extreme instability
   - Excessive lipid and/or debris
2. Evaluate lids and lashes to rule out:
   - Blepharitis
   - Meibomianitis
   - Tarsal plate inflammation
3. Evaluate cornea to rule out:
   - Neovascularization
   - Staining
4. Evaluate compliance:
   - Laziness is NOT an excuse
   - Extended wear means extended care

---

flection of the slit lamp beam, view the tear film for the presence of excess lipid (i.e., colored fringes with black spots that float by on the blink) or debris. A high level of lipid and/or debris in the unmolested tear film can signal problems with tear production or lid integrity. If you don't have a ground-glass diffuser on your slit lamp, a simple substitute is to create one by using two or three layers of translucent adhesive tape suspended over the light source. Be sure not to place the tape directly on any lenses or mirrors. Following assessment of the tear film with white light, view the closed lids and lashes, looking for signs of blepharitis (i.e., scales, crusts, or debris along the lash margins). With the patient's eyes open, inspect the openings of the meibomian glands to look for blockages, scarring, or unnatural secretions. Gently squeeze the lid against the globe and view the expression from the glands—it should express easily and be perfectly clear. Evert the upper lid to view the tarsal conjunctival surface, looking for unusual redness or bumpiness of the tarsal plate. Ignore bumps along the lid fold and in the far nasal and temporal areas (Fig. 9–1).

Following completion of the diffuse scan of the ocular surface, remove the diffuser and view the cornea in direct focal illumination with a moderately wide parallelepiped. Pay particular attention to the limbal area, because any significant vascularization is a contraindication to an extended wear schedule. Instill fluorescein and view the cornea in cobalt light with a yellow-gold barrier filter in place over the objective (Fig. 9–2) to identify any corneal staining that might indicate a dry eye condition.

The final assessment that must be made prior to fitting a patient for extended wear is the patient's motivation and compliance. This should include a discussion of the increased risks and responsibilities that are inherent in any extended wear regimen. The patient must understand that overnight wear of even approved lenses increases the risk of

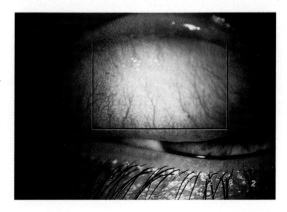

Figure 9–1. Tarsal conjunctival surface. The main area of concern for contact lens wear is the large rectangle outlined in black. The areas around the lid fold and canthi are of less importance.

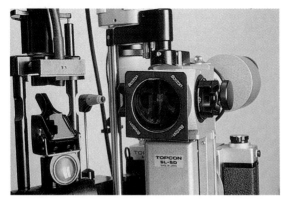

Figure 9-2. Wratten 2 barrier filter (Polymer Technology Corp., RGP Laboratories) placed over slit lamp objective to enhance appearance of fluorescein.

infectious keratitis, and that other complications, such as lid inflammation and corneal vascularization, may be increased with improper lens care or fitting. Additionally, the nature of soft lenses is such that changes may occur over time; adequate follow-up is required to continually assess on-eye performance.

After you have determined that your patient is suited to extended wear, you must select the appropriate lens to fit. As described in Box 9-2, the two most important aspects of lens fitting are adequate oxygen transmission characteristics of the lens and assuring lens translation to allow flushing of debris from behind the lens. With respect to oxygen transmission, both the water content of the material and its thickness are of importance. High-water-content lenses (≥ 50% water) pass oxygen more easily than low-water-content lenses, but they also must be made thicker for a given power. This means that the thinnest high-water-content lens will perform about the same as the thinnest low-water-content lens for standard low-minus powers, even though the average thicknesses are different. However, whenever thickness requirements for any part of the lens exceed the minimum possible for a given water content, as with high-plus or high-minus lenses, oxygen transmission will generally be superior with the high-water-content lenses.

There are other aspects of lens performance to consider. High-water-content lenses tend to be more fragile and require more frequent replacement than low-water-content lenses. The way in which the lenses deposit is also different; high-water-content lenses are somewhat more prone to deposition overall. However, low-water-content lenses tend to attract deposits primarily on the surface of the lens and may cause more irritation to the lid surface. In either case, frequent replacement of extended wear lenses can make either problem of little significance. Replacing the lenses every 2 to 4 weeks generally proves optimal in terms of material performance. Longer replacement intervals require

BOX 9-2. THINGS YOU SHOULD KNOW

1. Oxygen transmission
   - Low-H_2O lenses for extended wear must be THIN (<0.04 mm)
   - High-H_2O lenses better for thicker designs
     High minus powers
     Plus powers
     Toric designs (not recommended for extended wear)
2. Replacement frequency
   - More often is always better
     2 wk ideal
     3 mo maximum (with enzymes)
3. Lens diameter
   - Use minimum diameter to achieve limbal coverage
   - Try steeper base curve or alternate design with decentered lens
4. Base Curve
   - Fit as loose as possible without discomfort
     Primary gaze movement will be minimal with extended wear designs
     Use lag or finger-push assessment
5. Power
   - Determine by over-refraction of trial lens
   - Expected: spherical equivalent of spectacle prescription corrected for vertex distance

more attention to care, such as the addition of enzymatic cleaning. Following a decision on lens material, parameter selection is usually straightforward. Most lenses come in only one or two diameters and two or three base curves. To maximize tear exchange on the blink, use the smallest possible diameter and the loosest base curve that provides adequate limbal coverage. If trial lenses are available in all available base curves, the diagnostic fitting should be performed with the two flattest base curves available, unless the cornea is unusually steep (i.e., >45.00 D). Note that the middle base curve in a three-lens series will yield an acceptable fit in more than 80% of cases, with considerable overlap with the steeper and flatter bases.[1]

Allow the lens to settle for 15 to 20 minutes before making a final decision on fit. This time can be used for performing the over-refraction; discussing lens care, fees, and follow-up; and completing any necessary paperwork. A written informed consent document is recommended for extended wear patients and should be reviewed at this time.

When assessing lens performance, movement should be assessed in all positions of gaze. Primary gaze movement is usually minimal because of the thin lens profiles used for extended wear lenses. The lens should lag or slip slightly on upgaze or lateral gaze. The most useful assessment in most cases is finger-push movement. To perform this assessment, use your finger to pull the patient's lower lid to a point below the lens edge, push the lens up firmly, and quickly lower the lid. If the lens immediately returns to its normal position, finger-push movement is free. This is assurance that the lens will translate adequately during normal gaze excursions. If the return is sluggish, a looser base curve may be needed.

Power is determined by performing a spherical over-refraction over the trial lens, using the most plus or least minus power that yields best acuity. The sum of the trial lens and the over-refraction should be within about 0.25 D of the spherical equivalent of the vertex distance–corrected spectacle plane refraction, which is necessary if either meridian exceeds ± 4.00 D.

PROBLEM-SOLVING

Because of differences in material characteristics and lens designs, the base curve designation is of little help when comparing lenses of different materials or from different manufacturers. Therefore, if one type of lens does not provide acceptable movement or centration despite changing base curves, don't be afraid to try what appear to be exactly the same parameters from a different manufacturer. The most common mistake fitters make is increasing lens diameter to improve centration. A lens that decenters, causing limbal exposure, particularly in the superior temporal direction, is usually just too flat and not too small. Selecting a steeper base curve or alternate design will often improve centration without adversely affecting movement.[1] Similarly, if acuity is not optimal with one lens, simply changing the base curve (usually to a flatter curve) or lens type can yield surprising results. If acceptable acuity cannot be achieved using spherical lens designs and a toric lens is needed, it is best to return to a daily wear schedule. The increased thickness of most toric lens designs does not provide adequate physiologic performance for full-time extended wear.

The primary problems encountered with soft lens extended wear occur not during the fitting but during the follow-up period. Patients should be advised to wear their lenses no more than 6 nights per week, and less whenever possible, to minimize the cumulative effect of insufficient oxygen to the cornea. The lenses should be thoroughly cleaned and disinfected at the time of each removal and replaced at the appointed interval. If replacement frequency exceeds 2 to 4 weeks, enzymatic cleaning is usually indicated.

Complications related to hypoxia and inflammation are the most frequently encountered problems in patients on an extended wear regimen.[2-4] The most common hypoxia-related complications are striae, microcysts, and neovascularization. Because of the different thickness profiles for plus- and minus-powered lenses, the complications observed for each may be different. Plus lenses are more likely to cause central striae, whereas vascularization is more commonly seen with minus-powered lenses. Epithelial microcysts are seen in nearly all soft lens extended wear patients at some time and indicate the chronic hypoxia present with this modality. All edema-related complications require increasing the amount of oxygen available to the cornea. Increasing water content, decreasing thickness, or altering lens parameters to increase lens movement and tear exchange can have a small effect, but reducing the amount of overnight wear is by far the most effective strategy.

Managing hypoxia can also have an impact on inflammatory complications, because an edematous cornea seems to facilitate the movement of inflammatory cells into the cornea. Because the limbus is the most active area immunologically, avoiding insult to this area by maintaining a well-moving lens is key in managing these complications. The free movement of the contact lens during the open-eye period also facilitates the removal of debris, which may also act as a stimulus to inflammation, especially during closed-eye periods. The use of lubricating drops before retiring and upon awakening also assists in the removal of debris.

The fitting of soft lenses for extended wear is simple, requiring mainly good observational skills during the patient-screening and follow-up periods. Utilizing one of the many extended wear–approved frequent-replacement lenses provides the best balance of oxygen transmission and clean lens surface required for maintaining a healthy ocular environment. In no case should extended wear exceed the recommended 6 nights per week, and fewer nights are certainly desirable with currently available hydrogel materials.[5]

REFERENCES

1. Young G: Soft lens fitting reassessed. CL Spectrum 1992;7(12):56.
2. Efron N, Holden BA: A review of some common contact lens complications. Part 1: the corneal epithelium and stroma. Optician 1986;192(5057):21.
3. Efron N, Holden BA: A review of some common contact lens complications. Part 2: the corneal endothelium and conjunctiva. Optician 1986;192(5062):17.

4. Terry RL, Schnider CM, Holden BA, et al: CCLRU standards for success of daily and extended wear contact lenses. Optom Vis Sci 1993;70(3):234.
5. Schein OD, Buehler PO, Stamler JF, Verdier DD, Katz J: The impact of overnight wear on the risk of contact lens-associated ulcerative keratitis. Arch Ophthalmol 1994;112(2):186.

CHAPTER 10

Extended Wear: Rigid Gas Permeable Lenses

VINITA ALLEE HENRY

Extended wear contact lenses have decreased in popularity since their introduction, most likely as a result of the complications experienced with hydrogel extended wear. However, rigid gas permeable (RGP) extended wear lenses have been quite successful and have resulted in fewer complications. This is primarily because of the increased oxygen permeability and oxygen transmissibility of RGP lens materials. When a patient approaches the practitioner with a desire for extended wear lenses, RGP lenses should be a primary consideration. The first factors for the practitioner to evaluate are listed in Figure 10–1 and are discussed in the following sections.

THE EXTENDED WEAR CANDIDATE

The desire to wear extended wear contact lenses does not necessarily make the patient a good extended wear candidate. Although RGP extended wear lens wearers have experienced fewer complications than those using hydrogel extended wear lenses, complications are increased compared with daily wear lenses; thus, extended wear should be reserved for patients who find them a necessity because of refractive error, occupation, or hobbies. A thorough case history, including information about the patient's reasons for desiring extended wear lenses, visual acuity, occupation, hobbies, contact lens history, and medical history, is important in patient selection. A good extended wear candidate is a successful daily wear contact lens patient who needs to be able to wear contact lenses for longer periods of time because of his or her occupation or high refractive error. The patient should be extremely compliant in making follow-up visits and caring for his or her contact lenses. Questions to ask a potential extended wear patient are listed in Box 10–1 and described in detail in the following sections.

101

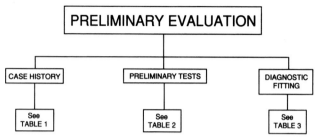

Figure 10-1. Preliminary evaluation of a rigid gas permeable extended wear candidate.

Why Do You Want Extended Wear Lenses?

Why a patient desires extended wear is important in establishing whether or not the reason is valid. A patient who desires extended wear lenses to decrease care or handling time generally is a patient who will demonstrate poor compliance. Extended wear lenses also require lens care and handling. The longer the lens is worn, the more deposits build up on the lens surface, requiring careful cleaning and disinfection on removal. Thus, a lazy, non-compliant patient is a poor candidate for extended wear. Conversely, a patient with a high refractive error who finds it difficult to function without visual correction or someone who works long or varying hours (e.g., nurses, doctors, emergency medical technicians) has a very real need for constant vision correction and may benefit greatly from extended wear. Patients who travel frequently or take camping trips and desire extended wear

---

BOX 10-1. PRELIMINARY CASE HISTORY QUESTIONS

1. Why do you want to wear extended wear contact lenses?
2. Have you worn contact lenses before?
3. Have you ever experienced any complications with contact lens wear?
4. What is your average wearing time?
5. How do you care for your present contact lenses?
6. Do you have spectacles you wear as a backup?
7. What are your occupation and hobbies?
8. Do you have any current medical or ocular conditions?
9. Are you taking any medications?
10. Do you experience seasonal or chronic allergies?
11. Have you experienced dryness of the eyes with or without contact lens wear?

lenses for these periods of time are other examples of patients who might benefit from extended wear lenses because of their occupations or hobbies. These patients will still need to be prepared to remove the lenses if there are any complications, but they may benefit from the ability to maintain lens wear during trips.

Have You Worn Contact Lenses Before?
Have You Ever Experienced any Complications With Contact Lens Wear?

Questions pertaining to the patient's contact lens history will aid the practitioner in determining the level of success of previous contact lens wear. A successful daily wear RGP patient likely will be a successful RGP extended wear patient, if all other ocular findings are normal. Likewise, a current RGP daily wearer experiencing contact lens–induced complications will most likely have increased complications with extended wear. Conversely, an unsuccessful hydrogel patient may be a good candidate for RGP wear if the reason for the lack of success is lens deposits, giant papillary conjunctivitis, corneal edema, or poor visual acuity. Other complications, such as dryness and lens adherence, will only be exacerbated by extended wear contact lenses.

What Is Your Average Wearing Time? How Do You Care for Your Present Contact Lenses?

These questions address current patient compliance. A daily wear patient should wear his or her lenses for an average of 12 to 14 hours. If the patient's wearing time is consistently longer than this either the patient's occupation or hobbies require longer hours, suggesting that extended wear is a good solution, or the patient is not compliant. If the patient wears daily wear lenses on an extended wear basis as a result of laziness, this suggests that he or she will also wear extended wear lenses longer than the recommended wearing period. This patient should be either thoroughly re-educated or considered a poor candidate and not fitted for extended wear lenses.

Do You Have Spectacles to Wear as a Backup?

All contact lens wearers should have backup spectacles in case of emergency complications. Because complications are more likely with extended wear, the need for backup spectacles and a willingness to wear them are important for continued success. Many daily and extended wear contact lens complications are exacerbated by continued wear of the lens because of a lack of backup spectacles or poor motivation to wear spectacles.

What Are Your Occupation and Hobbies?

This question has been covered in the first question's discussion; however, it is also important to remember that some occupations or hobbies may increase the risk of contact lens wear, such as a dirty, unsanitary environment (e.g., sand blasting, automobile mechanics, sanitation worker). In addition, some work environments prohibit contact lens wear (e.g., environments where chemicals and chemical fumes are present).

Do You Have any Current Medical or Ocular Conditions? Are You Taking any Medications? Do You Experience Seasonal or Chronic Allergies?

Patients with systemic conditions, such as diabetes, in which wound healing may be reduced, are at a higher risk with extended wear and are not good candidates. Likewise, pregnancy often affects the tear film, making it more viscous; thus, deposits are more prevalent, and the eye may be more dry, complicating extended wear. Patients with corneal dystrophies, keratoconus, post–radial keratometry or aphakia resulting in corneal compromise are also poor candidates for extended wear because of an already compromised cornea. Medications that can alter the tear film, thus creating a dry eye, include antihistamines, anticholinergics, anti-anxiety agents, phenothiazines, and oral contraceptives.[1] Allergies do not prevent extended wear of contact lenses if the allergies are seasonal and the patient realizes that reduced or no wear of the contact lenses may be necessary while the allergies are manifest.

Have You Experienced Dryness of the Eyes With or Without Contact Lens Wear?

Tear film abnormalities and dryness of the eyes are early predictors of lack of success with extended wear and are factors in causing complications such as corneal desiccation, lens adherence, and discomfort. In an early RGP extended wear study, 2 of 18 patients who discontinued wear within the first 3 months were patients with tear break-up times of less than 10 seconds.[2] Therefore, a patient exhibiting poor tear break-up times and less than optimal tear films should not be considered a good candidate for extended wear.

PRELIMINARY TESTING

When the patient is seated for the examination, some very basic testing should be performed after the case history is taken. The combination of the answers the patient provides during the case history and the results of the testing form a profile of the patient that is used in predicting patient success with extended wear. Preliminary tests, which should be performed prior to fitting with diagnostic lenses, are listed in Box 10–2.

Visual Acuity and Subjective Refraction

It is important to use baseline visual acuity and refraction as a gauge of the physiologic condition of the cornea throughout extended wear. Visual acuity should be 20/20 or, if reduced, an adequate explanation for the decrease in visual acuity should be determined. The predicted power of the final lenses is determined based on the subjective refraction and keratometry readings.

Keratometry

Keratometry readings are necessary to select diagnostic lenses. In addition, note any irregularities, mire distortion, or high amount of corneal astigmatism. Baseline values are also important so that it can be determined whether any changes occur in the corneal curvature during extended wear.

Slit Lamp Examination

A thorough slit lamp examination of the lids, lashes, conjunctiva, sclera, and cornea should be performed, not only to document baseline

---

BOX 10–2. PRELIMINARY TESTS

1. Visual acuity
2. Subjective refraction
3. Keratometry
4. Slit lamp examination
5. Lid eversion
6. Tear break-up time
7. Fluorescein evaluation
8. Slit lamp examination of any current lenses

values, but also to note any ocular abnormalities that may prohibit extended wear. Corneal dystrophies and pterygia are contraindicators of extended wear. Pingueculae will most likely not affect extended wear, but should be documented and monitored. Blepharitis or meibomianitis should be treated prior to initiating extended wear. Thorough documentation of corneal scars and lid position should be recorded as baseline values.

Lid Eversion

Although giant papillary conjunctivitis, also referred to as contact lens–related papillary conjunctivitis, is most common with hydrogel contact lenses, it has been noted on occasion with rigid lenses. Extended wear of rigid lenses, which increases the length of contact of the lens and lid compared with daily wear and possibly increases surface deposition, may increase this condition in rigid lens patients. Therefore, baseline documentation of the upper and lower lids should be obtained to determine whether changes occur with lens wear.

Tear Break-Up Time

By instilling fluorescein and having the patient hold his or her eye open for 10 to 20 seconds, the practitioner can scan the tear film for dark areas where the tear film is breaking up. The amount of time it takes for this to occur is termed tear break-up time (BUT). A tear BUT of 10 seconds or more is considered normal. In addition, observe the tear film for debris and oiliness to determine the quality of the tear film. Observation of the tear prism along the lower lid should reveal a straight and regular edge with a height of at least 0.3 mm in patients with an adequate tear film.[3] Other tests that aid in determining the patient's quantity of tear film are the Schirmer's tear test and the newer, more promising phenol red thread tear test.[4]

Fluorescein Evaluation

Baseline fluorescein evaluation should reveal little or no staining. If the patient is a current RGP daily wearer and reveals moderate corneal desiccation, it is unlikely they will be successful with extended wear unless the fit of the current lenses is poor.

Slit Lamp Examination of Current Lenses

Whether the current contact lenses are rigid or hydrogel, it may be helpful to observe the current fit of the lenses to determine if any previous complications are the result of a poor fit. The condition of the lenses can also be a clue to the patient's care and handling of the lenses.

DIAGNOSTIC FITTING

Diagnostic fitting of lenses is important in determining the final lens order. Empirical fitting, or fitting by using subjective refraction and keratometry readings to predict the final lens, has been found to result in more lens reorders, less patient confidence, and reduced patient compliance than fitting diagnostically.[5] Diagnostic fitting requires more time initially; however, in the long-term, this option produces a more satisfactory result. Experienced practitioners will verify that predicted lenses do not always perform as well as expected because of other factors, such as the tear lens and corneal topography. It is helpful to use diagnostic lenses of the same or very similar material and design as those to be ordered, because super-permeable lenses used in extended wear vary in specific gravity and flexibility. If a daily wear RGP lens material or a polymethyl methacrylate (PMMA) lens is used as a diagnostic lens, the final lenses may flex or decenter because of the differing lens mass and flexibility. By using the subjective refraction and keratometry readings, predicted lenses can be selected for the patient to try. The lens parameters that should be selected are listed in Box 10–3.

Lens Material

The early generation of RGP extended wear lenses were made of silicone acrylate (S/A) or polystyrene. To increase the oxygen permeability of the S/A materials, the amount of silicone had to be increased, which in turn increased the hydrophobic properties of the lens, resulting in a less wettable material. Polystyrene proved to be low in oxygen permeability and very prone to scratches. The polystyrene lens was approved

---

BOX 10–3. STEPS IN SELECTING LENS PARAMETERS

1. Lens material
2. Base curve
3. Power
4. Diameter
5. Center thickness
6. Final design

---

for only 36 hours of extended wear. Therefore, S/A and polystyrene materials are not currently used for extended wear.

To improve oxygen permeability and surface wettability, fluorine was added to silicone acrylate lenses. The primary extended wear lens materials used today are made of fluorosilicone acrylate (F-S/A). These F-S/A lens materials perform well when worn on an extended wear basis and provide deposit resistance, lens stability, and improved surface wettability. RGP extended wear lens materials that are approved by the United States Food and Drug Administration (FDA) are listed in Table 10–1 with the lens name, manufacturer, lens material, and Dk value.[6]

Oxygen permeability of a lens material is specified by the Dk value. Oxygen transmissibility of a lens must take into consideration the thickness of the lens; it is specified as Dk divided by lens thickness or Dk/L. It is important to remember that even if a high-Dk lens material is used, if the lens has an increased average thickness, oxygen transmission will be reduced. Thus, in the case of a hyperope, a high-Dk lens material must be used to achieve the same oxygen transmission as that of a lower-Dk myopic lens. In addition, if the lens is made thicker to decrease lens flexure, the oxygen transmission will be reduced.

Ideally, an RGP extended wear lens would result in an edema-free cornea. The Holden and Mertz criterion for an edema-free cornea upon awakening suggests that a Dk/L of 87 is required. To obtain a Dk/L of 75 to 100 and an equivalent oxygen percentage of 16%, the resultant minus lens would need a Dk of approximately 126 with an average thickness of 0.17 mm, and a low hyperopic lens would require a Dk of approximately 202 with an average lens thickness of 0.27 mm.[7–9] Lens materials are beginning to approach the necessary Dk values for the optimum lens; however, despite the lower than optimum Dk values currently approved, RGP extended wear lenses have been successful. In addition, it is important to realize that different corneas require different amounts of oxygen. Each patient must be monitored closely

Table 10–1. Rigid Gas Permeable Extended Wear Lens Materials

Lens Name	Manufacturer	Material	Dk
Polycon HDK	PBH	S/A	40
Paraperm EW	Paragon Vision Sciences	S/A	56
Fluoroperm 60	Paragon Vision Sciences	F-S/A	60
Fluorocon	PBH	F-S/A	60
Equalens	Polymer Technology	F-S/A	64
Fluoroperm 92	Paragon Vision Sciences	F-S/A	92

for symptoms and clinical signs of corneal edema to determine whether the lens provides sufficient oxygen for a given patient's cornea.

With this knowledge, which lens material is best for each particular patient? Extended wear lenses containing fluorine are superior to the other materials because they provide greater oxygen permeability and surface wettability; therefore, a fluorinated material is optimum. Occasional extended wear patients may require the medium-Dk lens materials (i.e., 60) to provide better durability when lenses are worn on a daily wear basis. Likewise, a previous PMMA or low-Dk RGP wearer may have acquired poor lens-handling habits, which could result in lens warpage of a highly superpermeable lens. These patients may benefit from beginning with a medium-Dk lens material and being re-educated on lens handling. They may be re-fitted at a later date into a higher-Dk material if the need arises. Hyperopic patients, full-time extended wear patients (i.e., 7 days of extended wear), and patients who exhibit corneal edema with medium-Dk lenses should be fitted with the high-Dk materials (i.e., ≥ 90).

Base Curve

Base curve radius (BCR) selection for extended wear lenses is very similar to that for daily wear RGP lenses. The optimal fit is a lens that centers well and tucks under the upper lid. To achieve this fit, the BCR selected should be equal to or slightly flatter than the flatter K reading. If the corneal astigmatism is greater than 2.00 D, it is likely that a bitoric lens design will be required to achieve an optimal fit. Hyperopic prescriptions require a slightly steeper BCR to maintain good centration. I subscribe to the fitting philosophy of Bennett, and his BCR selection guidelines are found in Table 10–2.[10]

Power

The predicted lens power is based on the subjective refraction and the tear lens. For example, if the subjective refraction is -2.50 D and the

Table 10–2. Base Curve Selection Guidelines

Corneal Cylinder (D)	Base Curve of Diagnostic Lens
0–0.50	0.50–0.75 D flatter than flat K
0.75–1.25	0.25–0.50 D flatter than flat K
1.50	On flat K
1.75–2.00	0.25 D steeper than flat K
2.25–2.75	0.50 D steeper than flat K
3.00–3.50	0.75 D steeper than flat K

BCR is 0.50 D flatter than flat K (i.e., "K"), the tear lens is equal to -0.50 D; therefore, the predicted lens power would be -2.00 D. If a -3.00 D diagnostic lens is fitted on the eye, the expected over-refraction would be $+1.00$ D. The final lens power is based on the diagnostic lens power plus the over-refraction; in this case, -2.00 D. If this final power differs from the predicted power, the diagnostic lens power and base curve should be verified. If the power and base curve are correct, a compromise can be made between the final lens power and the predicted lens power at the practitioner's discretion.

Diameter

The diameter of the lens should be large enough to provide good centration and prevent flare. A good starting point is a 9.2 mm diameter; however, diameters may range from approximately 9.0 to 10.0 mm. The diameter depends on the patient's palpebral aperture size, pupil size, refractive error, and lid tension.

Center Thickness

The higher the Dk value, the more flexible the lens becomes; therefore, extended wear lenses typically need a slightly greater center thickness to decrease the possibility of flexure and warpage. An increase in center thickness of approximately 0.02 mm over the lower-Dk materials is recommended. It is important to keep a careful thickness balance between making the lens more stable and reducing the oxygen transmission. A recommended center thickness chart is given in Table 10–3.[10]

Final Design

The final lens design should be based on the findings of the diagnostic lens fit. Once the BCR, power, and diameter have been determined, a

Table 10–3. Rigid Gas Permeable Extended Wear
Thickness Chart

Power (D)	Center Thickness
-1.00	0.19 mm
-2.00	0.18 mm
-3.00	0.16 mm
-4.00	0.15 mm
-5.00	0.14 mm
≥ -6.00	0.14 mm

lens design philosophy can be used to design the final lens. Such a design takes into consideration the edge lift and edge design to provide good tear exchange and comfort.[11]

Tricurve design
   Secondary curve radius: BCR + 1.0 mm/0.3 mm wide
   Peripheral curve radius: SCR + 2.0 mm/0.3 mm wide

Tetracurve design
   Secondary curve radius: BCR + 0.8 mm/0.3 mm wide
   Intermediate curve radius: SCR + 1.0 mm/0.2 mm wide
   Peripheral curve radius: ICR + 1.4 mm/0.2 mm wide

There are also computer programs that will design the peripheral curve systems after the BCR, power, lens material, and diameter are entered. Other factors to consider in the final lens order are blend and tint. I prefer a medium blend on the junctions of the peripheral curves. An example of a final lens design is as follows:

BCR: 7.8 mm
SCR: 8.6 mm/0.3 mm width
ICR: 9.6 mm/0.2 mm width
PCR: 11.0 mm/0.2 mm width
Power: − 3.00 D
Diameter/optic zone diameter: 9.2 mm/7.8 mm
Center thickness: 0.16 mm
Fluoroperm 60
Medium, or 'B', blend
Blue tint

FOLLOW-UP EVALUATIONS

After the lenses are dispensed and a good fit is achieved, the patient should be given a wearing schedule. Extended wear lenses should never be worn for more than 7 days without an overnight break. The patient may desire to alter this schedule. For example, some representative schedules include 3 days on with an overnight break, 5 days on with an overnight break, daily wear during the week and extended wear over the weekend, and extended wear only for business trips. Make sure the patient understands that the risks of extended wear increase the longer the lenses are worn. Extended wear lenses are FDA approved for 7 days of extended wear with an overnight break. To insure the lenses are removed weekly, it is best if the patient has a routine of removing the lenses each week on a set day or days: for example, every Saturday.

    The patient must be monitored on a regular basis. If the patient has never worn lenses, it is generally recommended that the patient build up to all day wear prior to wearing the lenses on an extended wear basis. The patient can be evaluated after 1 week of daily wear. If the patient is performing well with daily wear, the next visit would be the morning after the patient first sleeps in the lenses. Most symptoms and clinical signs of edema will disappear within the first 2 hours after awakening; therefore, a morning appointment will allow the practitioner to observe edematous signs. The next visit should be 3 to 7 days later. It is preferable for the patient to be evaluated after wearing the lenses for several days of extended wear rather than at the beginning of the weekly cycle; therefore, ask the patient to make each appointment after several days of wear. The follow-up schedule recommended for this first-time RGP extended wear patient is a 1-week daily wear visit, 24 hours after wearing lenses extended wear, 3 to 7 days later, and at 2 weeks, 1 month, and 3 months after first wearing the lenses extended wear. Thereafter, the patient should be evaluated every 3 months. If the patient is currently an RGP daily wearer, the visits are the same, except that the 1-week daily wear visit is not necessary.

At each follow-up examination, the following tests are recommended:

Subjective comments or complaints
Visual acuity
Over-keratometry
Over-refraction
Slit lamp examination with and without lenses
Lid eversion
Fluorescein evaluation with and without lenses
Keratometry
Subjective refraction

LENS CARE

As mentioned previously, increasing oxygen permeability of the lens is often accompanied by increased flexibility. This flexibility makes the lens more soft and fragile. The lenses are easier to warp and scratch. Because these lenses are worn longer, surface deposits may become more problematic. To properly care for extended wear lenses, the care system used should be one approved for RGP lenses and should consist of a wetting and soaking solution, surfactant cleaner, saline, lens lubricant, and most likely, an enzyme cleaner. The lenses should be cleaned on each removal in the palm of the hand with the little finger. Lenses cleaned between the index finger and thumb or in the palm of the hand with the index finger are more likely to become warped. In addition, cleaning between the index finger and thumb with an abrasive cleaner has been found to add minus power to the lens over time.[12] Therefore, although these cleaners can be very effective, they must be applied with a gentle digital pressure. After the lens is thoroughly cleaned and rinsed with saline, the lens should be stored overnight in a wetting and soaking solution to disinfect the lens. The following morning, the lens can be inserted. Lens lubricants are very beneficial for extended wear patients to use on awakening and at bedtime. This lubrication aids in flushing trapped debris and in rewetting the lens prior to sleep. An enzymatic cleaner, used either at every removal, every 2 weeks, or once a month, probably will be necessary to remove surface deposits, which commonly results because of the length of lens wear.

Poor initial surface wettability may be a problem with extended wear lens materials. Prior to being dispensed, the lenses should be soaked for 12 to 24 hours and the lens parameters verified. Often, the period of soaking alone will produce a comfortable, wettable lens. If the lens continues to exhibit poor wettability, even after soaking, use a laboratory cleaner such as Boston Laboratory Cleaner (Polymer Technology Corporation) or Fluoro-Solve (Paragon Vision Sciences). These cleaners cannot be used daily and should not be dispensed to the patient; however, they will aid in removing adherent substances such as residual pitch, waxes, and oils left from the manufacturing process, thus improving surface wettability.

COMPLICATIONS

The primary complications associated with rigid extended wear are warpage, flexure, corneal edema, corneal desiccation, lens adherence, vascularized limbal keratitis, and corneal abrasion. The following paragraphs discuss each complication in detail.

Warpage and Flexure

As suggested previously, the flexibility of these high-Dk rigid lenses can result in lens warpage or flexure. The symptom of either warpage or flexure is reduced visual acuity. Upon examination with the lenses on, it is difficult to differentiate between the two problems. Both may exhibit cylindrical over-keratometry readings and sphero-cylindrical over-refraction; however, when the lens is removed and the BCR verified on the radiuscope, the lens that is flexing will verify as a spherical lens on the radiuscope. Flexure is the result of the lens flexing or bending on the eye. To correct flexure, the lens may be fitted slightly flatter (i.e., 0.50 D or more) or the center thickness increased. Conversely, a lens that is warped will verify as spherical on the lensometer and as toric (2 base curve radii) on the radiuscope. Warpage is often the result of handling the lens with excessive pressure. Commonly, patients prone to warpage are previous PMMA or low-Dk rigid lens wearers. If the lens is cleaned in the palm of the hand with the little finger, warpage should not occur. The excessive heat and pressure of cleaning a lens between the thumb and index finger is the primary cause of lens warpage. If a patient continues to warp lenses while cleaning in the palm of the hand with the little finger, a hands-off type of cleaning, such as the Hydramat (PBH) can be used.

Corneal Edema

The early, acute signs of corneal edema are more difficult to observe in rigid extended wear patients than in hydrogel extended wear patients. Central corneal clouding, which is a faint circular haze seen in epithelial edema, is most easily observed by using sclerotic scatter or split limbal illumination. The patient may report morning blur for the first 15 to 30 minutes after awakening. If blur remains after 30 minutes, a change in lens is indicated. Vertical striae or fine white lines, typically in the pupillary region, appear when the stroma is swollen approximately 4% to 6%. Striae may be observed using a narrow parallelopiped.[13,14]

In chronic edema, microcysts can be observed as vacuoles or bubbles in the epithelium. Microcysts are cysts of cellular debris that migrate to the surface of the epithelium, resulting in fluorescein staining and mild to moderate discomfort. Microcysts can be viewed with marginal retroillumination in the area of the pupillary rim. Any observation of microcysts reveals an edematous condition requiring careful patient monitoring; however, more than 50 microcysts indicates a need for lens discontinuation.[15,16]

Another clinical sign of corneal edema is polymegethism. The endothelium is a layer of polygonal-shaped cells. With hypoxia, these cells become irregular and appear to vary in size and shape. This is known as polymegethism and polymorphism. The long-term effect of this phenomenon has not yet been determined. Polymegethism is best viewed with high magnification and specular reflection.[13,14,17]

Corneal Desiccation

Perhaps the most common complication with extended and daily wear rigid lenses is desiccation in the 3- and 9-o'clock regions of the cornea. This staining is a result of dryness in the affected areas. When the lens is removed daily, the lid has a chance to wet the areas of desiccation; however, with extended wear, this problem may be exacerbated because of the length of wear. The desiccation appears as areas of punctate staining that become coalesced and can eventually cause an area of opacification and vascularization if left unchanged. If an extended wear patient has areas of 3- and 9-o'clock staining that begin to coalesce, the patient should be reduced to a daily wear schedule. Methods of treatment include blinking exercises, lens lubricants, fitting fluorinated materials with improved surface wettability, a superior tucked-under-the-lid fit, and a lower edge lift. Obviously, blinking exercises and lens lubricants are secondary to providing a good lens fit and design.

Lens Adherence

Adherence of a rigid lens can happen with daily or extended wear; however, it is more common in extended wear. There are at least two reasons why adherence occurs with overnight wear: negative suction occurs with lid closure, and tears under the lens become more viscous.[14] An adhered lens will typically decenter peripherally and exhibit very little or no movement. If the lens is truly adhered, fluorescein will pool around the periphery but will be absent under the center of the lens. Trapped debris under the lens will form a circular pattern around the lens periphery. Upon lens removal, an indentation ring may be evident on the cornea. This indentation ring will typically disappear soon after lens removal. Frequently, superficial punctate staining will be observed where the debris was trapped against the cornea. If a lens has very little movement, punctate keratitis is present, the periphery of a lens appears very deposited, and a slight outline of the lens edge may be observed on the eye, it is apparent that the lens is exhibiting intermittent adherence.

Two methods of preventing lens adherence without changing lens design are the use of lens lubricants prior to sleeping and on awakening and keeping the lens clean and free of deposits. If these two methods do not prevent adherence, the following changes in lens parameters may be beneficial: (1) selecting a flatter BCR, (2) increasing the center thickness, (3) decreasing the diameter, and (4) flattening or blending the peripheral curve radii. A lens that occasionally adheres on awakening can be lubricated and the lens massaged through the closed lid to promote lens movement. If lens adherence is not corrected, it may lead to corneal distortion, edema, and even ulceration.[18]

Vascularized Limbal Keratitis

Vascularized limbal keratitis (VLK) can be observed in the 3- and 9-o'clock areas in both rigid daily and extended wear patients. Initially, the clinical signs include conjunctival hyperemia, staining, and peripheral infiltrates, which progress to an opaque elevated lesion and superficial and deep vascularization. VLK may progress through four stages: hyperplasia, inflammation, vascularization, and erosion.[14] Patient symptoms are lens awareness, pain, and redness. In the early stages, the lens may be re-designed by flattening the BCR or peripheral curves; in the later stages, however, lens wear must be discontinued until the condition has regressed.[13,19]

Corneal Abrasion

Corneal abrasions are not necessarily more common in rigid extended wear than in rigid daily wear, except in instances in which a patient may abrade the cornea upon awakening. Typically, the lens has displaced slightly or become slightly adherent during sleep. The patient forcefully pushes the lens in place, thus abrading the cornea. The use of a lens lubricant before sleep and upon awakening will lubricate the lens, preventing this from occurring. Foreign bodies (e.g., mascara, other cosmetic particles, dust) trapped behind the lens are the most common cause of abrasion in daily and extended wear rigid lenses. The use of a lens lubricant to flush the debris away or removal of the lens and thorough rinsing should prevent an abrasion from occurring.

SUMMARY

RGP extended wear lenses can be a successful modality for many patients. Careful patient selection, thorough testing, diagnostic fitting

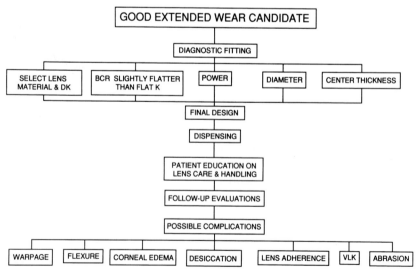

Figure 10–2. Nomogram of fitting and evaluating rigid gas permeable extended wear patients.

frequent follow-up, and patient compliance will enable most patients to enjoy wearing RGP extended wear contact lenses. A summary nomogram to highlight important points the practitioner needs to know is found in Figure 10–2.

REFERENCES

1. Bennett ES, Gordon JM: The borderline dry-eye patient and contact lens wear. Contact Lens Forum 1989;14(7):52.
2. Henry VA, Bennett ES, Forrest JF: Clinical investigation of the Paraperm EW rigid gas permeable contact lens. Am J Optom Physiol Opt 1987;64(5):313.
3. Lowther GE, Malinovsky VE: Dry eye: a clinical overview. Ft. Worth, Texas, Alcon Laboratories, 1988.
4. Sakamoto R, Bennett ES, Henry VA, et al: The phenol red thread tear test: a cross-cultural study. Invest Ophthalmol Vis Sci 1993;34(13):3510.
5. Bennett ES, Henry VA, Davis LJ, Kirby S: Comparing empirical and diagnostic fitting of daily wear fluoro-silicone/acrylate contact lenses. Contact Lens Forum 1989;14(3):38.
6. Thompson TTT: Tyler's quarterly soft contact lens parameter guide. 1993;11(1):48.
7. Holden BA, Mertz GW: Critical oxygen levels to avoid corneal edema for daily and extended wear contact lenses. Invest Ophthalmol Vis Sci 1984;25(10):1161.
8. Fatt I: The super-permeable rigid lens for extended wear. Contact Lens Spect 1986;1(1):53.
9. Bennett ES, Tomlinson A, Mirowitz MC, et al: Comparison of overnight swelling and lens performance in RGP extended wear. CLAO J 1988;14(2):94.
10. Bennett ES: Basic fitting. In Bennett ES, Weissman BA (eds): *Clinical Contact Lens Practice.* Philadelphia, JB Lippincott, 1991:1.
11. Bennett ES: Hard extended wear contact lenses. In Dabezies OH (ed): *Contact Lenses—The CLAO Guide to Basic Science and Clinical Practice.* Boston, Little, Brown & Co., 1990:1.
12. Carrell BA, Bennett ES, Henry VA, Grohe RM: The effect of rigid gas permeable lens cleaners on lens parameter stability. J Am Optom Assoc 1992;63(3):193.
13. Henry VA, Bennett ES, Sevigny J. Rigid extended wear problem solving. Int Contact Lens Clin 1990;17(5,6):121.
14. Schnider CM, Bennett ES, Grohe RM: Rigid extended wear. In Bennett ES, Weissman BA (eds): *Clinical Contact Lens Practice.* Philadelphia, JB Lippincott, 1991:1.
15. Zantos SG: Cystic formations in the corneal epithelium during extended wear of contact lenses. Int Contact Lens Clin 1983;10(3):128.
16. Holden BA, Grant T, Katow M: Epithelial microcysts with daily and extended wear of hydrogel and rigid gas permeable contact lenses. Invest Ophthalmol Vis Sci (Suppl) 1987;28:327.
17. Schoessler J: Endothelial polymegathism associated with extended wear. Int Contact Lens Clin 1983;10(3):148.
18. Morgan BW, Bennett ES: RGP lens adherence. Contact Lens Update 1989;8(2):17.
19. Grohe RM, Lebow KA: Vascularized limbal keratitis. Int Contact Lens Clin 1989;16(7,8):197.

CHAPTER 11

Frequent Replacement and Disposable Lenses

Neil B. Gailmard and Susan M. Gailmard

A breakthrough occurred in the contact lens field when Vista-kon introduced the first truly disposable contact lens under the brand name Acuvue; today, many manufacturers compete with variations on this theme. Prior to the commercially available blister-packaged lenses, some optometrists were already administering their own in-office planned replacement programs with vialed lenses; this was particularly popular with extended wear lenses.

The concept of frequent replacement of soft contact lenses was quickly accepted because it offered several advantages to both the patient and the practitioner. The fact that soft lens materials deteriorate with use, even with extreme efforts in cleaning, made this an excellent product to replace regularly. The lenses were introduced to the profession at a price low enough to allow the program to be presented to patients at a yearly cost not much greater than that of conventional lenses.

The manufacturers provided diagnostic trial lenses to doctors at no charge, which was a major investment by the companies. It paid off well, because these trial lenses were marketed to patients as free trial pairs. The practitioner needed to buy only the multipacks, which were, in turn, resold to patients. Lenses could be stocked in inventory or ordered as needed. The provision of contact lenses in "six-packs," offering the ultimate in convenience, was a marketing hit, but some doctors complained that it contributed to a trivialization of contact lenses. There was concern that this marketing strategy caused patients to not understand the risks of the medical device, possibly increasing non-compliance with professional care.

Disposable lenses were initially used only for extended wear. As clinical studies continued to document concern regarding the ocular health risks of extended wear, and as disposable lenses gained popularity, they began to be fitted more and more on a daily wear basis. As a matter of semantics, the daily wear use of lenses that were disposed of regularly became known as frequent replacement, programed replacement, or planned replacement. Technically, the United States

118

BOX 11-1. DO THESE FIRST

1. Discuss the options of conventional lenses versus disposable lenses. Review the patient advantages and yearly costs of each system. Consider limiting the number of programs offered within your practice and setting fees so that patients find disposables affordable.
2. Discuss extended wear versus daily wear; disclose the risks of extended wear to the patient; and weigh the risks against the convenience factors.
3. Tell patients what you recommend as best for them.
4. Trial fit good candidates with free disposable lenses and schedule a follow-up visit.

Food and Drug Administration (FDA) defines a disposable lens as a lens that is only used once—that is, whenever it is removed from the eye, it is discarded. With the maximum FDA-approved wearing time at 1 week, these lenses must be replaced at least weekly. Taking the concept of disposability to the maximum, manufacturers are now producing 1-day disposable lenses. Many lens brands that are actually disposable are prescribed and used on a daily wear basis, in which they are cleaned, disinfected, and reused by the patient. This technically makes them frequent replacement lenses. Many different programs exist under the description of frequent replacement, with various wearing schedules and replacement cycles of 2 weeks, 1 month, or 3 months. Disposable and frequent replacement lenses have been a tremendous improvement in the clinical management of the contact lens patient and have been good for the management and profitability of contact lens practice.

PATIENT ADVANTAGES

When compared with conventional lenses, many of the advantages of frequent replacement lenses can be related to the wearing of cleaner lenses. By disposing of the lens very often, the patient wears contacts with very little build up of proteins.

An advantage of frequent replacement lenses that is of primary concern to the optometrist is that of ocular health. Clinical evidence, as well as professional common sense, suggests that cleaner lenses produce fewer inflammatory responses from allergic or infectious processes. Disposable lenses have been successful in very sensitive patients and can reduce the incidence of red eyes, giant papillary conjunctivitis, and even dry eye complaints. A valid concern over eye health complications is prevalent with extended wear, but patients and practitioners must be careful to not automatically assign the risks of extended wear to the disposable modality in general.

Convenience is a major reason that disposable lenses have been so widely accepted. Patients enjoy the easy lens care, which may range from no care at all for the disposable extended wear patient to an easy rub and a soak overnight in a one-step solution for the daily wear patient. The daily wear patient may not need a separate surfactant cleaner or an enzymatic cleaner. Cleaner contact lenses can also contribute advantages to patients in the form of better vision and better comfort. Additionally, having a large supply of lenses on hand reduces bother if a lens is lost, torn, or damaged. Many doctors replace damaged lenses at no charge from their free trial supply. It is important that practitioners do not cancel out the convenience of disposables with office policies that are overly complex.

Depending on the fee structure of the practice, disposable and frequent replacement lenses can be more economical for patients than conventional lenses. Savings are realized by not buying replacement contacts for loss or damage, by buying fewer care products and cleaners throughout the year, and often, by not buying contact lens insurance or service agreements.

PRACTICE ADVANTAGES

One of the benefits doctors have enjoyed from disposable contact lenses comes in the form of better patient compliance: disposable lens wearers return for regular periodic examinations because they run out of contact lenses and need a new supply. Many practices dispense a standard number of lenses to last the interim between recommended visits and will only dispense more lenses after the checkup. Compliance with cleaning procedures is usually very good because the methods are so simple and inexpensive.

The use of disposable lenses can lead to fewer problem patient visits, because the cleaner lenses cause fewer complaints. Reduced problems caused by discomfort, blurred vision, and inflammation make examinations quicker and easier. These elements convert to greater patient satisfaction and increased word-of-mouth referrals of new patients.

Profitability is another advantage of frequent replacement systems, despite a trend for reduced prices on materials as a result of competition from alternate dispensing sources. The profit in this modality comes from the regular patient visits and the vast increase in the number of lenses purchased.

PRESCRIBING AND FITTING

Fitting disposable and frequent replacement lenses is exactly the same as fitting conventional soft lenses (see Appendix 1). A comprehensive eye examination, which includes a slit lamp examination before lenses are inserted, keratometry, and refraction, is always performed first. A good candidate is a patient with healthy eyes, good motivation, and a refractive error in the range available from manufacturers. Disposable lenses are indicated for questionably suitable patients, such as those who suffer from dry eye or allergies, because this system provides for lenses that are generally free of protein build up.

A trial lens is applied to the cornea so that centration and movement can be evaluated with the slit lamp. Some practitioners feel that disposable lenses tend to "look tight," even though base curves are relatively flat. Many of these cases still demonstrate excellent physiology after long-term lens wear. Practitioners may find different brands of lenses work better in different base curves; for example, our preference for most patients is the 8.8 base curve Acuvue, the 8.4 mm–base curve NewVue, and the 8.7 mm SeeQuence2. An over-refraction is performed to confirm the correct power.

Follow-up visits are scheduled as in any contact lens fitting; 1- and 3-week post-dispensing visits are typical. During these follow-up visits, a case history is taken, hygiene is reviewed, acuities and over-refraction are rechecked, keratometry is done with lenses off, and a slit lamp examination is performed. Resolving problems may include changing base curves or lens materials, changing wearing time if extended wear, changing lens powers, switching to toric designs, and changing lens care solutions.

Generally, disposable and frequent replacement lenses are easy to fit and present relatively few complications. Eye infections and corneal ulcers have been implicated with disposable lenses but seem to be more connected with extended wear rather than disposability. These problems are treated with topical therapeutic agents and temporary discontinuation of lens wear based on the diagnosis.

LENS DISCARD CYCLES

With so many different programs in practice, it is clear that a frequent replacement system can be quite successful *as long as the practitioner and staff are behind it.* Surveys show that the majority of throw-away cycles are at 2 weeks, but many others exist. The practitioner should consider many factors when deciding on a program. It may be practical to offer only one system of frequent replacement in a practice rather than to offer the patient a confusing array of options. This also prevents staff confusion over what fees to charge, the number of boxes to dispense, the timing of follow-up visits, and other details.

It is wise to dispense a sufficient number of lenses to last the interim between routine examinations, which may vary with daily wear or extended wear. Resist requiring superfluous visits of the patient, because this reduces convenience and raises patient costs. There is no need to see the disposable lens patient any more often than a conventional wearer.

The number of contact lenses in a box may have an effect on the throw-away cycle. Lenses are available in boxes of 6, 4, 3, and 30 (for daily disposal). Six-packs lend themselves nicely to discard cycles of 1 week, 2 weeks, and 1 month if the fitter intends to see the patient every 6 months, because the practitioner is able to dispense the proper number of lenses to be used in the interim. Four-packs are convenient for quarterly replacement programs because 1 box for each eye will last for 1 year, although this may remove the motivation for the 6-month check-up. Packs of 3 pairs of lenses work for any length program.

Keep in mind that the psychology of having a large quantity of lenses on hand can be significant for giving the impression of more value to the patient and for making it easier for them to actually part with lenses. Two-week discard cycles provide 26 pairs of lenses per year, compared to 4 pairs on a quarterly system, or only 2 pairs if dispensed in 6-month bundles. It also may be easier to remember the 2-week deadline rather than a 3-month deadline.

SPECIALTY LENSES

With the popularity of the disposable modality, manufacturers are offering most specialty contacts in this format. Toric lenses and bifocal designs are currently available, as are visibility tints, enhancement tints, and opaque lenses. All of these specialty lenses have been successful as disposable lenses, because the basic advantages for frequent replacement still apply. This has allowed a larger number of refractive conditions and cosmetic interests to be met. The lower price per lens has made these specialty disposable products very appealing to patients.

CLEANING AND DISINFECTING SYSTEMS

The same procedures apply to daily wear frequent replacement lenses as to conventional lenses. One-step multi-purpose solutions are quite popular, because they match the convenience theme of disposable lenses. Allergic and sensitive patients do well with non-preserved systems such as hydrogen peroxide–based products. It is generally not necessary to recommend the use of enzymatic cleaning except for lenses that are to be used for 3 months or longer.

An important step in the proper cleaning and disinfecting of all contact lenses is the friction rub with either a daily cleaner or the multi-purpose solution. Much debris and build up is removed with this rub, and a great deal of disinfection of microorganisms occurs during this step as well. Disposable lens patients often skip this step; therefore, the doctor and technician should take extra care to instruct the patient on its importance.

FEE STRUCTURE

Fee structures for disposable lenses are based on either professional fees plus materials or a global annual fee similar to a service agreement. Both methods work well, but the patient eventually comes to understand what the cost is for one multi-pack of lenses. This can easily be compared in cost to alternate sources, so a good strategy is to keep product price low and competitive. This allows higher fees to be charged for professional services, such as the fitting and ongoing examinations. It is hard to compare professional services, and you can increase the value of this aspect of care by providing excellent service and clinical care.

MANAGING REQUESTS FOR CONTACT LENS PRESCRIPTIONS

This is a matter of professional judgment, and also of state law; therefore, there is no one right way to handle requests for contact lens prescriptions. We believe the best philosophy is to treat contact lens prescriptions like drug prescriptions, which means we do release them to patients, but only when certain conditions important to safeguard eye health are met. The doctor can set an expiration date for contact lens prescriptions, and if the patient does not return for recommended follow-up care, the prescription becomes invalid or expires. Refusing to release the prescription may seem to patients like an abuse of their rights because they paid for the care. The ill will created can be detrimental to your practice. It may be better to tell the patient that you will release the prescription in writing but that a check-up is needed first if he or she is past due for one.

It is critical that patients be educated regarding the medical nature and risks of contact lens wear and the importance of regular examinations, even if the patient is asymptomatic. Many patients do intend to return for regular eye care as recommended but want their prescription for various reasons. It is unnecessary to force them out of your practice by refusing to release a prescription or by offering to transfer their entire record to another practitioner.

LENS INVENTORY

Because of the large number of lenses used by a disposable lens patient over 1 year, maintaining a stock of most lens brands and parameters is difficult for practitioners. Inventory is expensive to maintain, requires considerable staff time to manage, and takes up valuable office space. Some practitioners have used a "just-in-time" method, in which the manufacturer automatically ships a quantity of lenses just before the patient is due for a new supply. Office computer systems can also prompt the staff to place orders in anticipation of patient visits. These methods can cause problems when patients don't return when expected or if their prescriptions change.

Some practices find that having a stock of multi-packs on hand is a strong practice-building effort that continues the theme of convenience for disposable lens wearers. This practice can prevent the patient from having to return to pick up lenses by having them at the time of the visit. An inventory that is equal to the dollar amount of 1 month's billing with a company is an inventory that turns over every 30 days.

It is important for the contact lens technician to check the inventory and reorder frequently to keep the stock available. This can be aided by inventory control programs on computer systems, which may even include bar coding.

CHAPTER 12

Lenses for Sport Use

CAROL A. SCHWARTZ

Sports vision is considered by many to be an esoteric specialty applied to serious competitive athletes. Yet sports application of contact lenses is a subject with which all contact lens fitters should be familiar. The reason becomes obvious after a quick glance at the demographics of contact lens wearers: the majority are adults and young adults, who can be expected to participate in sports. In fact, more than two thirds of contact lens wearers are between 18 and 40 years of age. Considering the emphasis on physical fitness within this age category, it is reasonable to assume that the majority participate in at least one sport at the recreational level. Recreational athletes value optimal performance almost as highly as do professionals. A Harris Poll conducted in 1991 asked consumers why an individual would wear contact lenses; they found sports was the most common response, cited by 55% of respondents. This is an indication of a largely untapped potential market for contact lenses.

Contact lenses fitted for sport use are generally the same as those fitted for general wear. The fitting methods are typically the same as those with which you are familiar (see Appendix 1). However, differences exist in the manner in which contact lenses are used and may determine the type of contact lens chosen. Testing procedures for the fitting of athletic contact lenses is similar to the standard fitting procedure. Special attention must be given to the case history, material selection, and wearing schedule.

CASE HISTORY

Begin by taking a detailed case history not only of visual problems and general health, but also of sport history. Ask the patient in which sports they normally participate and at what level. In team sports, it is essential to know the position played, because this may be a factor in determining lens correction. To illustrate: a highly myopic patient with moderate astigmatism ($-5.00 -2.00 \times 170$) who plays offensive tackle at the college level needs to be corrected on the field. Yet this correction does not need to bring the patient to best visual acuity. This patient also is at risk for having lenses soiled, damaged, or lost during

125

play. A spherical disposable lens in their spherical equivalent power usually serves the purpose well for games, even if the same patient wears rigid gas permeable or soft toric lenses for general use. On the other hand, a quarterback with the same refractive error would find visual compromise of this type unsatisfactory.

It is important to be aware of the level at which the patient plays to determine the amount of interest they are likely to have for a sport-specific correction. An adult who plays competitive league tennis is more likely to value such correction than is one who plays "hit-and-giggle" doubles occasionally.

The fitter must be aware of the environmental and visual conditions under which the sport is played; he or she may consult one of several guides available, or he or she may simply ask the patient. It is important to know specific environmental factors such as exposure to dust, wind, and water for obvious reasons, but these conditions vary within sporting categories. Consider equestrian sports. A barrel racer is exposed to both wind and excessive dust; a show jumper experiences neither under normal circumstances. Canine competition includes several distinct types of sporting activity. You may assume the patient who tells you that their hobbies include showing dogs is participating in the better-known indoor kennel-club–style conformation trials. For this activity, any contact lens is appropriate. On further questioning, you may find the patient is actually working Newfoundland dogs in field trials and is required to jump into a lake and pretend to be drowning so the dog will rescue him or her. A disposable lens that can be discarded after exposure to stagnant lake water is appropriate for this use. Knowing the visual demands of each patient is also critical; as is knowing differences in visual demand that occur within categories of sport. Close-in sports such as judo are less vision-intense than are sports with a distance element, such as archery or field hockey.

LENS SELECTION

After the position, level, and conditions of the sport are ascertained, the choice of lens type is a matter of simple logic. As shown in Box 12–1, these elements will favor either soft, disposable, or rigid gas permeable lenses. The sports application, in addition to the patient's refractive error, health status, and lifestyle, will naturally lead to the correct choice. In some cases, the patient may need to adopt more than one type of contact lens (e.g., a patient who wears rigid gas permeable lenses for general use, but uses soft disposable lenses for scuba diving).

Sports that are highly kinesthetic, such as karate, basketball, or hockey, generally favor soft contact lenses. These include most contact sports and several others in which jostling or sudden impacts could

BOX 12-1. FACTORS IN CHOOSING TYPE OF LENS FOR SPORT USE

1. Factors favoring soft lenses

   - Contact or highly kinesthetic sports
   - Environmental conditions such as dust, wind, and debris
   - Part-time wear (i.e., sports-only applications)

2. Factors favoring disposable lenses

   - All soft lens indications
   - Water sports
   - Frequent, fast replacement probable

3. Factors favoring rigid lenses

   - V.A. critical to performance
   - Extreme ultraviolet exposure without dust or wind (e.g., fishing)
   - Full-time rigid gas permeable lens wear, part-time sports wear

cause a rigid lens to be dislodged. Sports such as rodeo expose the patient to excessive wind and air-borne debris, which may preclude rigid lens wear. Patients who will be wearing contact lenses part-time should also be considered for soft disposable contact lenses.

Disposable contact lenses are useful in all situations favoring soft lenses and also for aquatic sports because of the increased risk of water-borne contamination. Swimming is still considered a contraindication to soft lens wear; most patients who choose correction while participating in this activity must be advised of this. Disposable lenses are also the modality of choice when frequent loss is a risk or when immediate, on-site replacement of lost lenses is of great importance.

Rigid gas permeable lenses are chosen when the sport requires optimal visual correction and no contraindications (e.g., dust, water) exist. Archery, target shooting, and skeet shooting are all sports in which rigid lens correction is preferred. These patients should be made aware of the risk of lens loss and counseled to maintain a spare pair of contact lenses or spectacles at the sport venue.

One additional factor to consider is the probable exposure to ultraviolet (UV) radiation. The athlete may not be able to incorporate UV protection in a spectacle over-correction. Several rigid lenses and one soft lens contain UV filters. Because UV protection is more readily available in rigid lenses, they should also be considered when the exposure to UV light is extreme, as for avid fishermen.

There are several caveats the contact lens fitter should bear in mind when fitting athletes. The first is that patients must be made aware that visual correction is not equivalent to eye protection. For some sports, it may be necessary to wear both contact lenses and protective goggles. In the following sports, over-protection should be considered mandatory:

Racquetball
Target shooting
Squash
Motor sports (including any driving in an open vehicle)
Skiing

In many other sports, eye protection is advisable, although not mandatory (Table 12–1).

Another caveat is that athletes, trainers, and coaches can be very superstitious people. Most of us have heard stories about famous athletes who wear their lucky clothing, eat the same meals, and follow the same schedule before an important sporting event. Even those who do not go to these lengths are generally hesitant to change something in their training regimen before a crucial match. An athlete may insist on being fitted with contact lenses in the middle of a season. Sometimes this has occurred in the midst of a winning streak. No matter what the sport, winning streaks all have one thing in common—eventually, they come to an end. In these cases, the failure is almost always blamed on a change of equipment: possibly, the change from spectacles or no correction to contact lenses. Whenever possible, defer fitting until the off-season, particularly if the athlete is doing well.

For some sports, including tennis and racquetball, there is no off-season. How does one time the fitting of these athletes? The best approach to a seasonless sport entails three elements. First, schedule the fitting to allow at least 2 weeks before an important tournament or meet. Second, prepare the patient for the worst. This is a delicate balancing act for the contact lens fitter who must emphasize the eventual long-term benefits of contact lens correction while warning the athlete that in the short term their game may suffer from the change of correction just as it would from any major equipment change. Third, encourage the athlete to immediately begin practicing while wearing their contact lenses and perhaps to extend practice periods to allow them to adjust to their new visual status.

COMPLICATIONS

The most serious and unfortunately the most common sports complication is injury. It is advisable from a clinico-legal standpoint to be very cautious when dealing with minors: consider counseling the parent or coach in writing that eye protection is advisable for this patient despite the use of contact lens correction. Although this topic is outside the scope of this chapter, it should serve as another reminder that correction is not protection.

In many sports, drying of the lens may be a problem. The source is two-fold: the patient's blink rate may be reduced as he or she concentrates, and the environment under which the sport is played may also contribute to lens dehydration. Drying is most pronounced among wearers of thin, high-water-content soft lenses. The use of lubricating drops and increased attention to blinking may serve to relieve mild-to-moderate dryness; if symptoms persist, consider refitting the patient with a thicker, lower-water-content lens.

FITTING CONSIDERATIONS

In a few sports, the power of the contact lens may need to be adjusted for competitive use only. The primary example of this is the target shooter, particularly those who are presbyopic. These athletes have a unique visual demand in which they must be able to focus clearly on the distant target and also on the sights of the gun. One compromise is to fit the patient with a customized monovision correction. The dominant eye or sighting eye (most shooters are aware of the eye they prefer to use to sight) is fitted with a lens power sufficient to bring the front sights into clear focus. In some cases, both eyes are corrected to the distance of the sights and the target will appear slightly blurry. Because this type of correction is useful both to those who shoot pistols and those who shoot long guns and there are several arm-lengths (i.e., positions, stances) employed, it is useful if the patient can provide the exact measurement from their eye to the sight. They may also bring their unloaded competition weapon into the office so that trial lenses can be used to find an exact correction.

In rare instances, presbyopic patients who wear monovision or bifocal contact lenses may find that the near correction interferes with their performance. For monovision wearers, a third distance lens can be prescribed. If the sport requires protective eyewear, it may be prescribed with the opposite of the add power over the near eye. For example: A patient whose prescription is -3.50 D spherical OU with an add of 1.75 D is fitted with monovision lenses. His or her contact lens correction is OD, -3.50 D; OS, -1.75 D. This patient finds that the monovision correction hinders his or her performance when playing racquetball. A pair of prescription goggles with the following powers is dispensed to be worn over his or her contact lenses; OD, plano; OS, -1.75 D.

Table 12-1. Contact Lens Factors by Sport

Sport	Lens Type	Protection	Notes
Aerobics	Soft		Dryness
Archery	Any	Suggested	BVA, Wind
Baseball	Any	Suggested	
Basketball	Soft	Yes	
Bicycling	Any	Suggested	UV protection
Boating	Any		UV protection
Bowling	Any		
Dog trials	Any		UV protection
Equestrian	Soft	For some	Dust, wind
Field Hockey	Soft	Suggested	
Fishing	Any	Suggested	UV protection
Football	Soft or disposable	Suggested	
Golf	Any		UV protection
Gymnastics	Soft		Dryness
Hunting	Any	Suggested	UV, wind
Ice skating	Soft		Outdoor—UV, wind
Ice hockey	Soft	Suggested	
Martial arts	Soft		VA not a problem
Motor sports	Soft	Mandatory	
Parachuting	Soft	Mandatory	
Racquetball	Soft	Mandatory	
Rollerskating and rollerblading	Any		UV protection
Scuba diving and snorkeling	Disposable	Yes	
Shooting	Any	Mandatory	BVA or plus to front sights
Shopping	Any		Flying tag injuries

Table 12–1. Contact Lens Factors by Sport *Continued*

Sport	Lens Type	Protection	Notes
Skiing	Soft	Yes	Dryness, UV
Sledding and tobogganing	Soft	Yes	Dryness, UV
Soccer	Soft		UV protection
Softball	Any	Suggested	UV, dust
Squash	Soft	Mandatory	
Surfing and sailboarding	Disposable		UV protection
Swimming	Disposable		UV protection
Tennis	Any		Soft if competitive
Track	Soft		Dust
Volleyball	Soft		Dust, UV
Walking, jogging, and running	Any		UV protection

(BVA = best visual acuity; UV = ultraviolet; VA = visual acuity.)

If the patient is wearing bifocal contact lenses, he or she can be given single-vision contact lenses for sport use. This solves the problem for most athletes. If the sport has a minimal near component (e.g., golf or bowling, in which scores must be kept), the add may be prescribed as an over-correction. Again, this over-correction may be combined with protection. Some golfers have found that a small bifocal placed in the superior temporal quadrant of one spectacle lens is adequate for score-keeping and does not interfere with putting. These spectacles may be provided as sunglasses, thereby combining protection from UV radiation with the need for sporadic near correction.

Sports applications of contact lenses can provide a tremendous service to the patient and a refreshing change for the practitioner. All that is required is the willingness to discuss needs, apply logic, and creatively find a solution to each athlete's unique visual demands.

BIBLIOGRAPHY

1. Teig D: Contact lens care for your summer athletes. Contact Lens Spect 1994;(7):23.
2. Berman A: Sports vision for the primary care practitioner. Eyequest 1994;4(3):46.

3. American Optometric Association, Sports Vision Section: *Sports Vision Handbook*. St. Louis, American Optometric Association, 1993.
4. Teig D: How to prepare for emergencies. Contact Lens Spect 1994;(4):19.
5. Bennett ES, Allee Henry V: *Clinical Manual of Contact Lenses*. Philadelphia, JB Lippincott, 1994, p. 16.

CHAPTER 13

Pediatric Lenses

Karla Zadnik

It is estimated that almost 12% of school-aged children have visual problems that require referral from vision-screening programs.[1] The vast majority of these problems are correctable with spectacles and other treatments, but some unknown portion of them may require or benefit from contact lenses. Contact lenses should be considered in certain categories of pediatric patients. Regardless of age, unilateral aphakes necessitate contact lens fitting to minimize image size differences between the two eyes. High anisometropes require contact lens correction for the same reason, as do children with high, unilateral astigmatism. Children who have sustained ocular trauma often require a contact lens to correct irregular corneal astigmatism. Bilateral aphakes, high hyperopes, and high myopes can succeed in contact lenses, but spectacle correction should not be ruled out immediately.

In general, the problems encountered in children wearing contact lenses are the same ones encountered in fitting contact lenses in adults: major and minor physiologic complications, contact lens loss and damage, and the adequacy of visual correction with contact lenses. Superimposed on these problems are the difficulties of managing amblyopia, the special problems posed by adding the parent as an extra player in the contact lens compliance game, and the presence of an often-changing degree of refractive error as the eye grows.

BOX 13-1. DO THESE FIRST

1. Take off white coat
2. Obtain case history
3. Perform retinoscopy

Second visit, if necessary

4. Obtain Silsoft trial lens or lenses
5. Insert trial lens
6. Inspect contact lens fit (i.e., centration and movement)
7. Perform retinoscopic over-refraction

Different pediatric age groups require different approaches to contact lens fitting and continuing care. Young infants are easier to manage than toddlers. Motivated school-aged children are ideal candidates, whereas children whose parents want them to have contact lenses more than the child does do not perform as well. However, parental motivation—or at least a level of comfort with the idea of contact lenses—is important. Parents who understand the rationale behind their child requiring a contact lens following cataract surgery are far easier to work with than parents who observe the child's behavior based on the phakic eye and conclude that contact lens wear is largely optional. Special techniques and considerations are therefore tailored to the individual child based on two major factors: (1) the visual defect or refractive error underlying the need for contact lenses, and (2) the age of the child. This chapter presents techniques for the most frequently encountered, arguably most challenging, non-routine pediatric contact lens patient: namely, the child younger than 5 years of age who requires an aphakic contact lens or lenses.

THE APHAKIC CHILD

Although almost all adults undergoing cataract surgery in the United States receive intraocular lenses, this therapy is not the norm for post-operative care in young children. Because most young children's eyes grow by several millimeters up to 3 years of age and another 2 mm by puberty, intraocular lenses implanted at young ages will be optically obsolete by the patient's teens.[2] Therefore, most aphakic children, especially unilateral aphakes, are corrected with contact lenses. The most frequently used lens for the correction of pediatric aphakia is the Silsoft lens, a 100%-silicone lens manufactured by Bausch and Lomb.[3-6] This lens is readily available in the unusual pediatric parameters that correspond to infants' and toddlers' small eyes, steep corneas, and high aphakic refractive error (pediatric series: base curves, 7.5, 7.7, and 7.9 mm; powers, + 23.00 to + 32.00 D in 3.00 D steps; diameters, 11.3 and 12.5 mm).[7] The lens is easy to insert, difficult to displace, and provides high oxygen transmissibility.[8] It is well tolerated by infants and toddlers, and the child can be moved into the adult aphakic Silsoft lens when necessary (adult series: base curves, 7.5, 7.7, 7.9, 8.1, and 8.3 mm; powers, + 12.00 to + 20.00 D in 1.00 D steps; diameter, 11.3 mm).[9]

The fitting procedure for this lens may seem daunting to the practitioner who does not see large numbers of small children requiring contact lenses, but it is quite straightforward. The first office visit for the fitting of contact lenses is geared toward gaining the child's confidence and establishing rapport with the child and the parents. These children have undergone surgical procedures and are accustomed to examination by eye doctors with bright lights and stinging eye drops. Therefore, the first office visit may entail as little as a careful history of the child's ocular and systemic disease history, an assessment of visual acuity, if possible, and retinoscopy. Often, if these procedures have gone well and the child is happy and responsive, it is wise to defer the more invasive trial contact lens fitting for the second visit.

At the second visit, retinoscopy can be repeated and compared with the previous result. It is usually easier to perform retinoscopy with loose trial lenses and to calculate the resultant refractive error. For example, if the retinoscopic result is + 12.00 D in the vertical meridian (i.e., streak oriented horizontally) and + 13.00 D in the horizontal meridian (i.e., streak oriented vertically), the resultant lens cross is as depicted in Figure 13–1. The refractive error is recorded as follows: + 13.00 − 1.00 × 180, or + 12.00 + 1.00 × 90.

Vertex distance is an important consideration, especially because the goal is to convert the retinoscopic results to an approximate contact lens power. In the example illustrated in Figure 13–1, suppose the examiner thought he or she had been very successful in maintaining the trial lens at a vertex distance of 10 mm. Converting to the corneal plane:

Corneal power = 1/(1/Spectacle power) − Vertex distance in meters
Corneal power = 1/(1/+ 12.50) − 0.001 m = + 12.65 D

If the vertex distance were actually 20 mm, this would translate to a corneal power of + 12.82 D, which fortunately is an inconsequential difference.

The effect of vertex distance, however, is greatly emphasized with the high aphakic powers characteristic of very young infants. If, in-

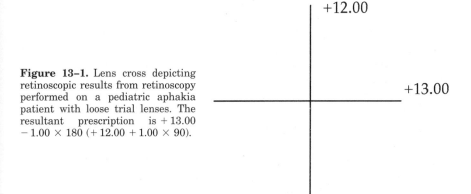

Figure 13–1. Lens cross depicting retinoscopic results from retinoscopy performed on a pediatric aphakia patient with loose trial lenses. The resultant prescription is + 13.00 − 1.00 × 180 (+ 12.00 + 1.00 × 90).

stead of a spherical equivalent of + 12.50 D, a 3-week-old baby with a post-operative refractive error of + 40.00 D is subjected to the same 10-mm error in vertex distance estimation, the calculated corneal power changes from + 41.67 D to + 43.47 D, an error of almost 2.00 D in a patient who cannot complain of the resultant blur. Sometimes, the possibility of such an error can be minimized by placing a high aphakic power contact lens on the patient and determining the total refractive error with a retinoscopic over-refraction.

After retinoscopy has been performed, keratometry can be attempted. Usually, keratometry will yield only an approximate corneal curvature value or a qualitative assessment of whether the cornea appears very steep or very flat. More likely, the performance of trial contact lenses on the eye will provide the most useful information on corneal curvature.

LENS INSERTION

At this point, trial contact lenses can be selected and applied. The younger the child, the more likely it is that the steeper Silsoft base curve will be needed. At approximately age 18 months, the flatter base curve should be selected as the first lens of choice. Initial lens insertion is one of the bigger challenges in fitting contact lenses in young pediatric aphakes. Figures 13–2 through 13–4 show the sequence of events I go through in inserting contact lenses.

Parents are often told to bring their child in for the initial fitting appointment when the child is "in a good mood," has just been fed, or is ready to take a nap. This imposes an unnecessary restriction on the

---

BOX 13–2. THINGS YOU NEED TO KNOW

1. Aphakic babies and toddlers have steep corneas and high plus refractive error
2. Contact lens insertion techniques do not require the child's cooperation
3. Silsoft lenses are effective in the management of pediatric aphakia
4. Contact lenses must be corrected by +3.00 D for near viewing
5. Contact lens–related complications are similar to those seen in adult contact lens wearers
6. Expect prescription changes between the ages of birth and 3 years, a period of rapid ocular growth

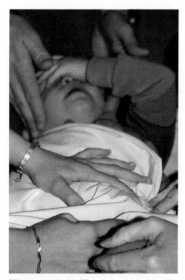

Figure 13-2. This wrapping technique uses a sheet and the examining room floor to immobilize a young patient for initial contact lens insertion.

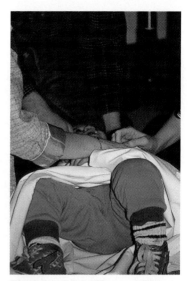

Figure   13-3. The   child   is wrapped in a sheet to allow the examiner to insert the contact lens.

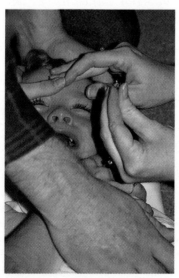

Figure 13-4. The aphakic contact lens is held with its inferior edge folded in anticipation of contact lens insertion.

parents. They can rarely predict such events with accuracy. The following technique does not require the cooperation of the child and does not require that he or she assume any particular mood or temperament.

Figures 13–2 and 13–3 illustrate an immobilization technique to keep the child from deflecting the examiner's, technician's, or parents' hands during lens insertion. The child is placed on his or her back on a clean sheet on the floor. His or her left arm is placed along his or her side, and the sheet is pulled across his or her body toward the right side to effectively pin the arm in place. This procedure is repeated in the opposite direction for the right arm. Topical corneal anesthetic is used to "wet" the lens before insertion. This eliminates the need to instill an eye drop prior to lens insertion, thereby avoiding traumatizing the child twice. The topical anesthetic takes effect just after lens insertion to facilitate initial adaptation.

The Silsoft lens is best held as shown in Figure 13–4, with the inferior edge pinched between the examiner's thumb and forefinger and the top portion fanning out from there. This keeps the heavy, high-plus aphakic lens from falling off the examiner's finger to parts unknown. A lid speculum is not used. The examiner and a technician assist each other in holding the child's lids open, often succeeding after the child has settled down a little. The fanned-out portion of the lens is placed on the superior bulbar conjunctiva, and the inferior pinched edge unfolds over the superior cornea as the lens is released onto the eye. When the eye closes, the lens centers, as long as it is not folded onto itself.

Typically, the parent is encouraged to comfort the child as the lens equilibrates, but the child cannot rub the eye for fear the lens will be displaced. Once the lens has equilibrated, the examiner can return to check its physical fit and the appropriateness of power by visual inspection of the lens centration and movement and by retinoscopy. If the first lens centers poorly or moves excessively, a steeper base curve or larger diameter lens is needed. If the first lens moves inadequately, a flatter base curve is warranted. Retinoscopic over-refraction provides the necessary information to order the correct power of lens. An extra + 3.00 D should be added to the distance refraction when the child is extremely young and near viewing predominates. Spectacles for use over the contact lens are prescribed in cases of high astigmatism (> 1.50 D). Spectacles do not usually incorporate an add, because the contact lens has been corrected for near viewing.

At the dispensing visit, the lens is inserted similarly. Parents are trained to handle the lens if possible, but often the lens is prescribed on an extended wear schedule at first so that parents can accustom themselves to lens insertion, removal, and handling gradually. A daily wear schedule should, however, be the ultimate goal. Sometimes, fitting the parents with disposable contact lenses for a period of time so that they can accustom themselves to lens handling will remove their fear of touching their child's eyes.

Occasionally, the contact lens fitting is best accomplished with the child under general anesthesia. If so, it usually takes place after the initial cataract extraction or trauma repair, no earlier than 1 week following surgery. Contact lens fitting techniques are similar to those described previously. Vertex distance during retinoscopy must be carefully monitored. It is sometimes difficult to remain a remote retinoscopic working distance when the child is supine on the operating table. The best technique is to position the table at its lowest setting and stand as high as possible. Contact lenses can be inserted and a retinoscopic over-refraction performed, but the influence of the lid and globe anatomy on lens centration and movement cannot be ascertained until the first lens insertion and inspection while the patient is awake. Occasionally, fitting while the child is anesthetized facilitates the fitting process, but it is by no means required for the fitting to take place.

If the lens is dispensed on an extended wear schedule, the child should be seen the following day, at 1 week, at 2 weeks, and thereafter on a conservative follow-up schedule. A switch to daily wear should occur as soon as the parents feel comfortable handling the lens that often. Each follow-up visit should consist of retinoscopic over-refraction, a visual check of lens centration and movement, a gross examination of the external eye, a slit lamp examination of the anterior segment, and a visual acuity assessment as soon and as often as the child's level of cooperation will permit. Amblyopia or strabismus therapy should follow as soon as the child has adequately adapted to the contact lens.

Lens care of the Silsoft lens is somewhat problematic. Cleaning with hydrogen peroxide–based systems results in a greasy precipitate on the lens after neutralization, so non-peroxide cold disinfection systems work best. Peroxide disinfection can be used in children on extended wear schedules whose lenses are cleaned in-office, but the resultant deposit must be removed with surfactant cleaner prior to reinsertion.

Parents should be instructed on the symptoms associated with complications in contact lens wear. As for any lens wearer, pain, redness, or decreased vision should prompt immediate lens removal and a call to the eye care practitioner. Parents need to be educated on the importance of having the child wear the lens according to the prescribed schedule, because not doing so can interfere with the patching schedule and, therefore, the visual rehabilitation. Parents should be supplied with several spare lenses in the event of frequent lens loss, so that the child's time out of his or her contact lens is minimized.

Children do quite well when fitted with the aphakic Silsoft lens. Complications are rare and usually manifest as mild ocular inflammations when they do occur. In the case of viral conjunctivitis, which is probably the most common complication, lens discontinuance until the condition clears solves the problem. Corneal complications should be treated as they would be in any other contact lens wearer. Other complications include torn lenses, deposited lenses, and seasonal lens intolerance. In short, any difficulty encountered in adult contact lens wearers also occurs in pediatric patients.

The degree of success of contact lens wear in aphakic children is debated.[10–13] Table 13–1 shows the results from three small case series of congenital cataract. Some children do well whereas others do poorly; there is some indication that factors such as age at surgery, time elapsed from surgery to visual correction, compliance with contact lenses or patching, and aggressive follow-up are important.[13]

For the infant or toddler who is unilaterally aphakic, contact lenses are the only viable treatment option. Fitting contact lenses on these patients is relatively straightforward, as described previously. Use of the Silsoft lens greatly facilitates the contact lens fitting and follow-up of these patients. These children's care and success often depends on the collaboration of many eye care practitioners: their surgeon, their contact lens practitioner, and the optometrist or ophthalmologist managing their post-operative amblyopia or strabismus treatment.

Table 13–1. Visual Results Following Congenital Cataract Surgery

Authors	Year	Number of Patients/Eyes	Visual Results
Pratt-Johnson and Tillson[11]	1981	6/9	20/30–20/400; 6 eyes at least 20/80
Beller et al.[12]	1981	8/8	20/30–20/80; all eyes at least 20/80
Robb et al.[10]	1987	12/12	20/70 to worse than 20/400; 5 eyes at least 20/80
Birch and Stager[13]	1988	19/19	20/30 to hand motion; 53% at least 20/80

REFERENCES

1. Blum HL, Peters HB, Bettman JW: *Vision Screening for Elementary Schools: The Orinda Study.* Berkeley: University of California Press, 1959.
2. Larsen JS: The sagittal growth of the eye. III. Ultrasonic measurement of the posterior segment (axial length of the vitreous) from birth to puberty. Acta Ophthalmol 1971;49:441.
3. Rogers GL: Extended wear silicone contact lenses in children with cataracts. Ophthalmology 1980;87:867.
4. Matsumoto EM, Murphree LM: The use of silicone elastomer lenses in aphakic pediatric patients. Int Eyecare 1986;2:214.
5. Levin AV, Edmonds SA, Nelson LB, Calhoun JH, Harley RD: Extended-wear contact lenses for the treatment of pediatric aphakia. Ophthalmology 1988;95:1107.
6. Cutler SI, Nelson LB, Calhoun JH: Extended wear contact lenses in pediatric aphakia. J Pediatr Ophthalmol Strab 1985;22:86.
7. Moore BD: Mensuration data in infant eyes with unilateral congenital cataracts. Am J Optom Physiol Opt 1987;64:204.
8. Fatt I: Gas-to-gas oxygen permeability measurements on RGP and silicone rubber lens materials. Int Contact Lens Clin 1991;18:92.
9. Moore BD: Changes in the aphakic refraction of children with unilateral congenital cataracts. J Pediatr Ophthalmol Strab 1989;26:290.
10. Robb RM, Mayer DL, Moore BD: Results of early treatment of unilateral congenital cataracts. J Pediatr Ophthalmol Strab 1987;24:178.
11. Pratt-Johnson JA, Tillson G: Visual results after removal of congenital cataracts before the age of 1 year. Can J Ophthalmol 1981;16:19.
12. Beller R, Hoyt CS, Marg E, Odom JV: Good visual function after neonatal surgery for congenital monocular cataracts. Am J Ophthalmol 1981;91:559.
13. Birch EE, Stager DR: Prevalence of good visual acuity following surgery for congenital unilateral cataract. Arch Ophthalmol 1988;106:40.

CHAPTER 14

Contact Lens Management of Keratoconus

Timothy B. Edrington

Keratoconus is generally managed with rigid gas permeable (RGP) contact lenses. In the past, practitioners fitted keratoconus patients with rigid contact lenses in an effort to slow the progression of keratoconus; currently, they are prescribed only when optically or cosmetically indicated.[1] Many fitting philosophies have been proposed for the management of keratoconus; most can be categorized as apical bearing (touch), divided support or three-point touch, apical clearance, and high-riding or lid-attached.[2–4] Except for the lid-attached philosophy, the lenses primarily position over the apex of the cone.

Concerns exist that flat or apical-bearing rigid contact lenses can lead to corneal scarring in keratoconus patients. Korb and colleagues reported 4 of 7 keratoconic eyes fitted with apical-bearing lenses developed scarring within 1 year, whereas none of 7 eyes fitted with apical clearance developed scarring.[5] Although this study raised concerns regarding flat-fitting contact lenses, it apparently did not alter the standard of contact lens care for keratoconus patients. In a multi-center survey of 1579 keratoconic patients, 75% of the eyes were habitually wearing an apical bearing or flat-fitting rigid contact lens.[6] The reasons offered for preferring an apical-bearing fitting relation for keratoconus patients are: vision is better; wearing time is increased; comfort is superior; and it is easier to achieve and maintain a keratoconic patient in a flat-fitting lens as the disease progresses.[7] Also, the degree of touch may be the factor behind corneal scarring (i.e., minimally flat lenses might lead to scarring less frequently than lenses fitted flat by a significant amount). A randomized prospective study must be conducted to answer this clinical question.

KERATOCONUS DIAGNOSTIC FITTING SET

I recommend a thirteen-lens diagnostic set to manage keratoconic patients; the parameters for the diagnostic lenses are summarized in

Table 14–1. Parameters for the diagnostic lens were determined as follows:

1. Base curve radii were selected to encompass the corneal sagittal heights for patients presenting with mild to severe keratoconus.

2. Contact lens powers were chosen to provide low-minus over-refractions for the majority of keratoconic patients.

3. The overall diameter (OAD) was set at 8.6 mm to provide an interpalpebral fit in which the lens positions over the apex of the conical area of the cornea.

4. The optic zone diameter (OZD) decreases in diameter for more advanced presentations of keratoconus to minimize areas of tear pooling and debris accumulation under the optic zone of the lens.

5. The secondary curve radius (SCR) ranges from 8.00 to 8.25 mm in order to obtain average peripheral clearance. Corneal curvatures beyond the base of the cone are similar to those of non-keratoconic patients.[8] Therefore secondary curve radii appropriate for non-keratoconic RGP contact lens fittings are indicated.

6. The peripheral or third-curve radius (TCR) for the tricurve lens design was set at 11.00 mm with a width (TCW) of 0.2 mm. This curve was selected to be a fitting curve as well as to start the posterior edge treatment.

7. Center thicknesses (CT) were calculated so that an edge thickness of approximately 0.10 mm was maintained for each trial lens. Center thicknesses in these lenses are thicker than those in cosmetic RGP

Table 14–1. Keratoconus Diagnostic Fitting Set

Base Curve	Power	OAD/OZD	SCR	TCR/TCW	CT
47.00 (7.18)	−5.00	8.6/7.0	8.25	11.0/0.2	0.14
48.00 (7.03)	−5.00	8.6/7.0	8.25	11.0/0.2	0.14
49.00 (6.89)	−5.00	8.6/7.0	8.25	11.0/0.2	0.14
50.00 (6.75)	−7.00	8.6/7.0	8.25	11.0/0.2	0.14
51.00 (6.62)	−7.00	8.6/6.5	8.25	11.0/0.2	0.14
52.00 (6.49)	−7.00	8.6/6.5	8.25	11.0/0.2	0.14
53.00 (6.37)	−7.00	8.6/6.5	8.25	11.0/0.2	0.14
54.00 (6.25)	−7.00	8.6/6.5	8.25	11.0/0.2	0.14
56.00 (6.03)	−9.00	8.6/6.0	8.00	11.0/0.2	0.14
58.00 (5.82)	−9.00	8.6/6.0	8.00	11.0/0.2	0.14
61.00 (5.53)	−10.00	8.6/5.5	8.00	11.0/0.2	0.14
65.00 (5.19)	−12.00	8.6/5.5	8.00	11.0/0.2	0.14
70.00 (4.82)	−15.00	8.6/5.5	8.00	11.0/0.2	0.14

All lenses ordered in polymethyl methacrylate material with a medium blend.
CT = center thickness; OAD = overall diameter; OZD = optic zone diameter; SCR = secondary curve radius; TCR = third-curve radius; TCW = third-curve width.

lenses of similar power because of the flatter secondary–to–base curve relation.

8. Polymethyl methacrylate (PMMA) material was chosen because of its machinability, dimensional stability, durability, and low cost. Lenses for patients should be ordered in the gas permeable material of choice.

SELECTION OF INITIAL DIAGNOSTIC LENS

The initial diagnostic lens base curve should be equal to or slightly steeper than the mean keratometric reading. In most cases, this lens will fit flat and touch the cone apex. Should this be the case, steeper lenses should be sequentially applied until apical clearance is obtained. If the initial diagnostic lens fluorescein pattern is steep or demonstrates apical clearance, sequentially flatter lenses should be applied until a flat-fitting relation is observed. The base curve of the steepest diagnostic lens that just touches the apex of the cone should be prescribed. The base curve that provides minimal apical touch is considered ideal. A sphero-cylindrical over-refraction should be performed with this final diagnostic lens in place to determine contact lens power. The following case report illustrates this fitting method.

Case Report 1

Subjective Data: A 23-year-old man presents with a history of reduced vision through his prescription spectacles for the past 2 years. He has never worn contact lenses. Ocular and medical history are unremarkable.

Objective Data: Presented for right eye only.

Habitual spectacles and distance visual acuity: $+2.75 -2.25 \times 105$ (20/40)

Keratometry: 44.25 at 110, 49.37 at 20, 2+ corneal distortion

Subjective refraction: $+3.25 -3.00 \times 95$ (20/40, +1/5)

Biomicroscopy:
   Vogt's striae
   Fleischer's ring
   No scarring

Assessment: Keratoconus.

Plan: Fit with a RGP contact lens.
    The following diagnostic rigid contact lenses were applied and their fluorescein patterns (FP) evaluated:

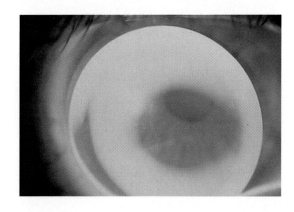

Lens 1. 47.00 D (7.18 mm)
base curve 8.6 mm
OAD; 7.0 mm OZD
FP, apical touch.

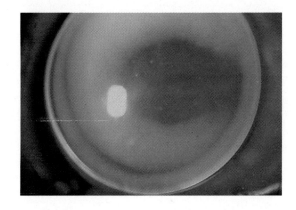

Lens 2. 48.00 D (7.03 mm)
base curve 8.6 mm
OAD; 7.0 mm OZD
FP, apical touch.

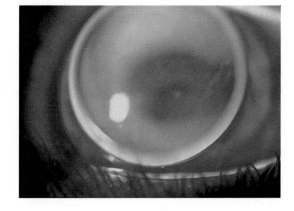

Lens 3. 49.00 D (6.89 mm)
base curve 8.6 mm
OAD; 7.0 mm OZD
FP, apical touch.

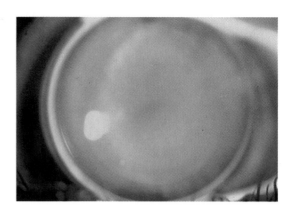

Lens 4. 50.00 D (6.75-mm)
base curve − 7.00 D
power; 8.6 mm OAD;
7.0 mm OZD FP, api-
cal clearance Over-re-
fraction: − 0.50
− 0.75 × 130 (20/20)

RGP Contact Lens Order: 49.50-D (6.82 mm) base curve; − 7.37-D power; 8.6-mm OAD; 7.0-mm OZD; 8.25-mm SCR; 11.0-mm TCR; 0.2-mm TCW; 0.13-mm CT; medium junction blend.

The base curve radius was determined by evaluation of the fluorescein pattern. This patient was fitted with a base curve mid-way between the steepest apical touch diagnostic lens and the first apical clearance diagnostic lens. An additional diagnostic lens of approximately 49.50-D base curve could have been applied if available.

In evaluating the fluorescein pattern of RGP lenses on normal corneas, the area of bearing is directly related to the amount of touch; that is, flatter fitting apical touch contact lenses exhibit smaller areas of bearing. However, the area of bearing with flat-fitting lenses on keratoconic corneas does not vary noticeably relative to the amount of touch. The fluorescein patterns shown in this patient illustrate this point. Therefore, to quantify the amount of touch, it is necessary to apply sequentially steeper lenses until a clearance fluorescein pattern is obtained.

The contact lens power was determined by adding the equivalent sphere of the over-refraction (− 0.87 D) to the diagnostic lens power (− 7.00 D) and compensating for any change of base curve between the diagnostic and ordered lens (+ 0.50 D). The OZD was determined by observing the width of the fluorescein pooling around the base of the cone. This width, as represented in Figures 14–1 through 14–4, is rather wide and could lead to staining of the corneal epithelium around the base of the cone after wear. If this occurs, the OZD must be decreased by modification. The peripheral curve system is evaluated by observing edge lift after fluorescein instillation. If edge lift is judged to be minimal, the SCR should be flattened. The lens should be ordered in a gas permeable material. I recommend using a material that is easy to modify.

MANAGEMENT OF
COMMON CLINICAL PROBLEMS

Two primary indications for penetrating keratoplasty (PK) for a keratoconic eye are: (1) decreased vision, generally caused by corneal scarring over the visual axis, and (2) contact lens intolerance leading to decreased wearing time. As previously mentioned, corneal scarring may be exacerbated by excessively flat-fitting contact lenses. This relation, however, has not been conclusively established.

Contact lens intolerance leading to decreased wearing time is often related to poor tear exchange. Excessively flat-fitting lenses overcome this problem because of their inherent excessive edge lift. Alignment fitting lenses provide minimal edge lift when standard cosmetic SCR-to-base curve radius relations are applied to a lens designed for a keratoconic patient. This standard cosmetic peripheral curve is approximately 1.0 mm flatter than the base curve radius. Therefore, SCRs are generally in the 8.00- to 9.00-mm range for a cosmetic RGP lens. Research indicates that the corneal topography beyond the base of the cone is similar to that of a normal cornea.[8] As the indicated base curve radius becomes steeper to manage the moderate or more advanced clinical presentations of keratoconus (e.g., base curve radii in the 6.00-mm range), the fabricated SCRs become too steep relative to the "normal" cornea beyond the base of the cone. This steep peripheral fitting relation leads to a tight-fitting lens, which provides limited tear exchange. For these reasons, ordering SCRs in the 8.00- to 9.00-mm range, regardless of the base curve radius, is recommended. A medium or heavy blend should be applied to the junction between the two curves. Unfortunately, it has been my experience that some laboratories disregard the ordered SCR and fabricate it relative to the base curve radius (i.e., generally 1.0 mm flatter). Therefore, it is beneficial to be able to perform lens modification procedures in your office if the dispensed lens exhibits minimal or no peripheral clearance during fluorescein pattern analysis. Also, because the peripheral curve system is so flat relative to the base curve, more material is removed than when fabricating a non-keratoconic lens. It is therefore necessary to order a lens with a CT sufficient to maintain a usable edge thickness after modification.

Another frequently encountered clinical sign is staining around the base of the cone. This staining often takes the appearance of swirl (hurricane) or dimple veil patterns. The patient is usually asymptomatic but may report reduced wearing time if peripheral clearance is not adequate. Reducing the OZD and blending the new junction between the base curve and the secondary curve decreases the amount of tear pooling around the base of the cone. This modification often diminishes the degree or severity of the epithelial staining. Fenestrations near the optic zone periphery may be considered as a second option. The following case report illustrates the common problems encountered in fitting or refitting keratoconic patients.

Case Report 2

Subjective Data: A 30-year-old man diagnosed with keratoconus 5 years previously presents with symptoms of reduced wearing time due to RGP contact lens intolerance. Visual acuity through the contact lenses is reported as good at both distance and near. No other significant history is elicited.

Objective Data: Presented for right eye only.

Distance visual acuity through RGP contact lens: 20/20

Over-refraction: $+0.50 - 0.50 \times 65$ (20/20)

FP (Fig. 14–1): Minimal apical touch; excessive clearance around the base of the cone (under the optic zone portion of the lens); minimal (1+) peripheral clearance

Biomicroscopy: 2+ staining of the corneal epithelium around the base of the cone

Assessment:

Excessive mid-peripheral lens clearance leading to staining around the base of the cone.

Binding of peripheral curve system leading to decreased tear pumping and decreased wearing time.

Plan: Reduce OZD and flatten the peripheral curve system. The OZD should be reduced by approximately 0.5 mm, and the secondary curve should be flattened by approximately 0.25 mm. A medium

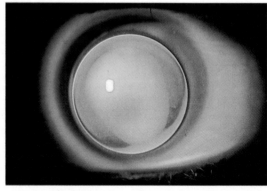

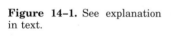
Figure 14–1. See explanation in text.

or heavy blend is then reapplied. These modifications can be performed in the office so that the lens can be reinserted and the fluorescein pattern re-evaluated. A follow-up visit in 1 week allows the practitioner to assess the effect on wearing time and corneal staining.

OTHER CONSIDERATIONS

I fit keratoconus patients with RGP contact lenses to provide good visual performance, not to retard the progression of the disease. If a keratoconus patient's vision needs can be satisfactorily met with spectacles or soft toric contact lenses, there are no contraindications to these forms of optical management. When corneal distortion limits the patient's ability to see adequately through a spectacle prescription, RGP contact lenses are indicated. Even after RGP lenses have been prescribed, a spectacle prescription should be considered for the patient to wear on a part-time basis after contact lens removal or if a corneal abrasion or infection occurs. As the disease becomes more advanced, spectacle refraction endpoints become more difficult to achieve, and refraction stability is decreased. Even so, a current spectacle prescription should be encouraged.

It is common to find oblique or against-the-rule residual cylinder on over-refraction; a spectacle over-correction can be prescribed to correct this cylinder. Even though measured corneal toricity is generally high, bitoric RGP contact lenses should only occasionally be prescribed.

It is common with moderate and advanced presentations of keratoconus for the corneal curvature to exceed the range of the keratometer (i.e., 52.00 D). To extend the range of the keratometer, a +1.25 D spectacle trial lens can be taped onto the objective side of the keratometer. Eight diopters are then added to the drum value to obtain the corneal curvature or k reading.

Aspheric back-surface RGP lens designs have been recommended for the optical management of keratoconus.[9,10] Even though an aspheric design can provide an excellent fitting relation for keratoconus patients, I feel that it limits the practitioner's ability to modify the lens or address a specific adverse sign or symptom without reordering a new lens. The practitioner is not always able to analyze or obtain from the laboratory the back-surface contour specifications. This makes it more difficult to determine the appropriate modification tool required to flatten the lens periphery or perform other modifications to enhance the fit of the lens.

I seldom prescribe rigid–soft hybrid lens designs because of the limited base curve parameters available for the rigid center portion of the lens.[11] These lenses are currently only manufactured in base curve radii appropriate for mild presentations of keratoconus. The steepest available base curve is too flat for the management of moderate and severe keratoconus patients. However, the rigid–soft hybrid lens design generally provides the patient with mild keratoconus a comfortable lens that centers well.

Lens centration can occasionally be improved by fitting the keratoconus patient with a piggyback lens system in which an RGP lens is fitted over a soft contact lens.[12,13] This design may also be contemplated when rigid lens wear creates a compromised corneal epithelium because of mechanical factors. To fit a piggyback design, apply a minus-power disposable soft contact lens to the patient's eye and perform over-keratometry. A minus-power lens is selected so that the new front surface of the lens–cornea is flatter and more regular than the corneal surface of the cone, and a portion of the refractive error is corrected by the soft contact lens. Utilizing the over-keratometry value as a starting point, rigid diagnostic lenses are applied. The endpoint is a rigid lens that centers without forming bubbles under the optic zone.

Presbyopia can be managed with a spectacle over-correction or monovision contact lenses; most RGP bifocal designs are not appropriate for keratoconic patients. Concentric or simultaneous designs do not generally succeed despite the limited lens movement obtained with keratoconus lenses because of the slightly inferior lens position. Alternating rigid bifocal designs position too low for adequate translation into the near optics.

REFERENCES

1. Kemmetmuller H: Corneal lenses and keratoconus. Contacto 1962;6(1):188.
2. Caroline PJ, McGuire JR, Doughman DJ: Preliminary report on a new contact lens design for keratoconus. Contact Intraocular Lens Med J 1978;4:69.
3. Soper JW, Jarrett A: Results of a systematic approach to fitting keratoconus and corneal transplants. Contact Lens Med Bull 1972;5(3–4):50.
4. Cohen EJ, Parlato CJ: Fitting Polycon lenses in keratoconus. Int Ophthalmol Clin 1986;26:111.
5. Korb DR, Finnemore VM, Herman JP: Apical changes and scarring in keratoconus as related to contact lens fitting techniques. J Am Optom Assoc 1982;53(3):199.
6. Edrington TB, Zadnik K, Barr JT, Gordon MO, CLEK Study Group: Scarring and contact lens fit in keratoconus: results from the CLEK (Contact Lens Evaluation in Keratoconus) screening study. Invest Ophthalmol Vis Sci 1991;32(Suppl):738.
7. Zadnik K, Mutti DO: Contact lens fitting relation and visual acuity in keratoconus. Am J Optom Physiol Optics 1987;64(9):698.
8. McMahon TT, Robin JB, Scarpulla KM, Putz JL: The spectrum of topography found in keratoconus. CLAO J 1991;17(3):198.
9. Lembach RG, Keates RH: Aspheric silicone lenses for keratoconus. CLAO J 1984;10(4):323.
10. Goldberg JB: The KAS keratoconic-aspheric corneal lens for keratoconus. Contact Lens Forum 1989;14(2):56.

11. Maguen E, Caroline P, Rosner IR, Macy JI, Newburn AB: The use of the SoftPerm lens for the correction of irregular astigmatism. CLAO J 1992:18(3):173
12. Baldone JA: The fitting of hard contact lenses onto soft contact lenses in certain diseased conditions. Contact Lens Med Bull 1973;6(2–3):15.
13. Polse KA, Decker MR, Sarver MD: Soft and hard contact lenses worn in combination. Am J Optom Physiol Optics 1977;54(10):660.

CHAPTER 15

Post-surgical Fitting: Refractive

BARRY WEINER

Radial keratotomy (RK) was introduced to the United States by Dr. Leo Boros in 1978, who learned the technique from Dr. Svyatoslav Fyodorov of Russia. Dr. Fyodorov based his techniques on the work of Dr. Sato of Japan, with the basic difference that Sato cut the cornea's epithelial and endothelial surfaces, while Fyodorov made his incisions on the epithelial surface only.

It has been estimated that 1,000,000 Americans have undergone this myopia-reducing procedure since the late 1970s, with many of them left either over-corrected or under-corrected and in need of some form of visual correction. The number of patients left with significant ametropia following RK varies with the preoperative degree of myopia. According to the Prospective Evaluation of Radial Keratotomy (PERK) study, 75% of those with myopia under 3.00 D will ultimately be corrected to within 1.00 D of emmetropia, whereas 67% of those between 3.25 and 4.25 D will achieve the same result. Only 49% of those over 4.50 D will be corrected within those parameters.

Many of these patients are reluctant to wear spectacles and may opt instead for contact lenses. Their reluctance for spectacle wear may be demonstrated in that they chose RK in the first place. Post-RK patients present the contact lens practitioner with numerous challenges and problems not present in the general population.

TESTS TO RUN

History

The most important test when fitting a post-RK patient is a good, complete history. A detailed history is invaluable in evaluating the direction you should pursue regarding lens type and the chances for a successful outcome.

RK patients have physical problems to overcome, such as abnormally shaped corneas and possible tear film complications. More importantly, these patients have psychological complications that may be more dif-

152

ficult for the fitter to overcome than the physical drawbacks. Many of these people were contact lens failures prior to surgery, which may have been their motivating factor for this procedure. They have paid a large sum of money to do away with the inconvenience of glasses or contacts. When they get to the contact lens practitioner, they are disappointed and often upset. The case history can provide clues to the practitioner regarding the patient's state of mind.

Previous optical history is vital to a successful fitting. If the patient was not able to wear contacts prior to surgery, it is essential to know why. Was the patient reluctant to put up with the inconvenience of cleaning and disinfecting his or her lenses, or was there some physical problem their previous doctor could not overcome? If the latter, what was that problem? This information guides the practitioner when choosing a lens modality.

A complete medical profile, including medications being taken, is necessary, because many medications have ocular effects that can hinder a successful conclusion.

A most important part of the history is the pre-operative refraction and keratometric readings. These readings are used as a starting point for the trial fitting evaluation. It may be necessary to contact the patient's prior eye care practitioner or the operating surgeon to obtain these findings. The patient's prior contact lens history should be obtained at the same time.

Refraction and Keratometry

It is essential to do a careful, complete refraction and keratometric evaluation for future reference. The time of day the refraction was performed should also be noted, because approximately 25% of post-RK patients exhibit diurnal fluctuations in visual acuity and refraction. It is advisable to re-do the refraction and keratometry at another time of day to evaluate diurnal variations if they are present.

Intraocular pressure variations cause less myopia or an increase in hyperopia in the morning, when the pressure is usually the greatest. The myopia increases or the hyperopia decreases as the day progresses and the intraocular pressure decreases.

Post-operative prescriptions and keratometry values are not necessary for the initial trial lens selection if the pre-operative readings are available, but they are useful in monitoring any lens-induced changes.

Slit Lamp Evaluation

A careful pre-fit slit lamp evaluation is absolutely essential. The surgical scars must be examined for any staining or wound gape (Fig. 15–1). Either of these events is a contraindication to lens fitting and

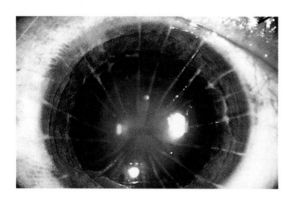

Figure 15–1. Post–radial keratotomy scarring centrally with inclusions noted at the 2-o'clock position.

must be resolved before a contact lens can be fitted. The incisions must be examined for inclusion cysts. These cysts can migrate to the corneal surface months or even years following surgery and cause delayed keratitis.

The cornea may also show other changes as a result of the surgery, such as stellate epithelial iron lines or fine corneal striae, which should be noted. The cornea should also be examined for vacularization into the incisions. Any abnormalities should be noted or, if possible, photographed.

Tear Film Evaluation

Irregularity of the corneal surface following RK may disrupt the normal tear flow across the corneal surface. A tear break-up time (BUT) test should be performed to evaluate the continuity of the tear film. The lipid layer of the tears can be evaluated using specular reflection from the slit mirror to check the integrity of the lipid layer on the surface of the tear film.

Negative staining over the incision lines is an indication that the scars are raised and is a red flag for careful post-fitting evaluation. Movement of the contact lens over these raised incisions may lead to corneal staining and possible corneal erosion.

A Schermer's tear test can be performed, but the results are not relevant to lens success in most cases, unless there is a complete absence of tears.

Computerized Corneal Topographic Analysis

If the fitter has access to a computerized corneal topography instrument, it can be very useful in fitting the post-RK eye and in subsequent follow-up evaluations to monitor lens-induced corneal changes.

Because the post-operative central keratometric readings are of little value in trial lens selection, a corneal map generated by a topographic analyzer can provide an initial starting point if the pre-operative findings are not available. A study by McDonnell, Garbus, and Caroline showed that a point in the mid-periphery, 3.5-mm superior to the optical axis, gives a good initial trial lens base curve in a large percentage of cases.

Changes in central keratometry caused by lens-induced edema or excessive lens bearing are evident in subsequent topography analysis when compared with the pre-fit photographs, and remediation can be initiated.

THINGS YOU NEED TO KNOW

It is important for the lens practitioner to make the patient realize that he or she is not dealing with a "normally" shaped cornea following RK surgery (Fig. 15–2). The fitter must explain to the patient that contact lenses are generally manufactured for a cornea that is steeper centrally with a gradually flattening peripheral area. Radial keratotomy changes that normal configuration, so that the central cornea is flat compared with a normal cornea. The mid-peripheral areas have steepened because of the weakening effect of the RK incisions, and the far periphery is close to normally shaped.

Contact lenses tend to center on the steepest area of the cornea. In the post-RK eye, this is no longer the center of the cornea as it was prior to the surgery, but it is now the mid-peripheral region. This will cause most lenses to decenter, with a tendency for most to move upward and nasally (Fig. 15–3).

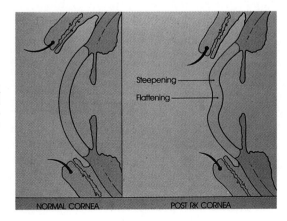

Figure 15–2. Central corneal flattening with mid-peripheral steepening following radial keratotomy. (Courtesy of J. Soper.)

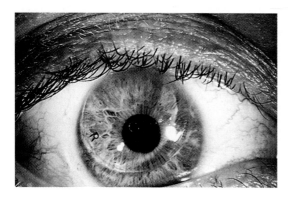

Figure 15–3. Superior lens decentration following radial keratotomy.

A major complaint of many post-RK patients is flare and glare following the surgery. It must be explained that this will usually resolve with time. Contact lenses can also induce flare and glare, and this must also be explained to the patient. Lens design should take this problem into consideration, which is why larger rigid gas permeable (RGP) lenses are preferred in most cases.

The lens prescriber must remember the state of mind of the post-RK patient; they must be handled delicately. Many of these patients are disappointed that surgery did not accomplish what they were told or hoped; they are upset and in many instances angry, not at the fitter but at the surgeon. The lens practitioner must be a good listener and a better communicator if he or she is to successfully fit these patients.

It is essential that all complications inherent in fitting these patients be explained prior to lens fitting. All possible complications must also be explained so that the patient does not experience any unpleasant surprises. A 10- to 15-minute consultation outlining possible pitfalls can save many hours of explanation later. An informed consent form is important and can save the fitter much aggravation later if complications arise.

LENS DESIGN

Rigid Gas Permeable Lenses

RGP lenses are the modality of choice for the post-RK patient. RGP lenses offer the advantage of good visual acuity with excellent physiologic response and the least corneal compromise. The initial trial lens selected can be of any design, usually that with which the fitter is most comfortable. It's best to begin with the simplest design first. The KISS ("keep it simple, stupid") principle truly applies in these cases. If this initial lens proves to be inadequate either physically, visually, or physiologically, then more complex designs can be utilized. RGP lenses in numerous standard designs can be adapted to the post-RK patient. Spherical and aspheric lenses have been used successfully by various practitioners. The OK™ series of orthokeratology lenses from Contex Contact Lenses adapt themselves well to some of these individuals. There are lenses specially designed to fit the unusual geometry of the post-RK patient, such as the Plateau lens from Menicon; others are available or in development.

Fitting. The base curve for the initial trial lens is selected by using the flattest K from the pre-operative keratometric readings, just as for a "normal" cornea. After applying this trial lens, the patient should be allowed to stabilize for 30 to 45 minutes to allow the lens to settle and any tearing to subside.

Slit lamp evaluation usually shows the lens decentering upward and nasally on most patients, but be prepared to find the lens in any quadrant of the cornea. Fluorescein evaluation should show a parallel fit in the mid-peripheral region with adequate edge lift. Central fluorescein pooling is noted in most patients because of the flat configuration of the cornea centrally (Fig. 15–4). No gross bearing areas should be seen. It is not uncommon to see air bubbles trapped under the central portion of the lens because of the flatter central corneal geometry (Fig. 15–5).

The lens must adequately cover the pupil. Any infringement of the lens edge or the peripheral curve junction will cause excessive flare and glare over and above that expected immediately after the surgery.

Centration is the main ingredient for a successful lens fit. Because of the altered corneal geometry from the surgical procedure, this is often difficult to achieve. Increasing the overall lens diameter while maintaining the base curve radius will help center the lens properly.

The criteria for a successful fit are the same as in a nonsurgical patient. There must be good centration with adequate tear interchange, minimal bearing on any area of the cornea, and adequate (1 to 2 mm) lens movement following the blink. The visual acuity should be crisp and stable.

An over-refraction of the trial lens will be necessary after proper fit has been ascertained. The final lens prescription will more closely reflect the pre-operative refraction than the post-operative refraction because of the lacrimal lens induced by the contact lens vaulting the flattened central cornea.

Because of the compromised nature of the cornea, a lens material that exhibits good oxygen permeability characteristics should be selected. Lenses in the Dk range of 28 to 60 are preferable because of their high permeability and good material stability. These lenses can-

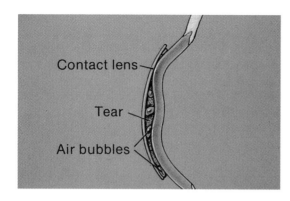

Figure 15–4. Central vaulting with trapped air bubbles as a result of post–radial keratotomy central corneal flattening. (Courtesy of J. Soper.)

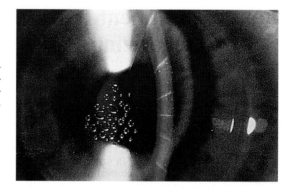

Figure 15–5. Trapped air bubbles following radial keratotomy, with a rigid gas permeable lens. (Courtesy of J. Soper.)

not be made excessively thin, because flexure may cause visual problems such as blurred or fluctuating acuity.

Hydrophilic Lenses

Soft lenses may be fitted on the post-RK patient if rigid lenses cannot be tolerated, but they must be used with extreme caution. A study by Shivitz and Arrowsmith showed that 33% of post-RK eyes fitted with soft lenses showed blood vessel ingrowth into the incision lines. The PERK study found neovascularization as a complication in 12 eyes during their 5-year study; all had been fitted post-operatively with soft lenses.

If a soft lens is to be used, there must be adequate lens movement to allow as little interference with tear film exchange as possible. There should be no impingement of the limbal vasculature, and the vision should be crisp and stable. Fluctuating vision is a sign that the lens is vaulting the central cornea excessively and is being deformed by the upper lid during blinking. If excessive vaulting is suspected, a K reading over the lens will show mire changes immediately after the blink.

A good rule of thumb for soft lenses would be to fit the flattest lens possible that does not drop off the cornea.

Hybrid Lenses

Hybrid lenses such as the SoftPerm lens seem to offer a good alternative to RGP or soft lenses, but they must be used with extreme care. The problem of vascularization into the incisions is even more pronounced with hybrid than with Hydrogel lenses. The low-water-content soft skirt and the low-Dk rigid center may not offer adequate oxygen permeability. This type of lens also has a tendency to tighten with wear and may cause corneal hypoxia with subsequent corneal edema. If all else fails, a trial with this lens type may be advantageous, but extremely careful follow-up evaluation is necessary. A base curve should be selected that closely matches the mid-peripheral curvature. Fluorescein evaluation is necessary to properly assess the alignment of this lens.

COMPLICATIONS

Surgical Complications

Radial keratotomy procedures are not as complication-free as many surgeons would have one believe. According to George Waring, M.D., the major complication of RK is its lack of predictability. The final outcome cannot be accurately predicted for any individual patient, which opens the door for the contact lens specialist.

Other complications have been reported in the literature. To date, only a small percentage of RK patients have had major complications that were sight-threatening, but the number of surgeons performing this procedure is increasing rapidly, as is the number of procedures being performed. RK is a surgeon-intensive procedure, and the final outcome is related to the skill of the operating physician. Good surgeons have good results, whereas marginal surgeons have marginal to poor results.

The complications noted during the PERK study were mainly refractive in nature. Three percent of 752 eyes had a decrease in best corrected acuity of 2 lines or more on the Snellen chart. Over-correction occurred in approximately 20% of the patients in the PERK study. Hyperopia is difficult to correct surgically with available procedures; therefore, a visual device, either glasses or contact lenses, becomes necessary.

Under-correction of the myopia is more common. Forty percent of the PERK study patients were left with some degree of myopia, and 12% were left with a significant amount, defined as 20/40 uncorrected acuity or worse. Other studies, including those by Deitz and Salz, showed similar results.

Other complications that have been reported include recurrent corneal erosions, map-dot fingerprint dystrophy, delayed-onset keratitis, epithelial cysts, and neovascularization. Endothelial changes have also been noted following corneal perforations when the surgeon has cut too deeply (Fig. 15–6).

Many of these complications preclude contact lenses as a rehabilitation device. Rare cases of cataracts, post-operative endophthalmitis, and traumatic corneal rupture along the incision line have also been reported.

The most common patient complaints following RK are excessive glare and fluctuations in visual acuity. The glare problem usually resolves with time as the surgical scars heal.

The diurnal visual acuity fluctuations have been known to last for years. RGP contact lenses are the modality of choice in this situation. As the central corneal curvature changes during the day as a result of the diurnal intraocular pressure change, the lacrimal lens formed between the anterior surface of the cornea and the posterior surface of the lens will vary to compensate for the corneal changes. As the central cornea steepens and the minus power increases, the lacrimal lens flattens proportionately and loses an equal amount of minus, so the visual result is constant.

Contact Lens Complications

Contact lens complications following RK can be similar to those found with a "normal" eye and are addressed in the same fashion.

Peripheral corneal desiccation, or 3-9 staining, may occur. Changing the edge configuration and edge lift may reduce this situation. Medium edge lift characteristics and a thin lens edge will minimize the staining. Reducing lens size is also an option, but a too-small lens will not center properly and may induce glare and flare.

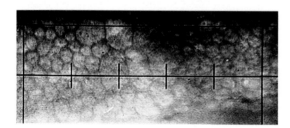

Figure 15–6. Endothelial cell changes along the incision line.

Poor tear exchange under the lens can induce corneal edema, even with high-Dk materials. This edema can cause a reverse orthokeratology effect, with the central cornea steepening and increasing the degree of uncorrected myopia. Loosening the fit by decreasing the optic zone diameter or reducing the overall diameter may relieve this situation. A higher-permeability material may also help.

Fluorescein staining of the incision lines may necessitate the removal of contact lenses until the scars have flattened. Bearing on a raised scar may lead to epithelial erosion and possible corneal infection.

The contact lens practitioner must bear in mind that he or she is working with a compromised cornea; therefore, caution must be exercised. The patient needs to be followed closely during the fitting process and routinely thereafter.

TROUBLESHOOTING

Flare and Glare

Many RK patients experience flare and glare during the post-operative period. If the post-RK contact lens patient reports these symptoms, the fitter must ascertain if it is constant or if it occurs only during lens wear. If it is constant, the patient merely needs to be reassured that the flare and glare will be reduced as the incision lines heal. If, on the other hand, the flare is seen only while the lenses are worn or if it is worse while wearing lenses, then some form of lens modification will be necessary. In most cases, increasing the overall lens diameter, increasing the optic zone diameter, or both will decrease or eliminate the problem.

When increasing lens diameter does not significantly reduce the glare effect, switching to an aspheric lens design may help. The junctionless back surface of many aspheric edge-to-edge lenses may reduce the flare and glare that originates at the peripheral curve junction of standard spherical lenses. It should be remembered that the rapid flattening from center to edge of an aspheric lens necessitates fitting the lens steeper than a standard spherical design. For example, a 0.65–eccentricity value aspheric lens should be fitted about 1.75 D steeper than a spherical design to achieve the same alignment fluorescein pattern.

Poor Centration

Because the post-RK cornea is steeper in the mid-periphery than centrally, a contact lens will tend to decenter toward the steeper area of the cornea. The norm is for the lens to ride upward and nasally, but this may vary from patient to patient.

The edges of high-riding lenses may infringe on the pupillary area and cause visual problems. Increasing the lens diameter will usually reduce this problem. Aspheric lens designs can be utilized if proper centration cannot be achieved by increasing the diameter of the lens.

Another approach for extremely high-riding lenses is to incorporate prism ballast to pull the lens down on the eye. Care must be taken that the lens shows good movement following the blink, or there is a danger of corneal edema caused by stagnation of tears under the non-moving lens. This situation can also induce neovascularization of the incisions if not corrected.

Specialty lenses may be utilized to improve centration. The Plateau lens from Menicon, developed by William Carter, Richard Eaker, and Joe Malinger, is a unique lens designed specifically for post-RK corneal geometry. This lens has a relatively flat central curve with a steeper secondary curve and standard peripheral curves. This lens is best fitted from a trial lens set, but if one is not available, the lens can be fitted empirically. The central curve selection is based on the flattest post-operative K reading, whereas the secondary radius is fitted to the flattest pre-operative K reading. The overall size is usually 10.0 mm with an 8.0 optic zone diameter.

The OK™ series of orthokeratology contact lenses by Contex Contact Lenses have also been utilized for the post-RK eye. In a similar fashion to the Plateau lens, these orthokeratometric lenses are relatively flat centrally with steepening in the mid-periphery.

Specialty lenses may improve centration and give a better lens-to-cornea relation than conventional lenses in some instances. Always try to start with the most simple design first, then go to the more complex lenses if necessary.

Low-Riding Lenses

Unlike high-riding lenses, low-riding lenses are more difficult to remediate. Decreasing lens mass by lenticulation or reducing lens size may be of some help. Changing to a lighter material such as polystyrene may also help raise the lens by reducing lens weight. Adding a minus lenticular configuration to the lens edge may allow the upper lid to more securely hold the lens in place and give a lid attachment type of fit.

As with standard lens fitting, low-riding lenses may induce peripheral corneal dessication and corneal edema, which can also lead to corneal neovascularization in the post-RK patient.

Specialty designs such as Plateau or OK-3 may improve centration, but if the lens remains low on the eye, a hydrogel lens may be the best choice.

Fluctuating Vision

Patients reporting visual fluctuations after blinking may have a lens that is either too steep, too flexible, or both. If the fluorescein pattern appears optimal, increasing the center thickness of the lens will decrease the lens flexure induced by the blink. A flatter base curve may also reduce the problem of flexure and visual distress. Careful assessment of the fluorescein pattern will guide the choice of remediation of this problem.

Fitting the post-operative RK patient is a challenge. The practitioner must deal with atypical corneal geometry and compromised corneal and tear film integrity. He or she must be able to handle the psychological barriers of the failed RK procedure as well as the physiologic complications. Post-RK patients need careful explanation and constant reassurance to get through the fitting process, but a successful conclusion is rewarding to both the patient and the practitioner. The three Ts—tact, time, and tenacity—are the necessary ingredients for a successful outcome.

BIBLIOGRAPHY

Ajamian PC: Radial keratotomy: an overview. Am Optom Assoc 1986;57:580.

Anderson AE: A fundamental approach to post-RK contact lens fitting. Contact Lens Forum 1988;13:46.

Arrowsmith PM, Marks RG: Visual, refractive and keratometric results of radial keratotomy: five year follow up. Arch Ophthalmol 1989;107:506.

Astin CLK: Keratoreformation by contact lenses after radial keratotomy. Ophthalmol Physiol Optom 1991;11:156.

Binder PS: Optical problems following refractive surgery. Ophthalmology 1986;13:739.

Buffington RD: Orthokeratology and the post-RK patient. Contact Lens Spect 1988;3:71.

DePaulis MD, Aquavella JV, Shovlin JP: Postsurgical contact lens management. In Silbert JA (ed): *Anterior Segment Complications of Contact Lens Wear*. Churchill Livingstone, 1994, p. 413.

Edwards GL: personal correspondence, 1994.

El Hage S: Controlled keratoreformation for post-operative radial keratotomy patients. Int Eyecare 1986;2:49.

Fleming JF: Corneal asphericity and visual function after radial keratotomy. Cornea 1993;12:233.

Goldberg JB: The RK-aspheric RGP corneal lens for radial keratotomy. Contact Lens Spec 1993;8:23.

Goodman GL, Troker SL, Stark WJ, et al: Corneal healing following laser refractive keratectomy. Arch Ophthalmol 1989;107:1788.

Harris WF, Malan DJ: Keratoreformation by contact lenses after radial keratotomy: a re-analysis. Ophthalmol Physiol Optom 1992;12:376.

Hoffer KJ, Darin JJ, Pettit TH, et al: Three year experience with radial keratotomy. Ophthalmology 1983;90:627.

Hom MM, Blaze P: An update on post-RK contact lens fitting. Contact Lens Spect 1986;1:46.

Houston JC: Management of refractive surgery failures. Contact Lens Spect 1987;2:33.

Insler MS, Ali Z: The effects of continuous soft contact lens wear after radial keratotomy in cats. J Refract Surg 1986;2:26.

Janes JA: Post-operative fitting of radial-keratotomy patients. Rev Optom 1983;120:59.

Janes JA, Reichel RN: Refractive surgery and contact lenses. Contact Lens Forum 1986;11:28.

Katz HR, Duffin RM, Galsser DB, Pettit TH: Complications of contact lens wear after radial keratotomy in an animal model. Am J Ophthalmol 1982;94:377.

Mallinger JC: Post-RK: a contact lens fitting methodology. Contact Lens Spect 1986;1:43.

McDonnell PJ, Garbus JJ, Caroline P, Yushinaga PD: Computerized analysis of corneal topography as an aid in fitting contact lenses after radial keratotomy. Ophthalmic Surg 1992;23:55.

Nelson JD, Williams P, Linstrom RL, Doughman DJ: Map-fingerprint–dot changes in the corneal epithelial basement membrane following radial keratotomy. Ophthalmology 1985;92:199.

Rowsey JJ, Balyeat HD, Monlux R, et al: Prospective evaluation of radial keratotomy, photokeratoscope corneal topography. Ophthalmology 1988;95:322.

Rowsey JJ, Balyeat HD, Rabinovitch B, et al: Predicting the results of radial keratotomy. Ophthalmology 1983;90:642.

Salz JJ, Salz JM, Salz M, Jones D: Ten years experience with a conservative approach to radial keratotomy. Refract Corneal Surg 1991;7:12.

Salz JJ, Villasenor RA, Elander R, et al: Four-incision radial keratotomy for low to moderate myopia. Ophthalmology 1986;93,727.

Shivitiz IA: Fitting contact lenses after radial keratotomy. Contact Lens Forum 1988;13:38.

Siegel IM, Cohen ML: Post-RK contact lense fitting. Contact Lens Spect 1992;7:41.

Vickery JA: Post-RK and the soft lens. Contact Lens Forum 1986;11:34.

Waring GO, Lynn MJ, Culbertson W: Three year results of the prospective evaluation of radial keratotomy (PERK) study. Ophthalmology 1987;94:1339.

Waring GO, Lynn MJ, Gelender H, et al: Result of the prospective evaluation of radial keratotomy (PERK) study one year after surgery. Ophthalmology 1985;92:177.

Waring GO, Lynn MJ, Gelender H, et al: Results of the prospective evaluation of radial keratotomy (PERK) study. Ophthalmology 1991;98:1164.

Weiner BM: Contact lenses for post-corneal surgery patients. Contact Lens Spect 1987;2:24.

Weiner BM: Troubleshooting clinical contact lens problems. Eye Quest 1993;3:36.

Werner DL: Refractive surgery: radial keratotomy. J Am Optom Assoc 1986;57:584.

Zadnik K: Post-surgical contact lens alternatives. Int Contact Lens Clin 1988;15:211.

CHAPTER 16

Aphakia

Edward Zikoski

Far and away, the majority of aphakic contact lens patients are infants and children. The success of intraocular lenses (IOLs) for adult aphakes has been such that the only remaining adult aphakes wearing contact lenses are those for whom IOLs have failed or those who became aphakic before IOLs became successful. This chapter therefore begins by discussing the more common patient: aphakic infants. Adult aphakic patients are discussed at the end of this chapter.

APHAKIC INFANTS

It has been estimated that one in every 200,000 infants is born with some form of lens opacity. Most often, this is discovered immediately by the pediatrician, and the infant is referred to a pediatric ophthalmologist for cataract extraction. Unlike adult cataract patients, in whom surgery is put off for as long as possible, in infants it is imperative that the cataract be excised as quickly as possible and visual rehabilitation started to avoid amblyopia.

IOLs have been used in infants since the mid-1950s. Concern regarding potential complications with posterior chamber IOLs and the ever-changing refractive status of the infant eye has limited their use. Researchers are also uncertain of the long-term effects of an IOL on the human eye; after all, these patients will have these IOLs for about 80 to 90 years. IOLs are contraindicated in patients with aniridia, infantile glaucoma, or a chronically infected eye. Therefore, IOLs are used only after contact lenses have been tried and discontinued.

PROBLEMS ASSOCIATED WITH FITTING INFANTS

Fitting an adolescent or an adult with contact lenses includes the intrinsic benefit of patient desire for contact lenses: they will do everything in their power to facilitate the procedure. When fitting an infant, the practitioner is dealing with a non-compliant patient who will literally fight every step of the way and do everything in their power to try to get the lens out of their eye. However, when successfully fitted, contact lenses offer the practitioner and parents several distinct advantages. Contact lenses are a non-surgical method of correction that can easily be modified as the child grows and their refractive status changes. With the advent of extended wear materials, the trauma of insertion and removal can be minimized.

When deciding what type of lens the infant should have, many factors must be considered. Usually, keratometric readings are unavailable; however, almost universally, the infant's cornea is extremely steep, and therefore steep base curves are required. High plus powers are needed, sometimes in excess of 30.00 D. Infants' palpebral fissures are tiny, requiring small-diameter lenses. It is preferable to be able to leave the lens in for as long as possible to avoid the trauma of insertion and removal. Ideally, what is required is a small-diameter lens that comes in steep base curves and is available in extended wear materials. Other extrinsic factors include the cooperation of the parents. Usually, both parents are necessary in the beginning for insertion and removal. The practitioner must also have a large inventory of lenses because of the high loss rate and the ever-changing refractive status of the infant.

Because of the extreme steepness of the neonate cornea and the thickness of high-plus lenses, care is advised so as to not fit the lenses too tightly. A lens fitted too tightly can lead to corneal edema, irritation, epithelial lesions, or iritis. Most of these problems can be eliminated through the use of highly oxygen permeable materials. Aphakic prescriptions are very thick, making oxygen transmission difficult. In addition, the children will be wearing the lenses on an extended wear basis. High oxygen permeability will reduce corneal edema and neovascularization. Silicone rubber offers the highest oxygen permeability available (Table 16–1).

Silicone rubber has many properties that render it a desirable material for pediatric contact lenses. The nature of the silicone material offers much more than oxygen permeability; silicone is an excellent

Table 16–1. Oxygen Permeability

Oxygen permeability with (cm 2/sec)
(ml O/ml × mm Hg)

Silicone = 7.90×10^{-10}
PMMA = 0.04×10^{-10}
CAB = 2.73×10^{-10}
HEMA = $0/186 \times 10^{-10}$

(CAB = cellulose acetate butyrate; HEMA = hydroxyethyl methacrylate; PMMA = polymethyl methacrylate.)

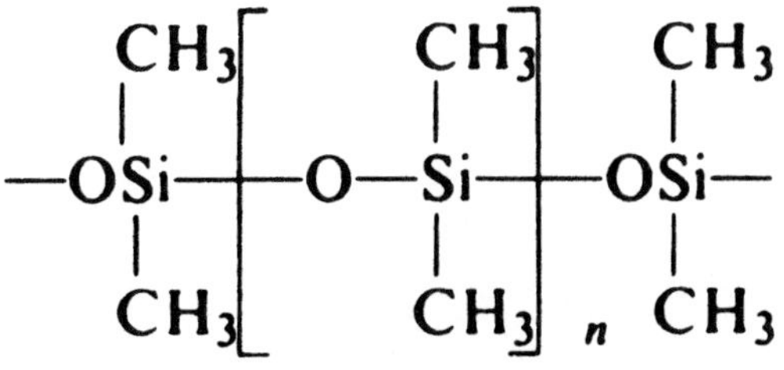

$$CH_3 \quad CH_3 \quad CH_3$$

Figure 16-1. The chemical structure of silicone.

$$-OSi\left[-O-Si\right]-OSi-$$

$$CH_3 \quad CH_3 \quad_n CH_3$$

thermal conductor, in that it does not allow heat to build up between the lens and the corneal epithelium. This reduces metabolic requirements and allows for better tolerance. Bacterial and preservation contamination are minimized as a result of the low water content of the lens. Ocular medications can be used with silicone lenses, because the preservatives in the medication will not accumulate on the lens (Fig. 16–1; Table 16–2).

The Silsoft lens manufactured by Bausch and Lomb is an excellent silicone lens. The pediatric version of this lens comes in three base curves (7.5, 7.7, and 7.9 mm) and two diameters (11.3 and 12.5 mm), and powers range from + 12.00 D to + 32.00 D (Fig. 16–2). Fitting the Silsoft lens is relatively easy and does not require keratometric readings. If the child is younger than 1 year of age, try the steepest base curve available (7.5 mm). Allow the lens to equilibrate on the eye for 30 minutes. The lens should move at least 1 mm (Fig. 16–3). If the lens does not move adequately, a flatter base curve is selected. Fluorescein may be used to highlight the movement of the lens. An alignment pattern is considered optimal. Obviously, a slit lamp examination is difficult with a pediatric patient. A penlight with a blue filter is usually sufficient to observe the fit of these lenses (Fig. 16–4).

After the proper base curve is selected, over-refract using loose lenses (Fig. 16–5). The Silsoft lens can mask up to 2.00 D of corneal astigmatism. If the child is younger than 2 years of age, add + 2.50 D to the final prescription to allow for the close proximity of the child's visual demands. Between the ages of 2 and 3 years, add + 1.75 D. After the age of 3 years, give the full distance prescription in the

Table 16–2. Physical Properties of Silicone

N = 1/435
Light transmission = 93% flat in visible range
Elasticity = 100%
Water = 2% on surface

(N = refractive index.)

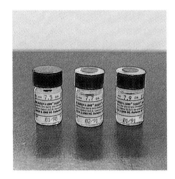

Figure 16–2. Base curves of the Silsoft lens.

Figure 16–3. Optimum centration of the Silsoft lens.

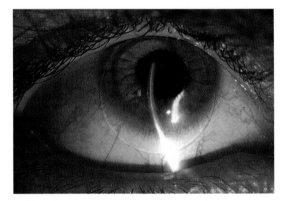

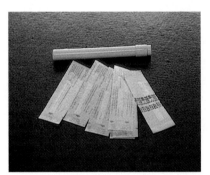

Figure 16–4. Penlight with blue filter and fluorescein strips.

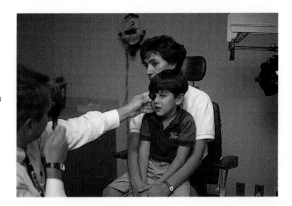

Figure   16–5. Over-refraction using loose trial lenses.

contact lens, and prescribe spectacles with an ultraviolet blocking agent and a + 3.00 bifocal.

There are many inherent problems with silicone lenses. They are hydrophobic, causing water to bead on their surface. To increase their wettability, the surface is either treated with chemicals or is subjected to ionic bombardment. Eventually, the silicone lens accumulates deposits from the tear film because of its permeability to large, soluble macromolecules in the tear film. This accumulation causes the lens to become cloudy. When this happens, corneal irritation is inevitable. Parents can usually see the build up on the lens when they remove it for cleaning. Deposits form at a much faster rate on silicone lenses than on other materials. Even with proper care, including regular enzymatic cleaning, these lenses must be replaced frequently. Care should be taken to not allow the lens to accumulate too many deposits. When a lens becomes coated with oil and mucous debris, it may stop moving on the cornea. The cornea will at first remain clear, but edema will follow, possibly accompanied by vertical striae. This can progress to an abrasion or iritis. Follow-up care is essential. Cost is another factor in silicone lenses. The practitioner's cost is 95 dollars per lens.

The patient should be evaluated 24 hours after the lens is dispensed, and again at 1 week, 2 weeks, and 1 month after beginning lens wear. If the patient is doing well with the lenses, they should be seen at 3-month intervals for the first year of life and at 6-month intervals thereafter. At each visit, an over-refraction with trial lenses is performed. The fit of the lens is assessed using fluorescein and a blue light. Parents are advised to return immediately if the child's eye becomes infected or if a discharge develops. Have the children wear the lenses continuously for 2 weeks to facilitate amblyopia training and minimize the trauma of insertion and removal. If the parents do not feel comfortable inserting or removing the lens, they may be told to return daily until they master the procedure. Some practitioners rec-

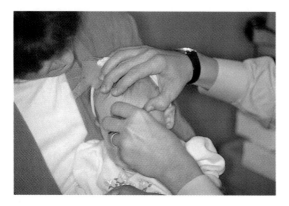

Figure 16–6. Insertion of a contact lens in a child under the age of 2 years.

ommend use of a lubricating drop prophylactically four times per day to increase surface wettability; however, I have not found this to be necessary.

Insertion and removal of pediatric contact lenses is usually a difficult task. The process can be facilitated by following a few simple procedures. If fitting an infant younger than 2 months of age or if dealing with a cooperative toddler, the parent can simply cradle the child in his or her arms while the lens is inserted (Fig. 16–6). I prefer the child to be drinking from a bottle or sucking on a pacifier during this procedure. With 2- and 3-year-old children, the procedure becomes more difficult. The toddler can be placed on a flat, comfortably padded table or on the floor. One parent holds the child's head still and offers support. The other parent holds the child's lower body and legs (Fig. 16–7). Hold the lens between the thumb and index finger, and bend it so that it looks like a taco (Fig. 16–8). With the other hand hold the child's upper lid tightly. A cotton-tipped applicator can also be used to hold the lid. Starting from an inferior position near the lower

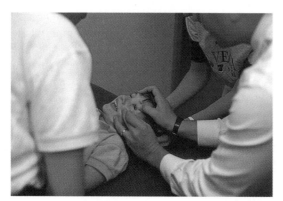

Figure 16–7. Insertion of a contact lens in a toddler or small child.

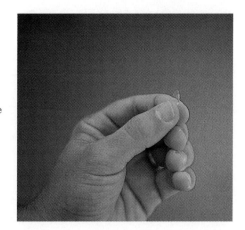

Figure 16–8. A method for holding the contact lens before insertion.

cul de sac, the lens is placed on the cornea in such a manner that the index finger can guide the lens into place.

Bear in mind that by this time the infant is probably screaming and thrashing, and his or her parents are probably quite distressed. Therefore, you have to be fast and aggressive. Unfortunately, an old saying is true in this case: "If force doesn't work, use more force." Hopefully, as the toddler becomes accustomed to the lens, the trauma of insertion and removal can be minimized.

Often, only one parent is available for the fitting process. To make the process of insertion less traumatic for the infant, an alternate way to hold the child is to have them sit on the parent's lap, facing the parent, with the child's legs straddling the parent's waist and with the child's head at the parent's knees. The parent holds the baby's arms down on their lap. If the child is thrashing, its head can be immobilized by holding it between the parent's knees (Fig. 16–9).

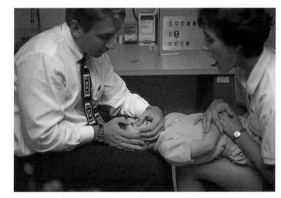

Figure 16–9. Insertion of a contact lens in an uncooperative child.

OTHER CONTACT LENS OPTIONS

Hydrogel Lenses

There are a number of hydrogel lenses available in pediatric parameters in daily and extended wear materials. When the Silsoft lens doesn't work or if there is an excessive loss rate, consider Lombart Lenses LL-79. Its base curves are similar to those of the Silsoft lens, but it has a larger diameter, which allows for more stability. Several companies custom-make lenses to any parameter. The largest drawback in dealing with these lenses is the problem of insertion. Most hydrogel lenses are flimsy and tend to fold back on themselves and on your finger. The fitting process is essentially the same as that with the Silsoft lens, with the exception that fluorescein cannot be used.

Rigid Gas Permeable Lenses

When all other options have been exhausted, fit the patient with a rigid gas permeable (RGP) lens. RGP lenses have several advantages over soft lenses. If the infant has a large amount of astigmatism, the optical correction and therefore the visual acuity will be better. For extremely steep corneas, the lens tends to center better. Insertion is also easier because the lens does not fold back on itself. RGP lenses can be custom designed, they have high oxygen permeability, an ultraviolet radiation blocker can be incorporated, and they are inexpensive. The negative aspects of RGP lenses include a higher loss rate. They are also more difficult to fit.

A diagnostic set is essential when fitting toddlers with RGP lenses. Usually, keratometric readings are not available. Start with a steep base curve and a small diameter. A lens with a 7.0-mm base curve and a 7.5-mm diameter is a good starting point. The child is positioned on the parent's lap as previously described, and the lens is placed on the child's cornea. Observe the fluorescein pattern with a blue light, not necessarily the slit lamp, and look for a central bubble. If an air bubble is observed, fit a flatter lens. Continue to fit flatter lenses until an alignment pattern is observed. Lid involvement is desirable but not essential. At this point, over-refract using loose lenses. When the final prescription is determined, add extra plus, as previously discussed, to compensate for the toddler's near visual demands.

With the introduction of fluorosilicone acrylate RGP lenses, we can now provide our patients protection from ultraviolet radiation. Remember, these patients do not have the protection that the crystalline lens offers. Also, the fluorocarbons tend to wet better, allowing for a more comfortable fit. I have found the Boston Cleaner and Conditioner to be an excellent cleaning regimen.

CRITICAL PERIOD

The timing of treatment for a unilateral congenital cataract is important. The critical period for vision deprivation in humans is still somewhat uncertain. Literature suggests that this period may end 2 to 6 months after birth. Therefore, it is most beneficial to initiate surgical treatment before 4 months of age.

The time the visual system is still "sensitive" to treatment may extend into adulthood. Although maximum effects can be expected of the unilateral congenital cataract patient treated before 4 months of age, the age at which treatment will not achieve positive results may occur well into childhood.

ADULT APHAKIC PATIENTS

Fitting adult aphakic patients is much simpler than fitting their infant counterparts, because typically, the patient is motivated and co-operative. Routine clinical testing can be performed as for any contact lens fitting; however, there are a few special considerations.

LENS POWER

The high-plus powers typical of aphakic correction are somewhat tricky to work with. The best bet is to trial fit using high-plus (about +12.00 D) diagnostic lenses. If such a trial set is unavailable, the fitter should use the most-plus lens accessible and carefully over-refract. The vertex distance between the corneal plane and that of the lensometer should be carefully measured. Using the vertex conversion chart (see Appendix 6), compute the patient's prescription by adding the vertex-corrected over-refraction to the trial lens power. Often, mistakes are made, even when the computations are done carefully. In addition, the aphakic lens will exhibit different flexure and masking behavior than did the trial lens. These differences will affect both the spherical and cylindrical components of the refraction. If the patient is being fitted with a soft lens, consider postponing the prescription of over-spectacles, which incorporate astigmatic and presbyopic correction, until the aphakic soft lens has been dispensed. The correction can then be fine-tuned, and compensation for differences made. If the patient desires toric soft lenses, monovision correction, or both, it is wise to order a high-plus trial lens, which will be exchanged after the trial fitting. Back vertex power is usually specified.

High-plus lenses, whether rigid or soft, will by necessity be very thick. When fitting soft lenses, consider choosing a design that includes lenticulation to reduce center thickness and minimize the potential for corneal edema. Rigid lenses in aphakic powers should also be lenticularized; even so, the lens will be heavy and tend to drop to an inferior position on the eye. Specifying a minus lens carrier and minimal optical zone diameter will aid centration. If the patient's pupils are irregular as a result of surgery, consider a lens with an artificial pupil. Because the eyelids of aphakic patients tend to be flaccid, a lid-attached fitting is probably contraindicated.

HANDLING DIFFICULTIES

Aphakic patients often find lens-handling difficult. Balancing the need to optimize oxygen transmission through a thick lens with the need to provide a lens strong enough to endure rough handling is arduous at best; compromise is necessary. The use of tinted lenses aids in handling and helps to minimize lens loss. Aphakic contact lens wearers must also maintain a spare pair of lenses. Because they no longer have the crystalline lens' natural protection from ultraviolet radiation, these patients should be counseled to wear sunglasses at all times when outdoors. Ultraviolet protection can also be incorporated into rigid lenses.

BIBLIOGRAPHY

Awaya, Sugawara, Miyake, Isomura: Form vision deprivation amblyopia and the results of treatment—with special reference to the critical period. Jpn J Ophthalmol 1980;24:242.

Awaya, Sugawara, Miyake: Observations in patients with occlusion amblyopia. Trans Ophthalmol Soc UK 1979;99:447.

Beller, Hoyt, Mary, Odom: Good visual function after neonate surgery for congenital monocular cataracts. Am J Ophthalmol 1981;95(5):559–565.

Birch, Stager: Prevalence of good visual acuity following surgery for congenital unilateral cataract. Arch Ophthalmol 1988;106:40–43.

Calhoun, Nelson, Cutler: Extended wear contact lenses in pediatric aphakia. J Pediatr Ophthalmol Strabismus 1985;22(3):86–91.

Calhoun, Nelson, Cutler, Wilson, Harley: Silsoft extended wear contact lenses in pediatric aphakia. Ophthalmology 1985;92(11):1529–1531.

Ching, Parks, Friendly: Practical management of amblyopia. J Pediatr Ophthalmol Strabismus 1986;23(1):12–16.

Drummond, Keech, Scott: Management of monocular congenital cataracts. Arch Ophthalmol 1989;107:45–51.

Eggers: Current state of therapy for amblyopia. Trans Ophthalmol Soc UK 1979;99:457.

Gurland J: Use of silicone lenses in infants and children. Ophthalmology 1979;86:1599–1604.

Hale: Unilateral pediatric aphakia: current treatment and lens choices. Contact Lens Forum 1986;11, 34–35.

Jastrzebski, Hoyt, Marg: Strabismus deprivation amblyopia in children. Arch Ophthalmol 1984;102:1030–1034.

Moore: The fitting of contact lenses in aphakic infants. J Am Optom Assoc 1985;56(3):182–183.

Pratt-Johnson, Tillson: Unilateral congenital cataract: binocular status after treatment. J Pediatr Ophthalmol Strabismus 1989;26(2):72–75.

Robb, Mayer, Moore: Results of early treatment of unilateral congenital cataracts. J Pediatr Ophthalmol Strabismus 1987;24(4):178–181.

Rogers: Optical corrections in congenital cataracts. Ophthalmic Forum 1984;2(3):139–140.

Sheets, Rogers, Parks, Hiles, Beauchamp: Round table discussion: congenital cataracts. Ophthalmic Forum 1984;2:141–148.

Taylor, Vaegan: Critical period for deprivation amblyopia in children. Trans Ophthalmol Soc UK 1979;99:432.

Watson, Sanac, Pickering: A comparison of various methods of treatment of amblyopia: A block study. Trans Ophthalmol Soc UK 1985;104:319.

Wright, Wehrle, Urrea: Bilateral total occlusion during the critical period of visual development. Arch Ophthalmol 1987;105(3):321.

CHAPTER 17

Orthokeratology

HARUE J. MARSDEN

The concept of orthokeratology has existed for many years. The ancient Chinese slept with sandbags placed over their eyes to reduce myopia. Today, contact lens practitioners use the programmed replacement of rigid contact lenses to modify the shape of the cornea. The use of hard lenses has shown success in the reduction of myopia, and the more recent designs have accelerated the rate at which this myopia reduction may be achieved. Research has demonstrated that myopia can be reduced between 2.00 to 3.00 D by such means.[1,4] Rigid lenses alter corneal topography; therefore, proper patient selection, lens fit, frequent follow-up, and lens changes are important. As shown in Boxes 17–1 and 17–2, a logical progression through normal fitting procedures, with slight modification, is effective in achieving orthokeratology.

PATIENT SELECTION AND EDUCATION

There are many variables to consider when screening patients. Each individual seeking myopia reduction has a unique motivating factor that may affect their level of success. Some of these patients include low myopes who do not require full-time correction, patients with vocational or avocational minimum visual requirements (e.g., peace officers, pilots), and even moderate to high myopes who would like to function better when uncorrected or utilize thinner spectacles when not wearing contact lenses. In identifying the patient's motivation, it is imperative that both the fitter and patient establish the endpoint (e.g., 20/15 unaided acuity, 20/40 unaided acuity, reduction of myopia as much as possible). The time frame must also be established if the patient must qualify for an employment physical in a limited period of time. These motivations and schedules will assist in determining how to proceed with the orthokeratology procedure.

Patient education is critical. The endpoint is the mutual goal of the patient and fitter; however, it is imperative that the endpoint be realistic. It is not feasible to promise 20/15 unaided acuity to a 4.00 D myope. Because each patient will have a different response to the procedure, it is impossible to promise all patients the same level of

---

BOX 17-1. DO THESE FIRST

1. Patient Selection

   - Determine patient motivation
   - Educate patient:
     Frequent visits are necessary
     Understanding financial commitment (no guarantees/refunds)
     Time commitment (follow-up visits)

2. Preliminary Testing

   - Case history
   - Baseline testing
     Unaided visual acuity
     Corneal curvature measurements
       Keratometry
       Corneal topography
     Objective and subjective refraction

3. Diagnostic Contact Lens Fitting

   - Empiric
   - Lens selection
     Conventional lens design
     OK™ series for accelerated ortho-K
   - Over-refraction
   - Fluorescein pattern assessment

---

success, especially if they have different sets of goals. An important aspect of patient education is that each patient understand that orthokeratology is a time-consuming procedure that requires frequent visits and lens changes. Because of the number of visits and lenses, the costs are high. Because there is individual variability, there are no guarantees and no refunds. It is important to establish these basic tenets prior to beginning the procedure.

PRELIMINARY TESTING

Begin preliminary testing with a thorough case history to determine whether any contraindications for rigid lens wear exist (e.g., corneal degeneration, medications). It is important to establish baseline findings, because they will be the reference point for refractive and unaided acuity changes. Because this test will be repeated on a regular basis, it is important to use a variety of acuity charts to eliminate memorization. Measurements of the cornea are also important, because it is the flattening of the central cornea that yields a decrease in myopia. Corneal topography is useful for a comprehensive assessment of a large area of the cornea; however, it is not always necessary. Accurate keratometry measurements are necessary for diagnostic lens base curve selection and establishing baseline corneal curvature measurements. This may be achieved via instrument calibration. Also note the mire quality; it is important to have good mire quality because poorly fitting lenses can affect the corneal surface, resulting in corneal distortion.

It has been postulated that comparing central and temporal keratometry readings will predict maximum endpoint of the orthokeratology procedure. To take the temporal keratometry measurement, the patient is instructed to look at the plus mire on the keratometer. Specifically, it has been estimated that the maximum change that can be achieved is one half of the difference between these findings. However, preliminary research shows little predictability in the reduction of myopia.[4]

Objective and subjective refractions are important baseline data that can allow the fitter to correlate unaided visual acuity and provide a reference for future changes in myopia. It is important that the refraction have a repeatable endpoint; one criterion is most-plus to best visual acuity. In correlating acuity and refraction, the fitter may detect pseudo-myopes or patients with accommodative problems; in these cases, orthokeratology may not be necessary. A slit lamp evaluation will identify any contraindications to rigid lens wear and establish baseline corneal appearance.

DIAGNOSTIC CONTACT LENS FITTING

If using a conventional tri-curve lens, the desired fitting relation of the first lens fitted is approximately 0.50 D flatter than alignment (Fig. 17–1). It is important that the lens center properly on the cornea. If the lens does not center properly, consider a larger-diameter contact lens, a prism ballasted contact lens, or truncation. The contact lens should be fabricated in a gas permeable lens material of mid to high Dk. Center thickness should be slightly thicker than a conventional lens design to assist in eliciting the orthokeratology affect.

The OK™ series lens is a unique lens design in which the secondary curve is steeper than the base curve; in a conventional tri-curve lens design, the secondary curve is flatter. Diagnostic lenses are essential to assess proper fit and centration. Fluorescein analysis is important to ensure adequate tear exchange with central bearing and mid-periph-

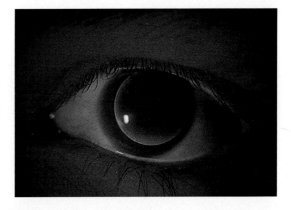

Figure 17-1. A conventional tricurve lens fitted for ortho-keratology. The design is fitted 1.00 D flatter than mean K.

eral pooling. The diagnostic lens base curve can be determined by selecting a lens that is 1.50 to 2.00 D flatter than the flattest central corneal meridian. If the patient experiences excessive tearing, allow them to blow their nose to eliminate the tears. Check the fit, evaluating the lens for adequate movement (1–2 mm) and centration. If movement and centration are not adequate, corneal health may be compromised, and the flattening of the cornea can lead to a displaced visual axis or irregular corneal topography. The fluorescein pattern should demonstrate moderate apical bearing (4–5 mm) and mid-peripheral pooling (2-mm-wide band). An appropriate fluorescein pattern is seen in Figure 17–2. After the base curve has been determined, over-refract to determine lens power.

The fitter must specify the base curve, contact lens power, and overall diameter if using an OK™ series lens. An example of an OK™ series lens order would be

Unaided visual acuity: 20/60
Keratometry: 42.00 × 44.00 @ 180

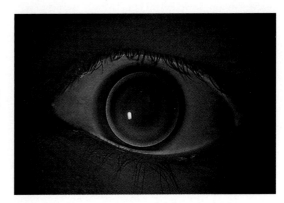

Figure 17-2. A well-fitting OK™ series lens. OK™-3 lens is fitted 1.50 D flatter than K.

Spectacle refraction: $-1.00 - 1.50 \times 180$ (20/15)
Diagnostic lens: 1.50 to 2.00 D flatter than K, or
OK™-3; 8.30/plano/9.6
Over-refraction: $+0.25$ DS (20/15).

If the base curve of 8.3 mm has an appropriate fluorescein pattern, the contact lens power that should be ordered is $+0.25$ (contact lens power plus over-refraction). The diameter of OK™ series lenses ranges from 9.0 to 11.5 mm, the 9.5-mm-diameter lens tends to provide good centration; however, if the tear reservoir (i.e., the area of mid-peripheral pooling) is deficient or if there is seal-off, a different diameter and flatter base curve lens may be necessary.

A lens designed with a secondary curve radius that is steeper than the base curve facilitates the orthokeratology process. Diagnostic fitting with this lens design is imperative to ensure controlled corneal changes. This lens design yields rapid changes; therefore, it is useful to allow the patient to wear the diagnostic lens for a few hours to determine how quickly changes occur and what the next appropriate lens should be.

DISPENSING

Dispensing lenses for orthokeratology is not much different than that for any other lens. With the lenses on the patient, check aided acuity, over-refraction, and fit. Application, removal, and re-centration should be taught as for conventional gas permeable lens wear. Lens care regimen is also the same as for conventional gas permeable lenses. If the patient has not previously worn contact lenses, he or she should begin wearing lenses on a limited wear schedule, gradually building to full-time wear.

The longer the patient is able to maintain lens wear, the greater the likelihood that the orthokeratology effect will occur. Within the first week, a patient who has never before worn lenses should be able to wear the lenses for a minimum of 8 to 10 hours, with maximum wearing time of 14 to 16 hours. As for any lens, the patient should be advised that lens wear should be discontinued if any pain or loss of vision occurs. If the patient experiences any irritation (i.e., burning, stinging, or scratchiness) or if the lens does not feel as if it is moving, he or she should call the office to schedule an appointment for a lens change or modification. The patient should also be informed to expect vision through spectacles to be affected by the orthokeratology procedure.

Depending on the time limitations of you and your patient, you may want the patient to wear the lens on the first day (or the fitting day) for 2 to 4 hours. Following lens wear, check aided acuity, comfort,

---

BOX 17-2. PATIENT MANAGEMENT

1. Dispensing

   - Lens assessment
     Aided visual acuity
     Over-refraction
     Fit assessment
   - Patient skills
     Wear schedule
     Insertion and removal training

2. Follow-up visit

   - Conventional lens design: 1 wk
   - OK-series design; 2–5 d
   - Follow-up testing (with lenses)
     Case history (incl. wear time now and maximum wear time)
     Aided visual acuity
     Over-refraction
     Fit assessment
   - Follow-up testing (without lenses)
     Unaided visual acuity
     Corneal curvature measurements
       Keratometry
       Corneal topography
     Objective and subjective refraction
     Slit lamp evaluation

3. Retainer Lenses

   - Final lens
   - Determine fit
   - Determine wear schedule

---

over-refraction, fit, unaided acuity, refraction, keratometry, and corneal health. If there have been rapid changes, follow the patient frequently to make appropriate lens changes.

FOLLOW-UP VISITS

In conventional orthokeratology, a follow-up visit should occur after 1 week of lens wear; if the patient is undergoing accelerated orthokeratology, the first scheduled visit should be within 3 to 7 days. A previous rigid gas permeable lens wearer on a full-time schedule should be monitored before 7 days, because corneal changes will occur sooner with longer wear. The fitter may want to order multiple pairs of lenses initially so that lenses can be switched as soon as possible; the second lens should be 0.50 D to 1.00 D flatter than the first lens. At all follow-up visits, the patient should be instructed to arrive wearing the lenses. Aided visual acuity and lens fit should be assessed prior to lens removal. If the fit has changed (i.e., if there is less central bearing), or if there is inadequate tear reservoir, inadequate movement, or lens adherence, the fit must be changed. Immediately after lens removal, unaided visual acuity, keratometry, and refraction should be assessed. With the OK™ series lens, the rapid corneal changes start to slow after the first 2 weeks. Weekly visits can become monthly visits as these changes start to slow down. If the patient no longer demonstrates change, going flatter with the next lens may no longer help. If the lens has a good apical bearing relation with a good tear reservoir, this may indicate that it is time for the patient to enter into retainer wear. In the case of a patient wishing to obtain 20/20 acuity, the fitter should try to obtain a refraction of low plus (+0.50–+0.75) to maintain acuity throughout the day.

RETAINER LENSES

To maintain the orthokeratology effect, lenses must be worn during some periods of the day indefinitely. In a conventional tri-curve lens design, the retainer is 0.50 D flatter than the central keratometry measurement. In the accelerated orthokeratology procedure, the retainer lens is the last lens worn as long as it provides adequate fit, is comfortable, and centers properly.

Wearing time of the retainer lens is dependent on the desired acuity and length of effect needed. It is recommended that the retainer lens be worn until the goal acuity is achieved throughout the day. The wear time may then be gradually reduced. For example, if the patient is wearing the contact lenses for 14 to 16 hours per day, he or she can decrease wearing time to 8 to 10 hours daily at first, and then continue decreasing wearing time by an additional 3 to 4 hours. After each reduction in retainer lens wearing time, the patient should measure the interval between last lens wear and first noticeable reduction in visual acuity. A home acuity chart and graph are helpful for this process. If orthokeratology occurred rapidly, regression may occur just as quickly after lens wear is discontinued. Most patients find it convenient to wear the lenses a few hours in the morning and a few hours before bedtime to maintain the orthokeratologic effect during the day.

The patient should chart his or her acuity following lens removal to determine the length of time that he or she can go without lenses.

Some patients have been able to wear retainer lenses successfully during sleep. Additional orthokeratology changes may occur during this period as a result of increased wear time. When used as an overnight retainer, it is of utmost importance to ensure that the lens is centered, that it fits properly, and that there is no lens-binding following sleep. It is also important to use a high-Dk lens material that is thin enough for safe wear during sleep and maintenance of the orthokeratology effect. The same risks involved with overnight wear of RGP lenses (e.g., edema, lens binding) exist; therefore, the patient should be advised accordingly. Aspheric lens designs have been suggested to alleviate the problem of lens binding in overnight wear.

The successful orthokeratology patient must be followed on a regular basis (every 3–6 months). Even during retainer wear, it is important to assess corneal health and regression of refractive changes. Patients may be encountered who have previously undergone orthokeratology who feel their vision with retainer lenses is not as sharp as it had been in the past. The use of corneal topography may be useful in these cases to establish whether uniform corneal re-shaping has occurred and further changes are possible. The OK™ series lenses may be an effective retainer when conventional tri-curve lenses have allowed regression.

In pursuing an orthokeratology practice, diagnostic fitting is important to ensure proper lens fit, vision, and success. Fee structures vary from practice to practice. This is a time-consuming procedure for the patient as well as the practitioner. Additionally, materials can be very costly, depending on number of lens changes required. Fees should reflect professional services and adequate materials for frequent lens changes (i.e., package the material fees as opposed to charging a fee per lens). With accelerated orthokeratology, changes occur quickly, and frequent office visits are necessary.

REFERENCES

1. Binder PS, May CH, Grant SC: An evaluation of orthokeratology. Ophthalmology 1980;87(8):729.
2. Cooper MD, Horner DG: Fitting manual for the OK lenses. Evansville, IN, 1991.
3. Contex OK lens fitting guide. Sherman Oaks, CA, Ortho-K, 1990.
4. Joe JJ, Marsden HJ, Edrington TB: The relationship between corneal eccentricity and improvement in visual acuity with orthokeratology. Optom Vis Sci 1993;70:139 Suppl.

CHAPTER 18

Cosmetic Lenses: Special Purposes

GARY G. GUNDERSON

The fitting of cosmetic lenses is among the most challenging and rewarding tasks encountered in contact lens practice. Several methods have been used to improve the cosmesis of patients with ocular disfigurement.

Prosthetic eyes are fitted after enucleation and are generally made of acrylics. Thinner scleral shells are used over a deformed blind eye (phthisical). The first stained scleral lenses for light protection in sighted eyes were tried in the early 1930s. With the development of polymethyl methacrylate (PMMA) and corneal lenses, it became possible for hard contact lenses to be painted and used for cosmetic purposes.

In the 1970s, soft lenses were introduced, and enhancing tints were developed for changing eye color in patients with lighter irises soon after. Since then, opaque soft lenses have been employed to change the appearance of darker irises.

Soft lenses are the most common method used for prothestic or cosmetic application.[1] Although this chapter concentrates on the application of soft lenses for patients with various disorders, a brief description of hard lenses is also included.

Box 18–1 outlines the procedure for fitting a patient with a cosmetic contact lens. It should first be determined whether the patient is a good candidate for cosmetic contact lenses. Factors to consider include initial and replacement lens cost, patient compliance, and most importantly, patient motivation. The practitioner must determine whether the eye to be fitted is sighted or non-sighted. An assessment of the location of the ocular problem (e.g., cornea, iris, lens) is made. The practitioner and patient must decide whether the lens will be worn full or part time. A refraction should be performed for sighted eyes. Keratometry should be performed on sighted and non-sighted eyes to aid in the initial lens fitting.

The practitioner must decide on a lens design. Rigid lenses are the oldest available modality, but they have fallen into disfavor because rigid gas permeable (RGP) materials are no longer being used for this

184

BOX 18–1. DO THESE FIRST

1. Establish:

   - Patient motivation
   - Patient compliance level

2. Determine:

   - Sighted versus non-sighted
   - Refraction and keratometry
   - Location of problem
   - Full- or part-time wear

3. Decide lens design:

   - Monocular versus binocular
   - Rigid versus soft
   - Standard design:
       Easier to match color
       Quicker delivery time
   - Appropriate color

4. Trial fit

   - Rigid
       Lens centration is critical
       Pupil size measured in dim illumination
       Color match (may require diagnostic lens)
   - Soft
       Less than 1 mm movement
       Minimal decentration
       Pupil size
         Match to other eye
         Dim or bright room illumination

5. Order lens

   - Investigate
       Re-tint policy
       Exchange policy
   - Take photos (optional)
       Color match (can be unreliable)
       Future reference

purpose. PMMA lenses can be painted to obtain desirable cosmetic results. PMMA lenses can be fabricated in a conventional size (9.0-mm overall diameter) or to cover the entire cornea (11.5-mm overall diameter). These lenses can be used to correct regular or irregular astigmatism or to provide greater iris detail if needed. Disadvantages of PMMA lenses include poor corneal physiology, longer adaptation time, and unsatisfactory iris color match. If the practitioner opts to fit a PMMA lens, centration of the lens is critical. Hard lenses may be more useful on dark irises, in which decentration effects are less obvious. It is suggested that lenses of various base curves be tried to obtain excellent centration and minimal but acceptable movement. Pupil sizes should be measured so that the eyes can be matched as closely as possible. Concise Contact Lens (San Leandro, CA) has various standard colors available. Lenses can be ordered with or without a light brown pupillary rim. Zadnik has reported that the color "dawn" is appropriate on many light blue irises.[2]

With the development of tints in soft lenses, most patients requiring cosmetic or prosthetic aid are fitted with this modality. Monocular fits are more appropriately handled with soft lenses for both physiologic and esthetic reasons. As in fitting rigid cosmetic lenses, minimal lens decentration is required for the soft cosmetic fit; optimal movement is less than 1 mm.

Pupil size determination is critical. For opaque black pupil lenses, the non-sighted eye's pupil must match the sighted eye in most settings. Pupil sizes can be selected by the practitioner to obtain the best results by measuring the pupil of the sighted eye in a variety of illumination levels. Because most practitioners do not have a trial set of specially tinted lenses, retinting and exchange policies should be investigated prior to ordering.

To obtain a satisfactory color match, the patient may need to be fitted binocularly; photography can be unreliable in matching iris color because of a color shift that takes place on many films. The best method for color matching is to have a tinted trial lens placed on the patient's eye.

Several examples using contact lenses for cosmetic or functional improvement are cited in the literature. Some of these include corneal defects,[3] pupil anomalies such as coloboma and aniridia,[4-7] leukocoria,[8-9] strabismus,[10-11] monocular polyopia,[12] glare related to albinism and iris abnormalities,[13-14] heterchromia,[15] diplopia,[16] and amblyopia therapy.[17]

Figure 18–1 shows the painted PMMA lens, which can be used to correct astigmatism or provide more natural iris detail than would a soft tinted or opaque contact lens. Figures 18–2 and 18–3 show three different Wesley-Jessen opaque lenses. The standard opaque lens can

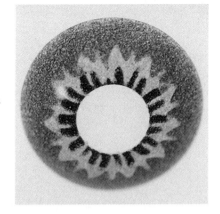

Figure 18-1. Painted PMMA lens with a light brown pupillary rim.

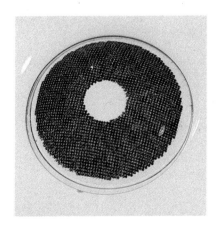

Figure 18-2. Wesley-Jessen hazel opaque lens underprinted with a 3.7-mm clear pupil.

Figure 18-3. Wesley-Jessen Complements brown ink lens underprinted with a 3.7-mm black pupil, and Complements brown ink lens double-printed with a 3.7-mm black pupil.

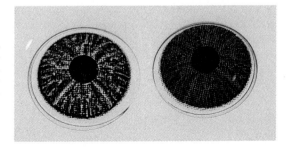

be used to hide corneal scars. These lenses are available in several standard colors and can be double-printed for more color or under-printed black for denser coverage. They normally have clear pupils but can be fabricated with opaque pupils 3.7 or 5.0 mm in diameter. Other variations and custom lenses are also available. These lenses can be used to hide pupil defects as well as iris and lens anomalies.

An alternative to Wesley-Jessen prosthetic lenses for similar anomalies are custom-tinted lenses designed by the practitioner. A black pupil lens can be used to mask a white pupil (Fig. 18–4). A peripheral, tinted zone can be created on a soft contact lens (Fig. 18–5). The central, tinted zone of these lenses is determined by the practitioner based on the patient's pupil size. Patients fitted with this design are often fitted binocularly with a clear pupil over the other eye to match iris color.

Patients afflicted by heterochromia can also benefit from custom lens design. Patients that have displaced pupils can be fitted with the lens design shown in Figure 18–6. This lens has a translucent black central zone that creates a central pupil and a peripheral tinted zone. The peripheral tinted zone masks the pupil anomaly and can reduce glare. The color can be selected by the patient. Patients who suffer from glare related to lens changes or vitreo-retinal changes may benefit from the lens design shown in Figure 18–7. This lens has an 11.5-mm solid tint. Lenses with lighter solid tints providing semi-transparent coverage can be used to allow some of the natural iris detail to show through the lens. This may give the appearance of better depth of the anterior chamber and a more natural overall look to the eye. Overall light

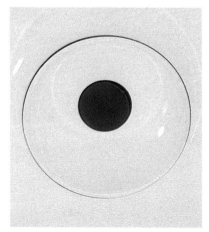

Figure 18–4. PBH (CTL) clear soft lens with a 4.5-mm black pupil.

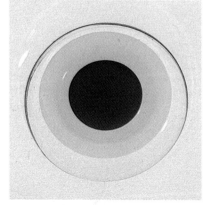

Figure 18–5. PBH (CTL) tinted soft lens with a 6.5-mm black pupil.

transmission should fall between 30% and 60% to reduce glare sensitivity.

The clinical use of cosmetic contact lenses in a patient with a corneal scar on the right eye is shown in Figures 18–8 and 18–9. A close-up photograph of the corneal opacity is shown in Figure 18–10. A Wesley-Jessen Durasoft 3 Flexiwear lens was sent to Adventures in Color for tinting. The patient was interested in a close eye-color match; therefore, lenses were ordered for both eyes. The darkest available brown tint was ordered with clear centers OU. A 4.5-mm clear pupil was selected for the right eye (Fig. 18–11) and a 6.0-mm clear pupil was selected for the left eye (Fig. 18–12). The smaller pupil was ordered on the right eye to ensure coverage of the opacity. Because the patient wanted to wear the lenses on a full-time basis, a larger pupil size was ordered for the left eye to prevent the patient from seeing the edge of the solid tint at night.

Most patients can be fitted with one of the lens designs described previously. Various companies can supply lenses to meet the needs of these patients. Box 18–2 lists the companies that supply cosmetic

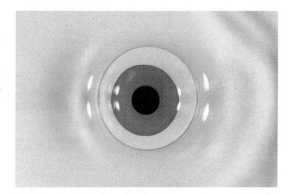

Figure 18–6. Brown-tinted lens with a translucent pupil.

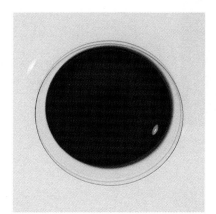

Figure 18–7. Solid brown lens with tint 11.5 mm in diameter.

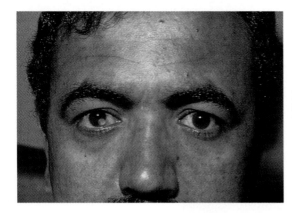

Figure 18–8. Patient with corneal opacity in the right eye with no contact lens.

Figure 18–9. Patient in Figure 18–8 with contact lenses placed on both eyes.

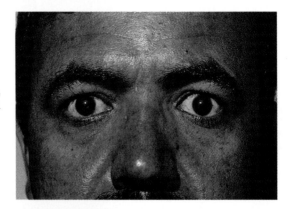

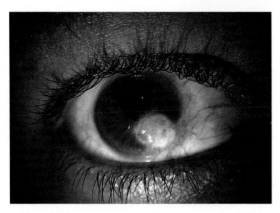

Figure 18–10. Close-up view of the corneal opacity in the right eye of the patient in Figure 18–8.

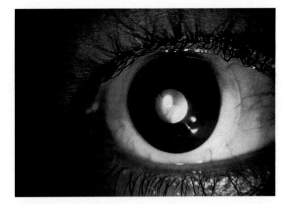

Figure 18–11. Cosmetic brown-tinted contact lens with 4.5-mm clear pupil on right eye covering corneal opacity of patient in Figure 18–8.

contact lenses. Manufacturers list recommended disinfection options with their products. The practitioner and the patient should be aware that tints may fade over time as a result of normal cleaning and disinfection. Some practitioners suggest using only chemical disinfection (without sorbates) rather than heat or hydrogen peroxide to minimize leaching of the dyes or discoloration of the lenses. Prices for cosmetic lenses vary among manufacturers.

When approaching a cosmetic fitting, the practitioner should try the simplest approach first. The easiest approach in many cases is similar to the case example presented previously. The practitioner obtains a successful fit by using clear diagnostic lenses, then determines the type of lens design needed and sends the lenses to the laboratory for tinting. High-water-content lenses are recommended, because these materials often maintain better corneal physiology. Additionally, low-water-content lenses do not absorb dyes as readily as do higher-water-content materials. It is often necessary to tint both sides of lenses requiring

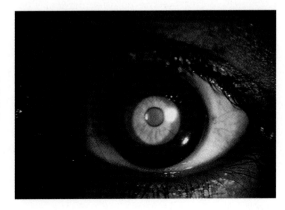

Figure 18–12. Brown-tinted contact lens with 6.0-mm pupil on the left eye of the patient in Figure 18–8 provides a better color match.

BOX 18-2. THINGS YOU SHOULD KNOW

1. Rigid lenses

   • Concise Contact Lens (1-800-772-3911)

2. Standard opaque soft lenses

   • Ciba Illusions (1-800-241-5999)
   • Pinkington Barnes Hind-Natural Touch (1-800-854-2790)
   • Wesley-Jessen (1-800-348-6859)

3. Prosthetic soft lenses

   • Wesley-Jessen special order (no sorbate solutions)
     Durasoft 3
     Durasoft 2
   • Narcissus Foundation (1-415-992-8926)

4. Custom-made soft lenses

   • Wesley-Jessen special order (no sorbates)
   • Pilkington Barnes Hind (CTL)
   • Alden Optical Laboratories (1-800-253-3669)
   • Kontur (1-800-227-1370)
   • Adventures in Color—send practitioner's lens (1-800-537-2845)
   • White Ophthalmics (Calgary, Alberta, Canada)
   • Igel Optics Limited (United Kingdom)

---

dark tints; this may lead to physiologic problems as a result of the presence of tint on the ocular surface. The practitioner should provide proper follow-up care, even for patients with non-sighted eyes, for this and other reasons. Lenses should always be removed and the cornea evaluated with fluorescein at each checkup.

Cosmetic contact lens fits are not common; however, fitting these patients is beneficial to both patient and practitioner. The greater amount of time and lesser economic reward of these fittings are outweighed by the pleasure the practitioner receives watching the cosmetic and psychological improvement in these patients. A case may initially appear difficult or complex, yet the information provided regarding various contact lens alternatives should encourage the practitioner to fit these patients. The future may hold more natural iris patterns and standardized designs.

REFERENCES

1. Cox ND: Pigmented contact lenses for prosthetic application. J Br Contact Lens Assoc 1991;14(4):145.
2. Zadnik K: Prosthetic hard contact lens for postsurgical, enlarged pupil. Contact Lens Forum 1987;12(4):24.
3. Barron C, Dishman A, Garafolo R, Akerman D, Bekritsky G: Opaque hydrogel prosthetic contact lens correction for the disfigured eye. Int Contact Lens Clin 1992;19(5,6):125.
4. Key JE, Mobley C: Cosmetic hydrogel lenses for therapeutic purposes. Contact Lens Forum 1987;12(4):18.
5. Zack MN: The cosmetic treatment of Adie's tonic pupil using subjectively tinted hydrophilic soft lenses. Contact Lens J Lond 1984;12(1):14.
6. Phillips AJ: Iris coloboma managed with a prosthetic contact lens: a case report and review. Clin Exp Optom 1990;73(2):55.
7. Spinell MR, Haransky E: The use of the new Wesley-Jessen opaque lens for a congenital aniridia patient. Int Contact Lens Clin 1987;14(12):489.
8. Higgins M, Spinell MR, Gonzales CM: A special contact lens design for a unique low-vision patient: case report. Contact Lens Specialist 1993;8(7):43.
9. Comstock TL: The use of tinted hydrogel prosthetic lenses. Contact Lens Specialist 1988;3(12):54.
10. Spinell MR, Bernitt D: Cosmetic occluder lens. Optom Monthly 1985;76(1):21.
11. Harwood LW: A "piggyback" PMMA occluder. Contact Lens Forum 1984;9(9):67.
12. Crews J, Gordon A, Nowakowski R: Management of monocular polyopia using an artificial iris contact lens. J Am Optom Assoc 1988;59(2):140.
13. Phillips AJ: A prosthetic contact lens in the treatment of ocular manifestations of albinism. Clin Exp Optom 1989;72(2):32.
14. Garcia-Kramer MY, Weissman BA: Use of tinted hydrogel contact lenses to reduce glare caused by iris abnormalities. Int Contact Lens Clin 1992;19(11,12):264.
15. Gunderson GG: The cosmetic treatment of ectopic pupils and heterochromia irides using tinted hydrophillic soft contact lenses. Int Contact Lens Clin 1993;20(1,2):40.
16. Reiser DE, Baldwin JB: Management of diplopia with a custom tinted soft lens in a patient with chorodial melanoma. South J Optom 1993;11(3):15.
17. Burger DS, London R: Soft opaque contact lenses in binocular vision problems. J Am Optom Assoc 1993;64(3):176.
18. Lutzi FG, Chou BR, Egan DJ: Tinted hydrogel lenses: an assessment of glare sensitivity reduction. Am J Optom Physiol Opthalmol 1985;62(7):478.
19. Greenspoon MK, Silver: Fitting cosmetic and prosthetic contact lenses. In Harris MG (ed): *Problems in Optometry.* Vol. 2, No. 2. Philadelphia, JB Lippincott, 1990.

CHAPTER 19

X-Chrome Lenses

GARY G. GUNDERSON

Red or magenta contact lenses have been prescribed as a means to help color-deficient patients discriminate colored signals in a variety of settings (e.g., to help differentiate traffic signals). Although such lenses are useful for some purposes, the practitioner must carefully screen patients during the fitting process.

Congenital red-green color deficiencies are thought to affect approximately 8% of the American male population and 0.05% of the female population. Three methods of testing for color deficiencies are available. Pseudo-isochromatic tests are designed to test color imbalance but not color discrimination. The Isihara color test, a screening procedure used in many offices, can give the practitioner an idea of the severity of the defect. The Farnsworth D-15 test isolates the 4% to 6% of the male population whose color vision defect is severe enough to cause problems in everyday situations. The Farnsworth 100 hue pattern test will give an even more detailed picture of the defect.

Information is lacking regarding the use of red or magenta contact lenses and their effect on specific types of color deficiencies. Normal individuals are trichromatic and possess three photopigments: red, green, and blue. Anomalous trichromats have three cone pigments, one of which is abnormal. The abnormalities vary, and a range of severity is present for each type of deficiency. This group comprise about 6% of the male population. Anomalous trichromats often have little awareness of their problems with colors although they fail color vision tests. Dichromats, who comprise approximately 2% of the male population, have only two cone pigments. Most commonly, the red or green pigment is missing. These individuals have more severely impaired hue discrimination and may show the most benefit from wearing a red or magenta contact lens in one eye.[1-3] Monochromats, who are very rare, have only one cone pigment and see only lightness differences. Visual acuity is usually reduced to 20/25 to 20/40 in these individuals.

Box 19-1 describes the procedures in screening a patient for a red or magenta contact lens. In discussing a color deficiency, a good case history is important to rule out ocular disease. Recent onset or monocular complaints should lead the practitioner to suspect a disease process; therefore, monocular color vision testing should be performed to

194

BOX 19-1. INITIAL SCREENING PROCEDURES

1. History

   - Rule out ocular disease
   - Establish prior contact lens use
   - Establish patient motivation

2. Standard examination

   - Refraction and keratometry
   - Good binocularity
   - Rule out presbyopic fit
   - Color vision
       Monocular to help rule out disease
       Determine severity of defect

3. Additional testing

   - Measure pupil size
   - Determine iris color
   - Evaluate tear quality and quantity

4. Optional testing

   - Repeat Isihara with Maddox rod
   - Loan anaglyphs without green filter for home tasks

---

help rule out pathology. A contact lens should not be used if disease is suspected; instead, an appropriate referral should be made. The more common red-green acquired deficiencies may result from progressive cone dystrophies, pigment epithelium dystrophies, or optic neuritis. Knowledge of previous contact lens wear may help in the design of the lens. It is important to establish the patient's motivation for wearing a red lens design.

After the case history, a standard eye examination for contact lenses is performed. It is critical to perform stereopsis testing and evaluate the binocular system. Patients with amblyopia or binocular vision problems are not suited for this lens design. Presbyopic patients interested in monovision, soft, or rigid bifocal contact lenses also should not be fitted with monocular red lenses. Iris color, pupil size in dim and normal room illumination, and tear break-up time should be measured. This information may be helpful in final lens design.

To demonstrate the effect of a red or magenta lens to a patient, a red filter such as the handle of a red Maddox rod or a pair of anaglyph glasses with the green filter removed can be shown to the patient. The filter is usually placed over the non-dominant eye. The red lens ana-glyphs can be sent home with the patient so he or she can try various tasks with the correction. The spectral transmission curves of various red lenses have been reported.[4] Because minimal differences exist be-tween these filters and commercially available red contact lenses, the patient can give the "filter lens" a real-life test. The patient should be told that this lens design may enhance color perception for certain tasks but will not cure the color deficiency. If both the patient and the doctor feel that a red lens design is appropriate, the practitioner must determine whether a soft or rigid lens is more appropriate. Previous history of contact lens wear may help to determine lens type; however, other variables should be kept in mind. A list of available lenses is provided in Box 19–2. Lens costs and fees for service should be deter-mined in advance and listed with other contact lens fees so the practi-tioner can inform the patient of the total cost at the initial visit.

Trial lenses should be evaluated on the patient at the initial visit. Some of the advantages of fitting soft lenses are listed in Box 19–3. For soft lenses, a 5- to 6-mm central red pupil generally supplies adequate coverage. Soft lenses may decenter slightly, requiring a slightly larger pupil size. If decentration is excessive and cosmesis is unsatisfactory because of the need for a larger pupil, select a different lens manufacturer. If a toric lens design is indicated, fit the lens according to standard procedures. Be sure to recheck the lens fit when the lens arrives at the office. This will avoid warranty and re-tinting problems. Kontur, Alden Laboratories, and the Narcissus Foundation

---

BOX 19–2. LENS AVAILABILITY

1. Rigid

   - Polymethyl methacrylate red #3 (many local laboratories)
   - X-chrome polymethyl methacrylate (many local laboratories)
   - Alberta II red gas permeable (Procon, Mountain View, CA; 1-415-968-8039)
   - Trans-aire pink gas permeable (Bentec, Sacramento, CA; 1-800-767-9175)

2. Soft

   - Narcissus Foundation (Daly City, CA; 1-415-992-9224)
   - Kontur Kontact Lens (Richmond, CA; 1-800-227-1320)
   - Alden Optical Laboratories (Alden, NY; 1-800-253-3669)
   - Adventures in Color (Denver, CO; 1-800-537-2845)

BOX 19-3. LENS CHOICE

1. Rigid

   - Binocular fit
   - Dark iris
   - Regular daily wear
   - Significant astigmatism

2. Soft

   - Monocular fit
   - Light iris
   - Occasional wear
   - Minimal astigmatism

will custom tint lenses to the fitter's specifications. Adventures in Color will tint any medium- or high-water-content lens with a red pupil. This is probably the most practical approach, because not all practitioners have red or magenta diagnostic trial lenses. Red-tinted soft lenses are shown in Figure 19–1. If cosmesis or centration continues to be a problem, tinting the peripheral zones of two lenses with matching colors and adding a central red pupil to one lens may eliminate the problem. This procedure may be more involved and require some creativity.

Red rigid lenses are shown in Figure 19–2. Spectral transmission curves for pink lenses differ from those for the darker red lenses. No study has compared the effect of the intensity of red tints. The darker red tint is recommended, if possible. Lens availability and advantages of prescribing rigid lenses are listed in Boxes 19–2 and 19–3. Normal diagnostic lenses without the red tint should be evaluated on the patient at the time of the initial visit to obtain a good fit. This should

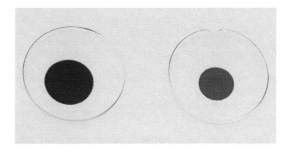

Figure 19-1. Red-tinted soft lenses with 7-mm and 5-mm red pupillary zones. The 5-mm lens has a lighter tint density. Darker densities are recommended.

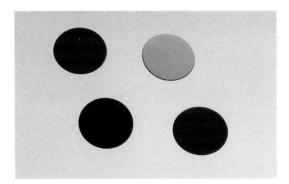

Figure 19–2. Red-tinted hard lenses. (Top, Alberta II and Trans-aire rigid gas permeable lenses; bottom, X-chrome and red #3 PMMA lenses.)

minimize re-order costs. Also, tear fluorescein patterns may be harder to evaluate on dark red lenses.

When dispensing soft lenses, thermal disinfection, hydrogen peroxide, and sorbate-containing solutions should be avoided.[5] These methods may change the color of the lens or leach the dye. Rigid lens care can be selected at the discretion of the practitioner. Standard contact lens dispensing procedures for the lens type prescribed should be followed. In addition, the patient should be warned that stereopsis may be influenced by lens wear.[6–7] The effect may be more apparent if the lens is worn only occasionally. Also warn the patient that wearing darkly tinted sunglasses over this lens design is not advised because of the low level of light transmitted to the eye wearing the red-tinted contact lens. Finally, remind the patient that color deficiencies are often an individual anomaly, and benefits of red lens designs will vary between individuals. The patient's color vision may be enhanced for certain tasks, but his or her color deficiency has not been eliminated.

REFERENCES

1. Richer S, Adams A, Little A: Toward the design of an optimal for enhancement of dichromat monocular chromatic discrimination. Am J Optom Physiol Optics 1985;62:105.
2. Sheedy JE, Stocker EG: Surrogate color vision by luster discrimination. Am J Optom Physiol Optics 1984;61:499.
3. Poknomy J, Smith VC, Verriest G, Pinkers AJLG: *Congenital and Acquired Color Vision Defects.* New York, Grune and Stratton, 1979, p. 357.
4. Gunderson GG: Comparison of transmission curves of commercially available red/magenta contact lenses. Int Contact Lens Clin 1993;20:23.
5. Greenspoon MK, Silver RL: Fitting cosmetic and prosthetic contact lenses. In Harris MG (ed): *Problems in Optometry.* Vol. 2 No. 2. Philadelphia, JB Lippincott, 1990.
6. Ciffreda KJ: Binocular space perception and the X-chrome lens. Int Contact Lens Clin 1980;7:36.
7. Matsumoto ER, Johnson CA, Post RB: Effect of X-chrome lens wear on chromatic discrimination and stereopsis in color deficient observers. Am J Optom Physiol Optics 1988;60:297.

CHAPTER 20

Post-penetrating Keratoplasty Lens Fitting

ARTHUR B. EPSTEIN

Helping people see better is what contact lenses are all about. This is especially apparent when working with patients who have had penetrating keratoplasty (PK). Although fitting contact lenses in these patients can be challenging even for the most experienced contact lens specialist, it is extremely rewarding for both patient and practitioner.

Working with corneal graft patients requires close interaction with the corneal surgeon; the contact lens specialist is an important part of the anterior segment team. Contact lenses provide the best, and sometimes the only, means of visual rehabilitation for the transplant patient. They are also a useful adjunct to secondary keratorefractive surgical procedures. PK has become increasingly common, especially in the elderly population. Problems with early anterior chamber intra-ocular lens implants caused significant endothelial damage in many patients. Because of this, pseudophakic bullous keratopathy is among the leading indications for PK.

In general, any condition that compromises central corneal integrity or clarity may be helped by corneal grafting. These include keratoconus, corneal scarring as a result of trauma or infection, and corneal degenerations such as Fuchs' dystrophy. Advances in surgical techniques and improvements in tissue collection, transport, and storage have also increased the number of procedures performed each year.

INDICATIONS FOR CONTACT LENS REHABILITATION

The precise percentage of post-PK patients who require contact lenses is uncertain. A reasonable estimate is that 20% to 30% of these patients will benefit from contact lenses.

High post-surgical corneal astigmatism is a frequent complication of PK. There is often a significant irregular component. This combination of high corneal cylinder and surface irregularity makes contact lens correction particularly advantageous.

199

Anisometropia is another important indication for contact lens correction. In cases in which aniseikonia induced by spectacles disturbs fusion, contact lenses can be a helpful adjunct. In some cases, a combination of contact lens and spectacle correction can be used to manipulate and equalize image magnification so that fusion can be achieved. It is important to remember that equal spectacle corrections do not necessarily result in equal image size.

PATIENTS, THEIR PROBLEMS, AND YOU

As with most surgery, PK is essentially a procedure of last resort. Even though the complication rate is small, most surgeons delay surgery for as long as possible. Although a conservative approach is usually a responsible one, many transplant patients live with severe visual problems for some time prior to surgery. Even after surgery, the healing process is protracted, and vision may remain poor for a considerable time.

No matter what the surgeon tells them prior to surgery, it is natural for patients to expect that this miracle of medical science will leave them with much-improved vision. Unfortunately, this is not always the case. Thus, many of the problems that the contact lens fitter faces in working with these patients are psychological.

Elderly patients usually have followed a long path before reaching your office. Many have had two or more prior surgeries. They have spent countless hours sitting in doctors' offices. Many do not see well, and their visual loss threatens their independence. They feel helpless and vulnerable. As a result of years of negative media coverage, many are afraid of wearing contact lenses.

BOX 20-1. DO THESE FIRST

1. Complete history: know the reason for the transplant
2. Complete external and slit lamp examination: make sure that the eye is healed and ready for fitting
3. Careful refraction
4. Keratometry: is the central cornea regular?
5. Photokeratoscopy or computed topography, if available
6. Trial lens fitting using an 8.2-mm base curve, 9.5-mm-diameter rigid lens
7. Make sure that a contact lens will improve the patient's vision

---

Patients with keratoconus often have a personality that can compli-cate the fitting process. Fortunately, they also seem to have better understanding and acceptance of their condition and are more tolerant of a complex and lengthy fitting process. Many have prior contact lens experience.

All post-PK contact lens patients require care and understanding. They may become angry at you or at the surgeon. Working with these patients is complicated and sometimes tedious. It can be a frustrating process even for the most skilled contact lens practitioner. However, if you think it is frustrating for you, imagine how the patient must feel. These feelings may be expressed as fear, depression, or outright hostil-ity. Some patients will act out, whereas others will seem meek and afraid to cooperate. I sometimes have to explain to patients that the efforts of even the most gifted surgeon will rarely duplicate the level of vision that existed prior to the onset of the condition. Sadly, many have expectations that plainly exceed the capability of their visual systems.

Being supportive is important, but maintaining a clinical distance is even more so. Try not to take intermediate failures personally. Today's failure can easily turn into tomorrow's success. Most patients re-member only the outcome, not how frustrating the process was or how long it took.

Another consideration is setting reasonable fees for this potentially time-consuming and costly process. Fees should be high enough to insure a profit but not so high as to make your services inaccessible. I use an income-averaging approach. With this method, I accept that I will lose money with the most challenging patients but make a profit fitting the less difficult ones. Overall, I try to maintain fees that insure a fair profit without excessive burden to any one individual. This is an incentive to hone your skills, because the better you are at fitting a patient, the more profitable the encounter will be. Also remember that major medical insurance provides coverage in many cases.

FITTING THE CORNEAL TRANSPLANT PATIENT

The first thing that you should know about fitting the post-PK patient is that it is nothing like fitting the normal contact lens wearer. Many of these patients have pre-existing ocular disease that can pose daunt-ing problems even after the transplant. Even in the best situations, the corneal topography is so drastically altered that it requires a com-pletely different fitting strategy. I've found that the greatest challenge for many doctors is abandoning the conventional techniques and doing things that may appear illogical to achieve a reasonable fit.

There are several factors that can complicate contact lens fitting in the post-PK patient. Physiology of the donor cornea is an important consideration. Although the host epithelium covers the entire transplanted cornea, endothelial function may have been compromised by the procedure. For that reason, oxygen permeability of the contact lens becomes an even more important factor than usual.

Existing corneal disease can be a tremendous problem. Corneal degenerations, such as Fuchs' dystrophy, produce an abnormal host cornea. The effect of the contact lens on the host cornea can be significant and may actually pose a greater threat to contact lens success than the effect of the lens on the transplant.

Patients requiring transplant because of inflammatory disease often have significant corneal neovascularization; this is commonly seen in patients with herpes keratitis. In the normal patient, visual disruption from neovascularization may occur through direct encroachment of the blood vessels within the visual axis or by leakage of blood or lipid. In the transplant patient, vascular ingrowth poses an increased risk of graft rejection. Vascularization may be stimulated by hypoxia or mechanical factors. To reduce this potential, contact lenses should be as permeable and as mechanically unobtrusive as possible. Thin, rigid lenses made of high-Dk materials, especially the fluorinated silicone acrylate polymers, are preferred by a majority of experienced practitioners. These lenses generally have excellent wetting characteristics, which are helpful in the post-PK patient.

Pre-existing or post-surgical corneal surface disease can present a special challenge to the contact lens fitter for several reasons. Tear film abnormalities are magnified by the abnormal corneal topography. The absence of an adequate tear film cushion can be especially problematic in fitting rigid lenses. Increased bearing in elevated areas, especially without an adequate tear film layer, can predispose the patient to corneal erosion. Abnormal tear film dynamics can also disrupt oxygen transmission and may make fitting hydrophilic contact lenses problematic.

Tear film stagnation combined with surface irregularity, especially at the host–donor interface or at suture tracks, may increase the likelihood of bacterial adherence. The possibility of corneal infection, although remote, remains a serious threat.

BEGINNING THE FITTING PROCESS

Although the patient would like to be able to see immediately after surgery, the cornea must heal sufficiently before the contact lens fitting process can begin. This is a frustrating time for many patients. I have found this to be especially true in the patient who has undergone

BOX 20-2. THINGS YOU NEED TO KNOW

1. A rigid lens has the greatest chance of success
2. Forget almost everything you know about fitting normal corneas
3. Rigid lens diameters will usually be large (>9.5 mm)
4. Rigid lens curvatures will often be unusually flat or steep
5. The lens should distribute bearing forces as evenly as possible
6. Some lens-induced staining is inevitable and is usually acceptable
7. If the central topography is regular and the eye is not inflamed, consider a soft lens, especially if the patient is sensitive
8. Watch out for neovascularization in the graft
9. Try a hybrid (SoftPerm) lens if centration cannot otherwise be achieved
10. A piggyback design should be used as a last resort because of poor oxygen transmission through the thick combination
11. Keep it simple—back-surface toric designs rarely work because of peripheral irregularity
12. Be patient—fitting post–penetrating keratoplasty patients is time consuming and challenging
13. Don't be afraid to consult the surgeon when you encounter fitting or other problems—you are both on the same team
14. Use caution with suction-cup removal devices
15. You must know how to recognize a graft rejection

the procedure more than once. Their recollection of the improvement that the contact lens provided is strong motivation to resume contact lens wear.

Contact lens fitting may begin as early as several months after surgery or not until more than 1 year later. Many factors affect wound healing: the age of the patient, the condition of the host cornea and donor button, the presence of ocular disease, the suturing technique, the individual healing factors, and the ophthalmic medications. Healing may be nearly complete in as little as a few months or may take more than 1 year. Stability of the cornea is an important but not absolute prerequisite for starting contact lens fitting. Consultation with the corneal surgeon is helpful in determining an appropriate starting date. Ultimately, the responsibility rests with the contact lens specialist (Fig. 20–1).

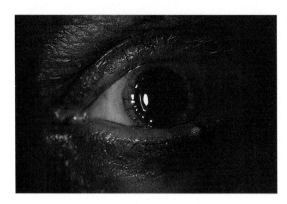

Figure 20–1. Not fully healed penetrating keratoplasty, several months before being ready for contact lens fitting.

Sutures, provided they are buried, are not a contraindication to contact lens fitting. Fitting contact lenses with sutures left in place is usually not a problem provided the lens does not disturb them. Exposed sutures are often successfully managed with a bandage soft contact lens. Obviously, corneal swelling surrounding sutures must be absent before lens fitting can be initiated (Fig. 20–2).

There are significant differences of opinion among surgeons regarding the appropriate time for suture removal. Sutures are generally removed earlier in younger patients. Many surgeons will defer suture removal when vision is stable and of good quality, especially in the older population. Significant visual degradation occasionally occurs after suture removal. This is often the primary reason for contact lens referral in these patients.

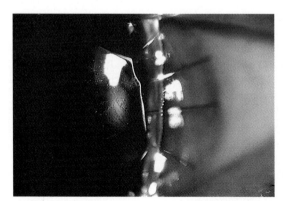

Figure 20–2. Swelling at the host–donor junction in a recently completed penetrating keratoplasty.

TOPOGRAPHY AND ITS MEASUREMENT

The normal cornea has an aspheric surface that flattens as it extends out to the periphery. This flattening process is typically gradual and generally symmetrical. The apex of the cornea is closely aligned with the visual axis. In patients who have undergone transplants, both corneal topography and symmetry are drastically altered. Often, a substantial and precipitous difference exists between central and peripheral topography. In the graft patient, the visual axis and corneal apex usually do not align.

Some grafted patients will have a perfectly regular, even spherical, central topography, with marked irregularity and distortion in the periphery. Other patients may have a highly toric central cornea surrounded by a generally spherical peripheral cornea. The central cornea is the most important determinant of the potential for spectacle correction. The corneal periphery is usually of greatest importance to the contact lens fitter.

The topography in most post-PK patients is at least somewhat irregular. In some cases, the irregularity is the result of surgical or postsurgical complications. A tilted graft can induce massive astigmatism and corneal distortion. A suture that breaks during healing can have a similar effect.

A protruding graft has a steep center and a flatter periphery. You can almost imagine that the donor button was too large, forcing it to bulge forward in its center. In many ways, this topography is similar to keratoconus, at least centrally. A tilted graft has a flat aspect, often with a steep, cliff-like drop off. The steep section can occur anywhere and will cause substantial edge lift with a rigid lens. Grafts can also have a flat center, where the central portion has collapsed inward, creating a plateau (Fig. 20–3). A raised junction is often present at the interface of the host and donor tissue.

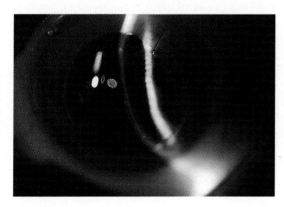

Figure 20–3. Plateau flattening of the central cornea in a penetrating keratoplasty patient. Note the sutures at the 2-o'clock position where a wound dehiscence was repaired.

The topographic variations among post-PK patients are nearly infinite. Unfortunately, conventional methods of assessing corneal topography are of little use in fitting the post-PK patient. The keratometer measures a circle far too small in diameter to provide useful information about the periphery. Keratometry may be useful in identifying patients in whom regular corneal curvature within the optical axis will permit correction with conventional spectacle lenses. Misunderstanding the value of keratometric readings can cause significant problems. Some contact lens fitters, fooled by the regularity of an astigmatic central cornea, will order a back-surface toric lens, only to find it a dismal and expensive failure.

Photokeratoscopy was for many years the standard for topographic analysis. Contact lens and cornea specialists became expert in interpreting the subtle vagaries of topographic anomalies. Computer-assisted topographic analysis has made photokeratoscopy obsolete. These devices produce a dramatic, full-color topographic picture.

Although I routinely use computerized topography, practitioners who do not have access to these expensive instruments need not feel deprived. I noticed long ago that essentially the same, albeit less colorful, picture is produced by the fluorescein pattern of a rigid trial contact lens. In cases in which a rigid lens ultimately will be used, the fluorescein pattern is of even greater use than computerized topography, because the fluorescein pattern incorporates real-time information about the effect of contact lens mass, bearing and flattening forces, lid interactions, tear film dynamics, and capillary attraction forces.

THE TRIAL LENS—THE MOST IMPORTANT FITTING TOOL

Because of the tremendous variability between central and peripheral corneal topography in graft patients, conventional keratometry is of little value in guiding the choice of a trial lens. Advanced computed topographic analysis is more helpful, but it provides no insight into visual potential and contact lens fitting characteristics. Using a trial lens is essential. I use a rigid lens for several reasons. Rigid gas permeable lenses are the preferred choice for most grafted patients. These lenses also provide a quick and simple way to evaluate visual potential. Perhaps the best reason is that evaluation of the fluorescein pattern is a great way to analyze corneal topography.

Many authorities suggest that the initial lens choice should straddle the keratometry readings. I have not found this approach especially helpful and recommend a much simpler method. I use a 9.5-mm-diameter lens with an 8.2- or 8.3-mm base curve. This choice is not arbitrary. It provides an excellent starting point for a majority of patients.

Because of diminished corneal sensitivity in most patients, the lens should be well tolerated. If the patient is extremely uncomfortable, topical anesthetic should be used. Over-refraction provides a good idea of how well the patient can expect to see. As in keratoconic patients, lenses that are poorly fitted, especially when fitted too steep, can substantially reduce acuity. Remember that some patients will have other eye problems that may reduce their quality of vision. The referring corneal surgeon should be informed of unexpectedly poor acuity, because it can be caused by cystoid macular edema, a sequela of the surgery.

Slit lamp evaluation of the contact lens with fluorescein provides a detailed view of the underlying corneal surface, particularly in the context of the lens–cornea relation. Topographic symmetry, lens centration, elevated or depressed areas, and most importantly, lens bearing are plainly evident. Evaluation of the fluorescein pattern yields much the same information that computed topography does, just without the color.

FITTING THE RIGID CONTACT LENS

Almost any type of contact lens that improves vision and does not harm the cornea is appropriate for use in the post-PK patient; however, some lenses are better than others.

Diminished endothelial capacity and the potential for neovascularization make high-Dk, rigid gas permeable contact lenses the first choice in fitting a grafted patient. Rigid lenses are also more effective in correcting the irregular astigmatism and corneal distortion commonly seen in these patients.

Most practitioners who are inexperienced in fitting post-PK patients are surprised by the large-diameter lenses that are often required. Typically, lens diameters will vary from 9.2 to 10.5 mm. Even larger lenses are sometimes needed to achieve a stable fit. Base curves will vary. A surprising number of patients require lenses that are much flatter or steeper than those normally used. Rarely, a symmetrically aspheric central cornea permits the fitting of a smaller lens design.

The actual fitting process is a matter of educated trial and error until a reasonably well-centered and stable lens fit is achieved. Experience makes the trial and error increasingly educated. Don't be discouraged. In time, what took weeks to achieve will take minutes.

The ideal lens design provides a balanced fit, with lens-bearing forces as evenly distributed as possible (see Fig. 20–4). In some pa-

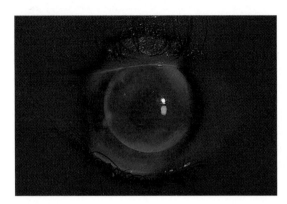

Figure 20–4. Fluorescein pattern of a rigid lens showing even bearing and a well-centered fit over a penetrating keratoplasty.

tients, uneven bearing is unavoidable. Focal areas of punctate staining in areas of high bearing are common. Provided the staining is not dense, does not cause scarring, and resolves rapidly with cessation of lens wear, some mild staining is acceptable in these patients.

Although larger-diameter lenses are often needed to achieve adequate centration, the smallest possible lens with the least mass is preferred (see Fig. 20–5). Thin lenses made of fluorinated silicone acrylate materials provide good bio-compatibility and excellent permeability. Conventional rigid gas permeable designs are readily available and easily modifiable and therefore are usually my first choice. Don't be tempted to get fancy. Back-surface toric designs may appear to be indicated, but peripheral corneal irregularity almost always makes them a poor choice (Fig. 20–6).

When a conventional spherical rigid gas permeable lens fails to provide good centration or acceptable bearing, aspheric and biaspheric designs should be tried. The Boston Envision, a biaspheric design, has

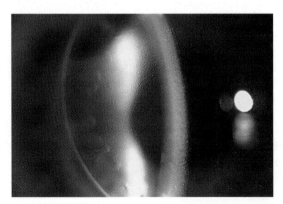

Figure 20–5. Well-centered rigid lens over a penetrating keratoplasty. Note the host–donor junction at the lens edge.

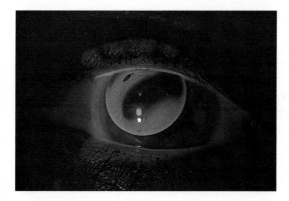

Figure 20–6. A high-riding, decentered bitoric rigid lens over a warped donor button. Note the irregular toricity of the central cornea. Neither a conventional spherical nor an aspheric rigid lens could be fitted.

been used in post-PK patients with good results. Fitting these lenses is similar to fitting conventional designs; trial fitting is essential.

When the central cornea is extremely flat relative to the periphery (i.e., the plateau graft), conventional lenses may not work. Special designs incorporating a flat central curvature with a steeper periphery are available. Although these patients are difficult to fit successfully, I have had reasonable success with Conforma's R-K Bridge lens.

A final consideration is lens handling. Many post-PK patients are elderly and may be terrified of contact lens wear. They are easily frustrated by lens insertion and removal and the demands of lens care. Patience and encouragement are especially important elements of successful instruction of these patients.

Patients who are afraid to touch their eyes, which is more common after surgery, are desensitized and trained using the following technique. They are given a supply of Celluvisc and instructed to place a droplet on the tip of the finger they will use to insert the lens. They are told to slowly bring their finger toward the eye until the Celluvisc touches the eye and runs in. Most return ready to proceed with their instruction.

For patients who have difficulty seeing a decentered lens, adding a ring of 10 to 15 (depending upon lens diameter) dots around the edge of the lens increases visibility and makes finding the lens in the eye much easier. The dots are difficult to see on all but the lightest of irises when the lens is properly centered. However, when the lens is off center, the dots make it stand out clearly. If you cannot make the dots yourself, ask the laboratory to do it. Incidentally, both techniques are helpful whenever patients or their assistants have difficulty with lens handling. This includes pediatric patients.

Lid laxity or dexterity problems, especially in the elderly population, may make use of a suction-cup removal device helpful. The patient must be absolutely certain that the lens is in place before the suction-cup is applied. Otherwise, serious corneal damage, including wound dehiscence, can occur. I advise patients to close the opposite eye to make sure that the lens is centered and that they see well through it before attempting removal.

Extended wear may be necessary when a patient or caregiver cannot safely remove a rigid lens. I have had good success using high-Dk materials for extended wear in post-PK patients. In these patients, rigid extended wear may be safer than soft lens wear in general.

Overly sensitive patients may not be able to tolerate rigid gas permeable lenses. For these patients, there are several other options.

HYDROPHILIC LENSES

Conventional or custom soft lenses can be used when the central corneal topography is regular. This is one of the few situations in which routine keratometry is useful in evaluating grafted patients. Keratometric mires should be undistorted, although significant astigmatism may be present. These patients typically have good vision with spectacle correction but require contact lenses because of significant astigmatism or anisometropia.

Fitting soft lenses on post-PK patients may be straightforward or complicated, and is sometimes both. In most cases, significant corneal cylinder necessitates the use of custom toric lenses. Corneal surface irregularity sometimes causes significant edge lift or bubbles to form beneath the lens. Although both findings are disturbing, neither is an absolute contraindication to soft lens wear. Soft lenses that look terrible often perform well, remain comfortable, and most importantly, produce no ill effects.

To minimize the potential for neovascularization, lenses with high permeability should be used in these patients. Extended wear lenses worn on a daily wear basis are preferred. In cases in which lack of patient dexterity precludes daily lens handling, extended wear is acceptable but must be monitored closely. Topical steroids have also been used to suppress neovascularization in post-PK soft lens wearers, although steroid-mediated immunosuppression in a patient wearing soft extended wear lenses can be a problem.

HYBRID LENSES

The SoftPerm lens, which has a soft skirt bonded to a rigid center, combines much of the comfort of soft lenses with the visual characteristics of rigid gas-permeable lenses. When fitted carefully, this lens provides excellent centration and stability. Visual acuity with the Soft-Perm lens generally lies partway between that of a rigid and soft lens.

Careful trial fitting must be performed. Fluorosoft, a high-molecular-weight fluorescein that does not stain the soft skirt, is placed into the lens bowl immediately prior to insertion. Fit is evaluated on the basis of fluorescein pattern and acceptable lens movement. The SoftPerm lens has shown a tendency to tighten and must be allowed to adequately equilibrate after insertion. Lens binding can lead to corneal edema and inflammation and must be avoided.

Limited fitting parameters and low permeability are currently the chief limitations of the SoftPerm lens. Although improved compared with earlier incarnations, the lens still has a tendency to separate at the junction of the hard and soft portions. However, comfort and excellent centration still make the lens potentially valuable in fitting post-PK patients. Pilkington Barnes Hind has recently received U.S. Food and Drug Administration approval for a wider range of SoftPerm parameters, which hopefully will make the lens more useful for these patients.

PIGGYBACK LENSES

Sometimes, a patient's corneal topography is too irregular to permit a stable fit with a rigid gas permeable lens. In other cases, a rigid gas permeable lens is needed for vision but is not well tolerated. In these situations, a piggyback design using a soft carrier with a rigid lens on top may be the only workable solution.

The soft carrier is selected to match the underlying topography of the graft. In a plateau graft, the flat central cornea is filled in by using a plus lens. The lens power is determined by the amount of fill necessary. The base curve of the lens is determined by trial fitting. In protruding grafts, a thin, high-minus lens usually works best. In both cases, using materials with the highest possible oxygen transmission is important because of the effective combined thickness of the lenses.

The soft lens is fitted first and allowed to equilibrate. Conventional fitting criteria of good centration and movement apply. After the lens has stabilized, keratometry performed with the soft carrier in place provides a good starting point for fitting the rigid over-lens. The use of Fluorosoft is helpful in determining an acceptable rigid lens fit. Again, the normal fitting criteria of good centration and even bearing are applicable. Although too much movement is not desirable, care must be used to avoid fitting the rigid lens too tightly.

A major problem with any piggyback design is its complexity for the patient, who must care for two different types of lenses, using different care products and techniques, which may be confusing. Lens handling is complicated, increasing the frequency of lost or damaged lenses. Reduced oxygen flux through the thick lens combination can also lead to complications, especially neovascularization. These patients must be followed closely.

TROUBLESHOOTING THE FIT

Resolving problems can be the most challenging aspect of fitting the post-PK patient. The problems are often complex, and the solutions sometimes counterintuitive.

When trying to resolve lens-related punctate (fluorescein) staining, it is important to remember that the ability of the cornea to tolerate bearing forces varies not just from patient to patient but between different areas of the same cornea. Excessive staining usually occurs on elevated areas of the cornea, often centrally or at the junction of the host–donor interface. Steepening the lens fit, either by decreasing the base curve, increasing the lens diameter, or both, tends to decrease the total area of any bearing force and shifts the area of contact toward the peripheral cornea.

When staining is primarily central, steepening the lens may reduce bearing forces sufficiently to reduce or eliminate any staining. Sometimes, steepening causes increased bearing on an even smaller surface area, and the problem may actually worsen. If this happens, flatten the lens to create a larger contact area and achieve more evenly distributed bearing.

Peripheral staining can be resolved by either flattening the lens or increasing its diameter. A flatter lens will place more load on the central cornea and less on the periphery. A larger lens will shift a greater proportion of the bearing load further out on the peripheral cornea. If these techniques fail to solve the problem, a smaller lens may clear the area of bearing in the periphery.

Achieving a well-centered, stable lens is difficult. Both centration and stability usually are improved by increasing lens diameter or steepening the base curve. When the central cornea is regular and the periphery extremely distorted, a small-diameter lens may center well.

If adequate stability cannot be achieved with a conventional (spherical) design rigid lens, try an aspheric lens. Plateau grafts, which have a flat center and steeper periphery, often require a specially designed aspheric lens like Conforma's R-K Bridge. When all else fails, a soft or piggyback design should be tried.

Poor vision due to irregular astigmatism or central corneal distortion may be improved by flattening the lens. This technique improves acuity by smoothing the optic zone, and it often works with both rigid and soft lenses. Unfortunately, increased central bearing may be a problem in some patients.

Trying to resolve problems in graft patients can be extremely frustrating. The solution to one problem may cause an entirely different set of problems to appear. Keep an open mind and be willing to try different approaches. Give your approach time to succeed. Most of all, keep the patient's feelings in mind. Be positive, but try to avoid creating unreasonable expectations, and later, disappointment, by being honest.

ADJUNCTIVE SURGICAL PROCEDURES

Advances in refractive surgical techniques have reduced the need for contact lenses in post-PK patients. When contact lenses are necessary, adjunctive surgery can be helpful.

Relaxing incisions reduce post-surgical residual astigmatism and surface irregularity. Arcuate incisions are made 180 degrees apart at both ends of the steep meridian. The effect of the incisions depends on their length, depth, and proximity to the visual axis. The effect increases dramatically the more central the incision.

Incisions are usually made at the slit lamp or operating microscope with the patient under topical anesthesia. A careful refraction and keratometry are performed. Computerized corneal topography is invaluable in planning the incision sites and characteristics. A relaxing incision can eliminate between 5.00 and 10.00 D of astigmatism. If additional reduction is required, augmentation sutures are placed 90 degrees from the steep meridian. Typically, six sutures are used— three on each side. The middle suture is made tightest for increased steepening along the flat meridian. The sutures are removed as the incisions heal and stabilize.

A corneal wedge resection is performed when higher amounts of corneal cylinder are involved. In this procedure, a wedge of corneal tissue is removed along the flatter corneal meridian at the graft margin. The edges are sutured tightly together and the wound allowed to heal over several months. The wedge resection can create a significant irregularity that may complicate rigid lens fitting. Relaxing incisions are preferred when contact lenses are to be worn.

The benefits of working closely with the corneal surgeon are clearly evident when an impossible contact lens fit is made easier by keratorefractive surgery. The surgery is uncomplicated, the patients do not mind it, and it can make your job as a contact lens specialist much easier.

GRAFT REJECTION

Every contact lens practitioner who works with post-PK patients must be aware of and able to recognize a graft rejection. Anything that causes corneal inflammation, including contact lens wear, may precipitate or exacerbate an episode of graft rejection.

Graft rejection is usually easily to recognize. It can involve the epithelium or the entire cornea. Epithelial rejection initially presents as a slightly elevated line that moves rapidly across the cornea. It may progress to endothelial rejection if left untreated. Sub-epithelial infiltrates, similar to those seen in adenovirus infection, may also occur. Epithelial rejection alone is a relatively benign condition that rapidly responds to topical steroids.

Endothelial rejection is far more serious. Disruption of endothelial function produces corneal edema and stromal thickening. Edema may be primarily central, with a relatively sudden onset, keratic precipitates on the endothelium, and a marked anterior chamber reaction. It can also occur at the host–graft interface, with engorgement of marginal blood vessels, fine keratic precipitates, and anterior chamber cell and flare. The keratic precipitates may form a Khodadoust (rejection) line on the endothelial surface.

Signs of corneal rejection include pain, injection, tearing, ocular discomfort, and reduced vision. These symptoms also occur as a complication of contact lens wear and can create confusion. It is extremely important to avoid confusing the two causes. Patients with corneal transplants should be advised to report such symptoms immediately. The clinician should consider the possibility of corneal rejection until the cause of the symptoms is definitively ascertained.

The prognosis is generally good if the rejection is recognized soon after it begins. Early treatment with topical steroids is critical. In severe cases, systemic and sub-conjunctival steroids can be used. If you encounter a possible rejection episode but are unsure, referral back to the corneal surgeon is wise. It is always better to err on the side of safety.

WOUND DEHISCENCE
AND LENS REMOVAL DEVICES

Suction-cup removal devices and plungers like the DMV lens remover are helpful for many patients; however, they must be used with extreme caution in patients with corneal transplants. It is very easy to mistake the outline of the graft border for the edge of the contact lens. This blunder can turn a decentered lens into a potential disaster. This is especially a problem for patients, but doctors are not immune from making this serious error.

The literature contains one report of a corneal wound dehiscence caused by the misapplication of a suction-cup removal device in a transplant patient. I am also aware of a case in which proper use of a suction device produced the same untoward result. Under certain conditions, a contact lens pulled by a suction device may generate enough force to severely traumatize the cornea.

Plungers should be used in transplant patients only when other removal methods fail. They should not be used routinely. Patients who do use suction-cup devices must be carefully trained in their use. To insure that the lens is in place before the device is applied, the opposite eye should be covered to confirm that the patient is seeing through the lens. A lubricating drop may help reduce lens adhesion. Doctors and technicians must also use these devices with caution.

SUMMARY

Fitting these difficult cases is especially gratifying. If you do wish to work with post-PK patients, it is my hope that this chapter provides a good starting point. This type of fitting stretches the limit of available lens design and technology. Hopefully, new materials and improved methods will make it increasingly easy to work with these complex patients.

Basic Fitting of Spherical Contact Lenses

CAROL A. SCHWARTZ

CASE HISTORY

Patient Motivation and Desire

When taking initial information from a prospective contact lens wearer, it is important not only to cover health and ocular history but also to question the patient about his or her motivations for wearing contact lenses and any previous contact lens experience. The information elicited will serve to begin the process of determining which contact lens modality will be most appropriate and what wearing schedule is best suited to the patient's needs. For patients who are current contact lens wearers, determine what type of lens is being worn, what the wearing schedule is, how they are caring for the lenses, the brand and parameters of the lenses (if known), what problems they are having, what they like about the lenses, and why they are changing providers. These answers will provide valuable information for your diagnostic fitting.

If they have had a previous failed experience, determine how long ago they wore contact lenses, what kind of lenses they were, why they discontinued lens wear, and why they are trying again. A patient who has failed with soft or rigid lenses may not necessarily need to be fitted with the other modality but may have a higher motivation with a different lens type. For example, patients who discontinued soft lens wear because they felt the care was too complicated may seem ideal for disposable lenses. Yet they may also succeed well with one of the newer, simpler care systems. A detailed and frank discussion will provide clues about the direction in which the initial diagnostic fitting should proceed.

It is also useful to determine whether the patient has unrealistic expectations of the benefits of contact lenses. For example, some athletes may believe that contacts will greatly benefit their performance. This may or may not be true but is very difficult for the fitter to guarantee. Such misconceptions or unrealistic expectations must be dealt with before the trial fitting. The final question, why they are coming to you, is very important. In the vast majority of cases, it is simply a matter of location, cost, or convenience. Beware of patients who report they couldn't get along with their last practitioner or have been to several practitioners, none of whom were able to satisfy them. If possible, contact the previous fitter to find out why the patient is leaving. Although the patient may have a legitimate complaint against their prior fitter, it may also be that the patient was severely non-compliant or so difficult

216

Table A1-1. Lifestyle Factors Affecting Choice of Lens Modality

Soft	Disposable	Rigid
Part-time wear	Occasional wear	Full-time wear
Contact sports	Water sports	Acuity-intense sports
Dusty environment	Dusty or smoggy environment	Controlled environment
Fear of rigid gas permeable lenses	Fear of rigid gas permeable lenses	Has no preconceptions
Willing to maintain	Wants no care	Wants minimal care

to work with that the practitioner suggested they find another doctor, or that the patient desires a level of perfection that is simply not achievable.

Contraindications and Lifestyle Factors

Very specific questions should be asked about the environment in which the patient lives and works, hobbies or sports that may have an influence on the type of lens selected, and how much time they are willing to devote to caring for their lenses. As shown in Table A1–1, some environmental and lifestyle factors will direct the fitting to a specific modality. Patients who wish to wear their lenses part time or sporadically should be directed to soft or disposable contact lenses. Patients who are often in dusty or smoggy environments or participate in sports in which flying debris is common should also consider soft or disposable lenses. Those for whom crisp, consistent vision is a necessity should be fitted with rigid gas permeable lenses.

Occupational factors that preclude contact lens wear include exposure to harmful fumes (e.g., a chemical worker). A beautician who is regularly exposed to fumes from hair spray and chemicals may not be able to wear contacts at the salon or may be best suited to a lens that can be disposed of easily when deposits form. Exposure to debris is also of concern; a mill worker may be better suited to soft lenses if sawdust is prevalent. Those who work in dry environments, such as airline cabins pressurized to 8000 feet, may need to be fitted with a low-water-content or rigid lens or may have to use lubricants. Despite the recurring myth of a spark welding contact lenses to the cornea and resulting in blindness, most other trades and professions are contact lens–friendly.

Health History

As part of the general case history, pay particular attention to conditions or medications that can complicate or contraindicate contact lens wear. Both prescription and over-the-counter medications should be taken into consideration, including decongestants, antihistamines, and birth control pills. Conditions such as thyroid deficiency or excess and rheumatoid arthritis may affect tear production and thus contact lens wear. Circulatory conditions such as diabetes should also be considered. As a general rule, these conditions, when controlled, do not contraindicate contact lens fitting but may restrict lens type or wearing schedule. After a careful case history has been performed, the following clinical tests will determine the parameters of the initial diagnostic contact lens.

REFRACTION AND CORNEAL MEASUREMENT

Computed topography is a wonderful tool for fitting contact lenses of any sort. However, the cost of such instrumentation has limited most fitters to the previous standard of central keratometry. Although imprecise, keratometry measurements are still the best indicator of the base curve of the trial lens. However, this is only a predicted base curve. The cornea is known to flatten beyond the approximately 3-mm central area measured by keratometry. Corneas do not all flatten at the same rate; therefore, central keratometry should be considered to be only a gross estimate of actual cornea shape, and therefore base curve. As a rule, eyes that are spherical, or nearly so, should be considered for soft contact lenses, because a rigid lens would have to be fitted extremely flat to assure tear exchange and reduce the possibility of lens adhesion.

The patient's refractive status should also be taken into consideration. Astigmatism can be managed with either rigid or soft contact lenses, as can most other conditions. Eyes with no astigmatism or with astigmatism limited to either refractive or corneal will generally be best fitted with a soft contact lens. Oblique astigmatism is usually best fitted with a rigid lens.

TEAR FILM VIABILITY

The quality and quantity of the pre-corneal tear film are of paramount importance to the success or failure of contact lens wear. Among rigid lens wearers, a dry-eyed patient may be more prone to increased deposit formation, discomfort, and 3-9 staining. Among soft lens wearers, dry eye symptoms can include discomfort, lens drying, deposition, and diffuse staining. There are several clinically useful simple tests of tear quantity; assessing tear quality in a clinical setting is more problematic.

Tests of tear quantity include: tear break-up (BUT), rose bengal staining, the phenol red thread test, observation of the height of the tear meniscus, and Schirmer's test.[1-3] Of these, BUT and Schirmer's test are the most commonly used; the BUT test has an added advantage in that it does not require anesthesia. To perform a BUT test, fluorescein dye is placed in the eye, and the patient instructed to blink to evenly distribute the dye throughout the tears. The cornea is examined under the slit lamp with the cobalt filter in place using a wide beam and low magnification. The patient is instructed to blink forcefully and then hold the eyes open without blinking. The tear film is observed and the time noted from the forced blink until dry or dark spots form. These dark spots indicate that the lipid layer has reached the mucin layer. The test may be repeated several times, particularly if the first test demonstrates a short BUT. An average BUT is 15 to 20 seconds; a BUT of 10 seconds is considered a borderline dry eye, and a BUT of 5 seconds or less indicates a clinically dry eye, for which contact lenses are contraindicated.[4]

The tear meniscus can also be evaluated at this time. The height of the tear prism from the top of the inferior lid to the point at which the tear film first touches the cornea (seen as a dark line) is noted. A height of approximately

0.3 mm is considered normal. A meniscus that is very slight or has scalloped or uneven edges may be indicative of a dry eye.

The phenol red thread test was developed by Hamano and colleagues in Japan.[2] It is performed by placing a high-quality thread treated with phenol red dye in the inferior cul-de-sac. It is similar to Schirmer's test but can be performed without anesthesia. The thread is placed so that one end is in the inferior cul-de-sac and the remainder of the thread is allowed to drape over the lid and cheek slightly temporal to the midline. After 15 seconds, the thread is removed and the portion that has been turned red by the presence of tears measured. A value of 23.9 mm is considered normal; any value under 9 mm is considered diagnostic of dry eye.[3]

The tear film should also be evaluated for debris from cosmetics, pollution, or metabolism. Such debris may indicate poor tear quality, low tear quantity, meibomian gland dysfunction, or improper use of cosmetics. Any baseline corneal staining should be noted. In some environments, slight corneal staining is common among non-wearers of contact lenses. Significant staining may be a contraindication of contact lens wear. A line of diffuse horizontal stain slightly below the corneal midline may be indicative of lagophthalmos and a contraindication to extended wear.[5]

PHYSICAL MEASUREMENTS

Several anatomic measurements should be made: horizontal visible iris diameter, pupil size, and fissure height. These are generally measured with a small (pd) rule; several contact lens manufacturers also supply these with pupil templates. The iris is measured across the midline; 10 to 13 mm is considered normal. Pupil size is measured under both dim and bright illumination. Fissure height is measured at the widest point. These measurements are used as general guidelines in determining which lenses will best suit the patient. Typically, larger eyes require larger lens diameters. Patients with very small fissures are best fitted with rigid lenses to aid in lens handling. Patients with large pupils will require lenses with large optic zones to avoid flare at night.

Iris color and blink rate should also be noted during this gross inspection. The position of the patient's lids should be diagramed on their charts; this may have a bearing in fitting spherical lenses but is most often taken into consideration when fitting bifocal or toric lenses. The practitioner should also note lid tension; very tight lids may displace contact lenses, whereas very loose lids may not provide adequate support for specialty designs requiring lower lid involvement. During slit lamp evaluation, the lids should be everted for examination and to detect any vernal or allergic changes that may be aggravated by contact lens wear.

DETERMINATION OF APPROPRIATE LENS TYPE

The preceding tests should provide some clues regarding the appropriate lens type for the patient. For example, a patient with an essentially spherical prescription who suffers from seasonal allergies can be best fitted with a disposable lens. A patient with borderline dry eye who travels frequently may require a rigid gas permeable lens. A patient with astigmatism who wants to wear lenses for sports and works on a computer can be fitted with any lens modality. With the advanced lens materials and designs available, most patients will be able to be fitted with virtually any type of lens. Experience will help make lens type selection easier.

SOFT LENS DIAGNOSTIC FITTING

Soft lenses are extremely easy to fit, which may account for their approximately 85% market share.[6] For more than 25 years, soft lens manufacturers have refined their spherical lenses to make them as foolproof to fit as possible. There are three basic fitting parameters the practitioner must specify: base curve, diameter, and power. Unlike rigid lenses, however, soft lenses must be fitted from a diagnostic lens that is identical in every parameter other than power. Each manufacturer uses its own proprietary design. In soft lens fitting, factors such as thickness, optic zone diameter, and lenticulation will affect the overall fit of the lens. Because these may not be specified or changed by the fitter, it is important to verify that these parameters will be acceptable by using the appropriate diagnostic trial lens.

It is critical that a soft contact lens cover the cornea fully to avoid staining and desiccation. Sizes ranging from 13.5 to 14.5 mm in diameter are common, and those approximately 14.5 mm in diameter are most often used. If the patient has a large pupil, a lens with a large optic zone should be chosen to avoid flare in scotopic conditions. Flare occurs when the edge of the optic zone encroaches upon the pupillary zone; the patient will report seeing lights or images shooting off to one side of the field of view. This effect will be in the opposite direction of the encroachment.

Base curve is selected from the central keratometry readings. Most manufacturers offer two or more base curves in each lens diameter. For a 14.5-mm-diameter lens, base curves of approximately 8.6 to 8.7 mm are generally able to accommodate most moderately shaped corneas. Very steep corneas (≥ 45.00 D) generally will be best fitted with a steeper base curve lens; most manufacturers offer a base curve of approximately 8.3 to 8.4 mm to accommodate these patients. Very flat corneas (≤ 41.00 D) can be fitted using a base curve of approximately 9.0 to 9.1 mm.

Because the lens must be fitted using a lens of the same material and manufacturer as the lens to be ordered, lens material must be selected before a diagnostic lens is placed in the eye. The water content of the lens is related to the amount of oxygen it transmits to the cornea; the higher the water content, the greater the oxygen transmission. The material itself is also a factor in the amount of oxygen that passes through the lens. The amount of oxygen that will diffuse through a specimen of the material is known as its oxygen permeability, or Dk. This is a characteristic of the material, just as is color or hardness. However, Dk is of limited use to contact lens practitioners, because it fails to take the thickness of the lens into consideration. The Dk divided by the thickness of the lens is known as its oxygen transmissibility, or Dk/L. This value is of much greater importance to the fitter because it describes the amount of oxygen that can travel through the lens to be metabolized by the cornea. These measurements must be carried out on sophisticated equipment in a laboratory setting. Various charts, including promotional brochures supplied by the manufacturer, will provide Dk and Dk/L for a given brand of soft lens. It is important for the fitter to remember that these may not be representative of the lens they are fitting. For example, if the Dk/L is calculated for a low-minus lens, it will overstate the amount of oxygen available to the cornea behind a thicker high-plus lens, even though they are both manufactured of the same material. Another method of expressing the amount of oxygen available behind a lens is the equivalent oxygen percentage.[4] For practitioners, it's generally enough to remember that the higher the water content, the more oxygen permeable the material. Thickness of the lens should also be taken into consideration; a very thick, high-water-content lens may be as permeable as a thin, low-water-content material.

On the surface, it might seem that the optimal lens for any patient would be that offering the highest water content and the thinnest design. This is not always the case. High-water-content materials tend to be more fragile than their mid-water-content counterparts. Very thin, high-water-content lenses tend to dry out more quickly and may be very uncomfortable in patients with borderline dry eyes or in those who work in low-humidity environments. High-water-content materials may attract deposits more quickly, and because they may not be able to be cleaned using one of the more aggressive regimens, will exhibit increased spoilage. Taking these factors into consideration, the fitter will find that for daily wear use by the average individual, there are many moderate-water-content lenses (i.e., those containing from 45%–60% water) that will serve the majority of patients well. The goal is to find a lens that provides enough oxygen for normal metabolism (more is not necessarily better) and that the patient can handle and clean without an excessive number of damaged lenses. Even so, frequent replacement of these lenses is recommended.

Lens tint is a matter of patient and practitioner preference. For presbyopic or highly hyperopic patients, a visibility tint should be considered mandatory, because these patients may not be able to see the lens to insert or remove it. Cosmetic tints can be used for trial lenses, even if the patient will be ordering a clear or visibility tinted lens. Practitioners who routinely use cosmetically tinted diagnostic lenses have found they often dispense a higher than average number of cosmetic lenses and second pairs.

After diameter, material and design, and base curve have been determined, the trial lens is selected. The power of the diagnostic soft lens is immaterial unless it is significantly different from that of the patient's prescription. Bear in mind that to reduce thickness, and thus increase oxygen transmission, manufacturers design plus-powered soft lenses with an anterior optic, or lenticular, zone. As lens power increases, the diameter of this zone may decrease. If possible, when fitting extremely high-powered plus or minus lenses, it is preferable that the lens have a power relatively similar to the predicted prescription power. The predicted power of the lens is the spherical equivalent prescription corrected for vertex distance (see Appendix 6).

After the diagnostic lens has been chosen, it is placed on the patient's eye, and the eye is allowed to adapt. When excess tearing has subsided, the patient can be considered adapted. The lens should first be examined for proper fit using the biomicroscope. Assessment of fit is performed first, because if the patient is still slightly unadapted, visual acuity and over-refraction will be affected more than will the slit lamp examination.

Fluorescein dye is not used to assess the fit of soft lenses because it is absorbed by the material and will ruin the lens. Rather, the fitting relationship is determined by making judgments about the movement of the lens on the eye. Setting up a moderately wide optic section, the fitter should first determine that the lens is relatively centered on the cornea and covers it completely, extending out onto the sclera slightly in a full 360-degree range. Some spin-cast lenses have a slight tendency to decenter somewhat, but a lens that is significantly decentered is indicative of a too-flat base curve. After determining that the lens provides adequate coverage, evaluate lens movement.

Lens movement is judged in one of three ways: the "guesstimate," use of a measuring reticule within the slit lamp eyepiece, or by comparing it with something of a known width. Most practitioners judge movement by guess and experience; however, those with limited experience may wish to measure the width of the slit lamp beam, rotate it to the horizontal position, and compare the movement they observe with this. Soft lenses typically move approximately 0.25 to 0.50 mm with the blink. Some lenses, particularly disposable or ultra-thin designs, may show less movement. However, minimal movement is a requirement of all soft contact lenses. If no movement on the blink or upward gaze can be seen, a flatter base curve should be fitted. The fitter should then return the slit lamp beam to the vertical position and study the edge of the lens as the scleral vessels pass under it. The edge of the lens should never impinge on these vessels, causing them to seem to disappear at the lens edge; nor should the lens drag the vessels as it moves on the blink. Either of these is an indication that the lens is too steep or too large.

Last, the fitter should examine the lens for esthetic purposes. Does the tinted portion of the lens extend beyond the limbus, creating a halo effect? If so, the lens will not be cosmetically acceptable, and a lens with a smaller tinted area or smaller overall diameter should be considered. Is the lens edge visible with the naked eye? Again, a smaller lens will provide better cosmesis. A well-fitting soft lens is shown in Figure A1–1.

After the lens has been deemed to be physiologically satisfactory, the fitter must concern himself or herself with visual performance. Visual acuity through the lens is measured and a spherical over-refraction performed. If acuity through spherical lenses is adequate for the patient, the lens can be ordered as follows: material, base curve, and diameter same as those evaluated. Power is determined by adding the spherical over-refraction, corrected for vertex distance, to the power of the diagnostic lens.

Dispensing and Follow-Up

Dispensing of the patient's lenses should include verification of fit and visual function and instructions on proper lens care and handling (see Appendix 2).

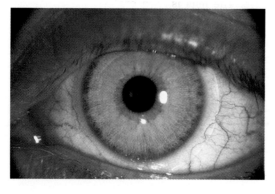

Figure A1–1. A well-fitting soft contact lens. There is full corneal coverage, extending onto the sclera, without blanching of vessels as they travel under the edge. (Courtesy of CIBA VISION.)

After the practitioner is assured that the patient understands all care and wearing instructions and is proficient in inserting and removing the lenses, he or she can be released. Daily wear patients are generally seen at approximately 1 week post-fitting and thereafter as needed to ensure the fitting is progressing as expected. At each follow-up, a case history is taken, visual acuity through the lens is checked, and an over-refraction is performed. The fit of the lenses is checked. With the lenses removed, a slit lamp examination and keratometry are performed. Extended wear patients are often instructed to begin by wearing their lenses on a daily basis. After their first return visit, if all is as expected, they are allowed to sleep with their lenses in and told to return the following morning for evaluation.

After patients are stable in their contact lenses with no changes in fit or prescription, they may be released to routine follow-up. Soft daily wear patients are generally seen at 6-month intervals; extended wear patients more often.

RIGID LENS DIAGNOSTIC FITTING

One of the simplest and most effective rigid lens fitting methods is that taught at the Illinois College of Optometry. The computations are extremely uncomplicated: the base curve of the rigid diagnostic lens is determined by computing the average keratometry reading and subtracting an amount determined by overall lens diameter (Table A1–2).[7] Lens diameter is determined by visible iris diameter (smaller eyes accommodate smaller lenses), steepness of the corneal curvature (steeper eyes receive smaller lenses), fitting relation desired (smaller diameter interpalpebral lenses or larger lid-attached fitting), and most importantly, fitter preference. Bearing in mind that larger lenses tend to be more comfortable than their smaller counterparts, 9.0- to 9.5-mm-diameter lenses are most commonly used.

The intermediate curve is approximately 1 to 1.25 mm flatter than the base curve and is 0.2 mm wide. The peripheral curve radius ranges between 10.50 and 12.25 mm; steeper base and intermediate curves have steeper peripheral curves. The peripheral curve is 0.4 mm in diameter; all curves are treated with a medium blend. If a variety of powers are available in that base curve, the power closest to the spherical component of the patient's vertex-corrected prescription is used as the diagnostic lens.

The lens is placed on the eye and the patient allowed to adapt; fluorescein dye is placed in the lower cul-de-sac, and the patient instructed to blink several times to distribute the dye. The lens is then evaluated with the slit lamp and cobalt filter. After the blink, an interpalpebral lens should re-center quickly. Ideally, a wide slit lamp beam passed slowly from edge to edge should

Table A1–2. ICO* Rigid Lens Fitting Parameters

Overall diameter	8.5 mm	9.0 mm	9.5 mm
Base curve radius	mean K	mean K − 0.50 D	mean K − 1.00 D
Optic zone size	7.3 mm	7.8 mm	8.3 mm
Peripheral curve	10.50/0.4 mm	11.25/0.4 mm	12.25/0.4 mm
Intermediate curve = base curve + 1 mm/0.2 mm width			

* Illinois College of Optometry.

reveal no areas of bearing (dark areas indicating that the lens is touching the corneal surface). Neither should there be large areas of clearance (a wide bright area between the lens and cornea). When the beam of the slit lamp is opened fully, the observer should note an even distribution of fluorescein under the entire lens surface with more obvious clearance under the peripheral and intermediate curves. In reality, this is almost never the case. As shown in Figure A1–2, a well-fitting lens is considered one in which the areas of bearing or clearance are minimal and viable edge clearance is provided in a full 360-degree range. A lens that is too steep will exhibit a large central area of pooling and may move sluggishly on the blink; if this is the case, a diagnostic lens at least 0.50 D flatter in base curve should be evaluated (Fig. A1–3). A flat lens will be less comfortable, show excessive fluorescein dye in the intermediate area, show central bearing, and may move in an erratic manner (Fig. A1–4). A diagnostic lens at least 0.50 D steeper should be employed. If the fluorescein dye shows a marked pattern of bearing in one meridian and clearance in the other, resembling a bowtie or dumbbell, the patient may require a toric or aspheric lens. A lens that fits adequately under the optic zone but does not provide 360-degree edge clearance should be ordered with the same base curve and diameter, but with flatter peripheral and intermediate curve radii.

A lid-attached lens should remain securely under the upper lid with little lateral movement. The lens, which is fitted large and flat by design, will show a great deal more tear pooling under the entire surface; the greatest amount at the inferior edge, diminishing gradually until the lens tucks under the superior lid (Fig. A1–5). It is important to ensure that the lower edge of the optic zone remains below the pupillary zone to avoid flare.

After the lens fit has been deemed to be acceptable, an over-refraction should be performed, first with spherical lenses only, then in sphero-cylindrical form. If vision is adequate through the spherical over-refraction, the lenses may be ordered as follows: the parameters identical to those of the trial lens with power adjusted for the over-refraction. As with soft lenses, when the power of the over-refraction exceeds ±4.00 D, a vertex conversion must be made. Unlike soft lenses, the power ordered in hard lenses may not be identical to the spectacle refraction because tears under the rigid lens form a liquid lens that has a positive or negative effective power. Tears under a lens fitted 1.00 D steeper than the flattest keratometry reading will form a +1.00 D lens; conversely, the tears under a lens fitted 1.00 D flatter than K will form a −1.00 D lens. When this lacrimal lens is added to the contact lens power, the

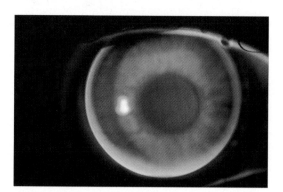

Figure   A1–2. A   well-fitting alignment contact lens. (Courtesy of Polymer Technology Corp.)

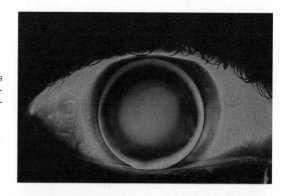

Figure A1–3. A too-steep lens showing central fluorescein pooling. (Courtesy of Polymer Technology Corp.)

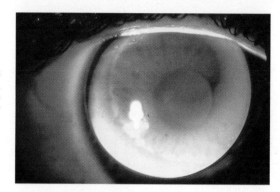

Figure A1–4. A too-flat lens showing excessive peripheral pooling and bearing zone. (Courtesy of Polymer Technology Corp.)

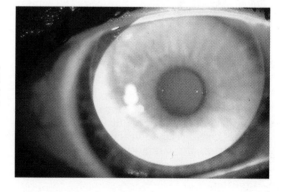

Figure A1–5. Lid-attached fitting requires the lens to be fitted flat and tucked under the upper lid. (Courtesy of Polymer Technology Corp.)

sum should approximate the spherical equivalent spectacle refraction. If the lens appears to fit well, yet the patient requires an astigmatic correction to attain acceptable acuity, a toric lens should be considered.

Minor adjustments to the fit of the lens can be made when ordering. Most commonly, this entails ordering a flatter or wider peripheral curve system. It may be wise to make such changes in small increments. Altering peripheral curves is a very simple in-office procedure explained in Appendix 3. Because the procedure is so simple, small changes can quickly be made to avoid over-correcting and thus spoiling the lens. Care should be taken when widening peripheral curves, because the change in optic zone size will affect the fit of the lens. While holding the base curve constant, making the optic zone smaller will loosen the fit of the lens; making the optic zone larger will tighten the fit. Excessive edge clearance has been indicated as a cause of 3-9 staining; an edge treatment that allows mobility and adequate tear exchange is all that is needed.

Center thickness is determined by consulting a table prepared for the type of material you wish to order, or it may be left unspecified for the laboratory to compute for ease of manufacture. Typically, rigid gas permeable lenses range in thickness from 0.12 mm to 0.25 mm. An optimal center thickness for moderate-Dk lenses is 0.15 mm; for high-Dk materials, the optimal center thickness is 0.17 mm. Thicker lenses are obviously heavier and therefore may not center well. Excessively thin lenses may flex on the eye, causing variable vision; in some materials, the lens may be excessively fragile. To reduce the center thickness of a high-plus lens and avoid knife-like edges, a lenticular design with a minus carrier may be required. For high-minus lenses, edge thickness may be extreme; this may be uncomfortable for the patient or interfere with proper lens positioning as the lids manipulate the lens. There are two possible remedies: a lenticular design or a CN bevel. The CN bevel is a long, tapered anterior bevel that trims away excess material. It can be added at any time in-office or can be included in the original lens order.

A lenticular lens is one in which there is an optic zone on the anterior surface. This is done to control edge and center thickness in the higher powers. For plus lenses, it reduces center thickness and increases edge thickness; for minus lenses, center thickness remains constant and edge thickness is minimized. The thickness of the lens at the junction of the two anterior zones should be approximately 0.13 mm.[8] The diameter of the anterior optic or lenticular zone for a plus-powered lenticular lens should be as small as possible to reduce center thickness. However, the zone should also be sufficiently large that the patient does not experience flare. For the sake of structural integrity, the diameter of a lenticular lens should never equal that of the posterior optic zone and is usually at least 0.2 mm smaller.

In the majority of cases, the material of the diagnostic lens is inconsequential to that ordered. The exceptions are very high-Dk or flexible materials. Typically, diagnostic lenses are manufactured in a very durable material, usually a low-Dk silicone acrylate. When ordering a higher-Dk material, the practitioner should be aware that center thickness may need to be increased; the laboratory can guide the fitter regarding this parameter. Lenses should be ordered from a reputable laboratory authorized to manufacture the material desired to ensure a quality product.

Dispensing and Follow-Up

Dispensing and lens care are critical to the patient's success and long-term satisfaction with contact lens wear. Appendix 2 provides step-by-step instructions for dispensing and lens care. Prior to dispensing rigid lenses, they should be verified for base curve, diameter, optic zone diameter, center thickness, and power. Particular attention should be paid to verifying the edges; they should be well rounded rather than sharp or excessively blunt. After verification, the lenses should be carefully cleaned to remove residue from manufacturing and handling and then soaked in the appropriate storage solution for at least 4 hours prior to dispensing. Dispensing and follow-up visits are performed as for soft lenses. Small changes in fit and power may be made in-office, as described in Appendix 3.

REFERENCES

1. Basinger K, Johnson Y: No-nonsense solutions to the tear dilemma. Contact Lens Spect 1994;(4):20.
2. Hamano T, Mitsunaga S, Kotani S, et al: Tear volume in relation to contact lens wear and age. CLAO J 1990;16(1):57.
3. Sakamoto R, Bennett ES, Henry VA: The phenol red thread tear test: a cross cultural study. Poster presented at the Annual Meeting of the American Academy of Optometry, Orlando, FL, December 1992.
4. Bennett ES, Allee HV: *Clinical Manual of Contact Lenses.* Philadelphia, JB Lippincott, 1994.
5. Schwartz CA. Take a deeper look at ocular surface disease. Rev Optom 1993;130(9):71.
6. Health Products Research, Inc: *Vision Care Survey.* 1992.
7. Jurkus JM: Personal correspondence. 1994.
8. Mandell RB. *Contact Lens Practice.* 4th ed. Springfield, IL, Charles C Thomas, 1988.

Lens Care and Dispensing

David P. Libassi

Many patients perceive contact lens fitting, dispensing, and follow-up care to be trivial. The application and care of this optical device, which the United States Food and Drug Administration (FDA) considers to be an ophthalmic drug, must be properly presented to the patient. In addition, practitioners must properly document contact lens data, including patient instruction on handling, wearing hours, and care.

Before handling lenses, contact lens wearers should be instructed to wash their hands with a mild soap that is free of oil, lotion, and perfume. Substances found on the surface of the hands, such as oil, perfumes, lotion, and dirt, can contaminate lens surfaces. Several manufacturers of hypo-allergenic soaps have labeled their products as being safe for use with contact lens wear (Box A2–1). Thorough rinsing with clean running water should be followed by the use of a lint-free towel to dry the hands. If lint-free towels are unavailable, wringing the hands damp dry is preferable to the use of a fluffy towel. In addition, patients should understand that keeping fingernails smoothly trimmed and round will reduce the possibility of lens damage during removal and cleaning. The possibility of corneal or conjunctival abrasion is also reduced when fingernails are trimmed and clean.

The patient should work over a clean dry surface, placing a towel over counter surfaces or stoppers over sink drains to minimize the chance of lens loss. Patients should be instructed to establish a routine of handling the right lens first and left lens last to reduce the possibility of confusing lenses. However, presbyopic patients who have been fitted for monovision should habitually insert the near lens first and remove it last to ease the lens-handling process.

Before insertion, each lens should be placed on the tip of the index finger of the inserting hand for visual inspection. Patients should re-rinse the lens if necessary to remove apparent lint or debris. Lenses that appear to be damaged

---

BOX A2–1. HAND SOAP PRODUCTS FOR CONTACT LENS WEARERS

1. Eyecare Special Hand Soap (Channel Laboratories)
2. Eyecare Lint-Free Towels (Channel Laboratories)
3. Contact Lens Wearer's Glycerin Soap (Lobob Laboratories)
4. Optisoap (Optikem International)
5. OptiNaps (Professional Supplies)
6. Pure and Natural Soap (Dial Corporation)

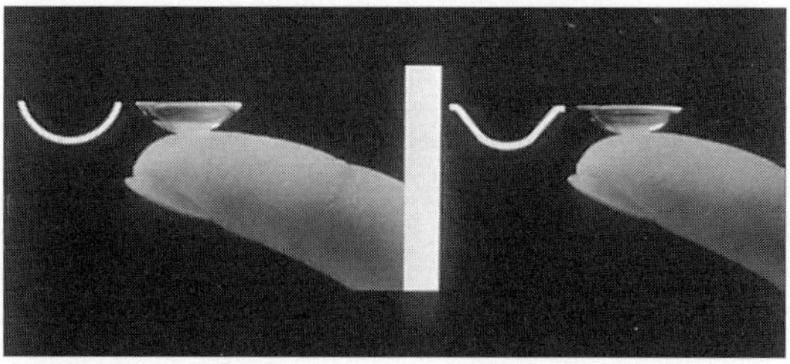

Figure   A2–1. Correct   lens edge profile *(left)*. Inverted lens edge profile *(right)*.

or torn should be replaced. In addition, soft contact lenses must be inspected for correct orientation before insertion.

There are several different methods of lens inspection for correct orientation:

1. *Lens profile technique:* place the lens on the tip of the dry index finger. As shown in Figure A2–1, when the lens is oriented:

   • "Outside out, inside in," lens edges sweep upward
   • "Inside out, outside in," lens edges flare outward

2. *"Taco test":* place the lens along a crease in the palm of the hand and slowly close the palm. When the lens is oriented:

   • "Outside out, inside in," lens edges reach toward each other
   • "Inside out, outside in," lens edges flare outward

3. *"Pinch test":* pinch the lens between the tip of the index finger and thumb. As shown in Figures A2–2 and A2–3, when the lens is oriented:

   • "Outside out, inside in," lens edges reach toward each other (see Fig. A2–2.)
   • "Inside out, outside in," lens edges flare outward (see Fig. A2–3.)

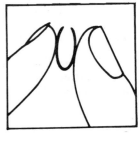

Figure   A2–2. Two-finger   pinch   test   demonstrating proper lens orientation.

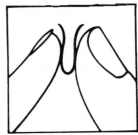

Figure A2–3. Two-finger pinch test demonstrating inverted lens orientation.

Rigid lenses should also be inspected to assure they are free of debris and damage. The lens should be removed from the case in which it has been soaking in wetting or conditioning solution and placed on the tip of the index finger. A visual inspection should be performed. Lenses that appear coated should be cleaned; damaged lenses should be discarded and replaced. The clean lens should be placed on the tip of the index finger for insertion and receive one drop of wetting agent on the inside surface.

Many different techniques exist for insertion and removal of rigid and soft contact lenses. The practitioner must observe the patient's comfort and dexterity with lens handling and coach the patient accordingly.

UNIVERSAL CONTACT LENS INSERTION

1. With the lens placed on the tip of the index finger of the dominant hand, the patient should fix his or her gaze in a mirror in the straight-ahead position. The mirror or target may also be on a flat surface as long as the patient works directly over it. The middle finger of the inserting hand should pull down the lower lid. If necessary, the middle finger of the free hand can raise and immobilize the upper lid by reaching across the forehead and grasping the lid margin and lashes.
2. While maintaining a fixed gaze, place the lens gently on the cornea. If the patient looks away at the last moment, the lens may be placed on the temporal or inferior bulbar conjunctiva. The patient should look downward and release the lower lid first, followed by the upper lid.
3. Lenses placed on the inferior or temporal conjunctiva must be centered. The lens should be trapped by finger pressure through the lid at the far edge of the lens. The patient should then turn his or her gaze into the trapped lens to accomplish centration.

SOFT LENS REMOVAL

1. To facilitate lens removal, place a drop of soft lens wetting solution or saline in the eye.
2. The middle finger of the lens-removing hand pulls down the lower lid as the patient fixates on a target in upward gaze. The patient may see the tip of the index finger as it pulls the lens onto the inferior conjunctiva. The patient will notice a reduction in vision.
3. The patient places the fleshy part of the thumb of the same hand against the lower lashes. The index finger continues to drag the lens toward the thumb, pinching the lens off the eye.

Note: removal of the soft lens directly from the cornea is not recommended because of the possibility of corneal irritation.

RIGID LENS REMOVAL

Blink Technique

1. Working over a flat surface, the patient should fix his or her gaze at a straight-ahead target. The patient should open his or her eyes as wide as possible.

2. Place the middle and index fingers of the hand on the same side as the lens about to be removed on the outer edges of the upper and lower eyelashes. The free hand is placed below the open eye to catch the lens.
3. As the lens wearer gently pulls the eyelashes toward the ear, a forceful blink is made to "pop" the lens off the eye.

Two-Hand Technique

1. With the patient's gaze fixed in the straight-ahead position, the index finger of one hand is placed on the lower lid lashes directly below the bottom of the contact lens. The index finger of the free hand is placed on the upper lid lashes above the top of contact lens.
2. With gentle finger pressure keeping the eyelids against the globe, the lid margins are brought together, catching the edges of the lens and forcing it from the eye.

Suction-cup removal should be presented only to patients who are in need of a back-up removal device to be used after their primary technique has failed. The patient must maintain straight-ahead gaze as the suction cup is placed gently against the rigid lens surface and pulled off the eye. This method of lens removal is not to be relied on as a primary technique because of the risk of eye injury and the likelihood of suction-cup loss or deterioration.

Especially for the new patient, it is possible for lenses to become displaced when looking into extreme positions of gaze or during excessive eye rubbing or tearing. It is the eye care provider's responsibility to instruct the patient and observe his or her ability to re-center the lens. The first step in this process is to locate the lens by looking in a mirror or by touch.

SOFT LENS RECENTRATION

Once located, the soft lens is easily re-centered by looking in the direction of the lens and blinking several times. On occasion, the lens wearer may need to gently massage the displaced lens through the eyelid while looking in the direction of the lens.

RIGID LENS RECENTRATION

Once the lens is located, the index finger can be used to apply gentle pressure through the lid to the lens edge farthest from the cornea. With the lens trapped in place, the patient should then look in the direction of the decentered lens. When the bony structures of the nose and brow interfere with recentration, an alternate technique requires moving the lens to the temporal conjunctiva by gently massaging the lens through the lid.

Ultimately, the decision about releasing contact lenses for home use depends upon the patient's ability to remove the lens from the eye on the first or second attempt. At the time of dispensing, the patient may need practice for lens insertion but must show proficiency with lens removal.

CONTACT LENS CARE

Lens care systems often play an important role in determining a patient's success or failure in lens wear. FDA guidelines stipulate that contact lenses must be cleaned and disinfected after each wearing. There are an overwhelming number of lens care systems available to patients; confusion over which solutions to use and how to use them may contribute to a patient's inability to wear his or her lenses. Part of the dispensing doctor's responsibility is to select and prescribe a lens care system that meets the following three important criteria:

1. A lens care system must be an effective FDA-approved regimen not likely to produce allergic or toxic ocular response.
2. The care system should be convenient, fitting into the patient's lifestyle and lens wear schedule.
3. The care system must be cost-efficient, allowing for economical solution or lens replacement.

When deciding which of the many care systems to provide, the practitioner's options are narrowed by the type of lens worn. Knowledge of the preservative within a solution and the patient's potential for sensitivity are key elements in care system selection. Contact lens manufacturers and solution manufacturers provide package inserts with their products stating safety and compatibility of products. Solutions intended for rigid lenses are usually incompatible with solution-absorbing soft lenses because of their chemical preservatives and viscosity. Chemical preservatives such as thimerosal, benzalkonium chloride, chlorhexidine, and chlorobutanol do not bind to rigid lens materials but will accumulate within soft lens materials and can cause ocular irritation by leaching out during lens wear.

Effectiveness of a care system can be a significant factor in determining lens performance. Selection of lens care systems should be individualized for the patient, depending on the quality and quantity of the tear film, lid function, completeness of blink, and lens wear environment. Attention to lens-cleaning efficiency and frequency of enzyme cleaning can be key elements in comfort and vision.

Convenience in lens care is a second consideration when selecting a solution system. The FDA approves lens care packages as complete systems requiring cleaning, rinsing, and disinfection. Simplicity of steps and rapid recycle time are appealing to both patient and doctor. Simplicity and ease of use may help reinforce patient compliance.

Lens care cost and availability can be important factors when choosing a lens type and frequency of replacement. The practitioner may be wise to calculate the cost of lens care per month and per year for several different care systems. The cost of lens care versus the cost of frequent lens replacement must be analyzed. Of equal concern should be patient's access and ability to purchase replacement lens care solutions. If patients are unable to replace the solution samples that were provided at the time of dispensing, they may be forced to purchase an alternate product or discontinue lens care altogether. The selection of an unknown solution leads to a breakdown in compliance, possible adverse solution interaction, or possible hypersensitivity reactions.

When determining which lens care disinfection system is right for your patient, keep in mind that the system must be compatible with both the lens material and the patient. Contact lens material and water content are the variables that determine compatibility with disinfection systems.

Every lens care system for rigid or soft lenses can be viewed as having three simple steps: cleaning, rinsing, and disinfection. It is the provider's legal responsibility to instruct the patient to perform these steps each time the lens is removed. The only exception to this rule is one-time-use contact lenses that are discarded on removal.

Cleaning

The role of any contact lens cleaner is to solubilize and remove surface protein, lipid, mucus, inorganic deposits, eye makeup, airborne contaminants, and the bulk of micro-organisms found in the tear film. Omission of this critical lens care step may lead to poor lens comfort, poor vision, poor fit, and an increased risk of eye infection.

Conventional lens-cleaning technique requires digital rubbing of the lens in the palm of the hand in a non-circular pattern with an appropriate cleaning agent. Many lens care instruction booklets recommend 20 seconds of cleaning per side to insure sufficient debris and contaminant removal. Hands-off lens cleaning devices are also available for those patients with a persistent history of lens damage or poor compliance. These manual or electronic devices agitate the lens in cleaning solution to solubilize surface debris.

There are several types of lens cleaners available.

1. Simple surfactants are most commonly used for daily rigid and soft lens cleaning.
2. Abrasive particles plus surfactant daily cleaner (white suspension) are often used to scrub rigid and soft lens surfaces to remove stubborn deposits.
3. Isopropyl alcohol and surfactant daily cleaner (approved only for soft lenses) can be used to dissolve lipid deposits on soft lens surfaces.
4. Enzyme tablets are cleaners that, when dissolved in solution, soften protein deposits found on the surfaces of both rigid and soft lenses. Enzyme cleaning is performed in addition to or in conjunction with digital lens cleaning. Frequency of enzyme cleaning varies from daily to weekly depending on the patient's needs.

The selection of a lens cleaner can be directed by the patient's present ocular health or past contact lens history. Patients demonstrating oily or debris-laden tear film, blocked meibomian gland orifices, or heavy makeup use may be directed to a care system including a combination-type lens cleaner (abrasives or alcohol in conjunction with surfactant) and frequent enzyme soaking.

Rinsing

The second step in the lens care sequence provides for the rinsing of all lens surfaces. After the physical process of cleaning and enzyme soaking has been completed, the cleaning agent and free-floating debris must be rinsed away in preparation for disinfection. Rigid contact lenses can be rinsed with clean, drinkable tap water. If concerns exist about the quality of tap water, sterile preserved or non-preserved saline should be used.

Unlike rigid lenses, soft contact lenses should never be rinsed with tap water. Due to the larger pore size and surface bio-film, soft lens materials are more likely to be contaminated by foreign substances found in tap water. Consequently, they are to be rinsed only with pre-packaged sterile solutions.

Disinfection

Disinfection is fully effective only after proper lens cleaning and is critical to insure the inactivation of all microorganisms remaining on the lens surface and surrounding fluid. All lenses should be disinfected after removal from the eye prior to reinsertion. The selection of an appropriate disinfection system is important in minimizing sensitivity reactions. The selection of an appropriate disinfectant is based on the lens material and the patient's ocular condition, hygiene, lifestyle, and economics. At present, there are two FDA-approved methods of contact lens disinfection: thermal and chemical.

Rigid Lens Disinfection

As a rule, rigid gas permeable lens materials are not compatible with thermal disinfection because of the potential for lens warpage. Rigid lenses are routinely disinfected by use of preservative-based chemical disinfectants, which require a minimum 4-hour soak time following cleaning.

Soft Lens Disinfection

Thermal Methods. Thermal disinfection of soft lenses is a very safe, effective, and inexpensive method of lens care, but it has limitations. Thermal disinfection inactivates microorganisms on lens surfaces by raising the temperature of the lens and saline solution to 80°C for a minimum of 10 minutes. A major advantage of thermal disinfection lies in the fact that patients who have experienced solution-sensitivity reactions can safely care for their lenses using preservative-free products. Unfortunately, the compatibility of soft lenses and thermal disinfection is limited to low-water-content ($<50\%$) lens materials. Repeated thermal disinfection is contraindicated for use with moderate- ($>53\%$) to high-water-content ($>79\%$) lens materials because of potential damage to the lens polymer. Thermal disinfection has fallen into disfavor because of its tendency to bake protein onto lens materials of any water content. Thermal disinfection is most often recommended for use by children or adults in whom hygiene and solution sensitivity have been problems. The use of the microwave oven for thermal lens disinfection has been investigated by various researchers. Microwave disinfection of low-water-content soft lenses has been effective in deactivating microorganisms but has not become an approved process because of the lack of a commercially available microwavable lens case.

Chemical Methods. The most common means of soft lens disinfection is the use of either preservative (chemical) or hydrogen peroxide (oxidative) disinfection. A perceived advantage of the preservative disinfection systems is convenience. A minimum number of solution bottles (all-in-one cleaner/disinfecting solution) and freedom from electricity make preservative disinfection desirable for travel. In the case of some preservative disinfection systems, the FDA has approved long-term continuous disinfection and storage of lenses when placed in a disinfectant-filled, unopened case. ReNu Multi-Purpose Disinfecting Solution (Bausch and Lomb) has been approved for up to 7 days continuous disinfection; Opti-Free (Alcon Laboratories) is approved for up to 30 days.

The disadvantages of preservative disinfection systems include longer soak times and possible patient allergic reactions. To provide anti-microbial effectiveness, these preservative systems require a minimum 4-hour to overnight soak time. For patients who have a history of environmental allergies, careful thought must be given to the choice of a preservative disinfectant. Although preservatives such as thimerosal and chlorhexidine have the strongest history of producing ocular allergic or toxic sensitivity reactions, a patient may become sensitive to any preservative. To help minimize sensitivity reactions, patients should rinse lenses with a sterile, non-preserved saline before insertion.

Potential hypersensitivity reactions can be avoided by the use of hydrogen peroxide disinfection. Oxidative disinfection systems are safe and effective and contain no sensitizing preservatives. In addition, evidence suggests the expansion and contraction of the lens matrix during peroxide disinfection may help maintain cleaner lens surfaces. The soak time for peroxide disinfection varies from 10 to 55 minutes, depending on the system selected. The neutralization phase ranges from 10 minutes to 6 hours. Although hydrogen peroxide does not bind to or accumulate within the soft lens material, neutralization of surface peroxide is necessary before lens insertion. Insertion of a soft lens containing residual peroxide will cause hyperemia, tearing, chemosis, photophobia, and superficial punctate keratitis. Disadvantages of oxidative systems include their relatively high cost and complexity of use.

In addition to lens care and disinfection instructions, practitioners should emphasize the need for periodic replacement of the contact lens storage case to patients. Recent clinical studies of contact lens case contamination point out the need to replace lens storage cases on a monthly schedule or perhaps with each purchase of replacement lens solutions. Several contact lens solution manufacturers have embraced this practice by packaging replacement storage cases with retail replacement solutions.

In-office disinfection and storage of trial contact lenses is an issue that has been addressed by the Centers for Disease Control and Prevention, the American Academy of Optometry, and the American Academy of Ophthalmology. These governmental and professional agencies agree that rigid and soft trial lenses should be exposed to full-strength 3% hydrogen peroxide for a minimum of 10 minutes to ensure safe storage. Heat disinfection of low-water-content soft lenses is known to be very effective as well. Guidelines for in-office trial lens disinfection are available from each of these agencies.

PATIENT MANAGEMENT

When dispensing contact lenses to a first-time wearer or a new lens modality to an experienced patient, a written record of an adaptive wear schedule is necessary. Patients should be directed to the lens care guide in the solution system to reinforce the doctor's discussion on lens care, handling, and wear time. The new lens wearer should be educated about the importance of gradually increasing lens wear to allow for comfort, vision, and lens-handling adaptation. The practitioner should educate the patient about common symptoms of lens adaptation and the need to alert the doctor should he or she become concerned (Box A2–2).

The adaptation schedule prescribed by the practitioner should serve as a guide for the contact lens patient. Patients should be informed that not all lens wearers adapt at the same rate and that one schedule does not necessarily work for all patients. The key elements of all lens adaptation schedules are

---

BOX A2-2. COMMON SYMPTOMS OF LENS ADAPTATION

1. Lens awareness on blink
2. Increased tearing
3. Increased light sensitivity
4. Glare at night
5. Readjustment to spectacle wear
6. Lens dryness

---

consistency of lens wear, a gradual daily increase in wearing time, and careful self-monitoring of eye condition.

For the new contact lens patient, initial lens wear time may be shifted to evening hours or weekends to accommodate the patient's daily work routine. For the experienced contact lens patient with a successful past history, the practitioner may choose to accelerate the lens wear schedule. For the new patient fitted for flexible or extended lens wear, a follow-up visit documenting successful daily lens wear is desirable before overnight wear is initiated. A corneal examination should be scheduled for the first morning after overnight lens wear (Table A2–1).

DOCUMENTATION OF THE DOCTOR–PATIENT RELATIONSHIP

Pre-printed contact lens documents are available in a multipage carbonless (NCR) format from many office suppliers. As with any contract, the signed and dated original document remains in the patient's chart, and the copy is provided to the patient.

Table A2-1. Typical Rigid or Soft Lens Adaptive Wear Schedule

Day	Daily Wear Hours	Flexible or Extended Wear Hours
1	4	4
2	6	6
3	8	8
4	10	10
5	12	12
6	14	14
7	14	16
8	14	Overnight wear with morning office visit

Contact Lens–Fitting Contract

The establishment of a written contract explaining the responsibilities and commitments of the practitioner and patient is a vital step to ensure that the patient fully understands the scope of the doctor–patient relationship. This written contract should specifically state the length of the lens fitting period and the importance of daily lens care and follow-up office visits. This document should describe the general risks and benefits of contact lens wear and the need for appropriate long-term follow-up care. Finally, the contract should state the requirements that need to be completed before the doctor can provide the patient with a written contact lens prescription.

Documentation of Lens Handling and Lens Care

A formal lens-dispensing document should be completed at the time of lens dispensing. This document should serve as a helpful reminder of the training the patient received in contact lens handling and care. Completion of this form documents the fact that the patient demonstrated proficiency in lens insertion, re-centration, and removal. This document should clearly state the components of the FDA-approved contact lens care system the patient has been instructed to use. Finally, this document should advise the patient to read the package insert and lens care guide enclosed with the starter package.

Documentation of Lens Wear Schedule, Follow-Up Appointment, and Emergency Care

Patients should leave the office with a written copy of the prescribed wearing schedule and brief description of lens adaptation symptoms. This form should contain the time, date, and instructions for the first follow-up office visit. A brief description of future follow-up visits should also be listed, as well as instructions for obtaining emergency eye care.

Precautions for Monovision Patients

This contract should serve as documentation of the discussion between doctor and patient concerning the limitations of daily lens wear, eye health risks of lens wear, possible reduced distance visual acuity, and compromised depth perception. This notice should advise the patient to initiate monovision lens wear in casual, familiar surroundings before driving or working. This contract signed by patient and doctor will document the patient's understanding of the possible adverse effects and his or her informed consent to proceed with monovision therapy.

Precautions for Monocular Patients

After careful consideration and discussion with the monocular patient concerning the eye health risks and rewards of lens wear, it is advisable to obtain formal documentation of the patient's understanding, justification, cooperation, and motivation for lens wear. This document should contain the boundaries of lens wear, such as conservative daily wear, the use of full-time protective eye wear, and strict compliance in follow-up care as stated by the doctor.

BIBLIOGRAPHY

Bennett ES, Grohe RM: Lens care and patient education. In Bennett ES, Weissman BA (eds): *Clinical Contact Lens Practice.* Philadelphia, JB Lippincott, 1991.

Harris MG: Legal issues in contact lens practice. In Bennett ES, Weissman BA (eds): *Clinical Contact Lens Practice.* Philadelphia, JB Lippincott, 1991.

Mandell RB: *Contact Lens Practice.* 4th ed. Springfield, IL, Charles C Thomas, 1988, pp. 326–351.

Mandell RS: Lens handling, care and storage. In *Contact Lens Practice,* 4th ed. Springfield, IL, Charles C Thomas, 1988, p. 568.

Steel JA: Lens care, patient management, and follow-up. In Barr JT (ed): *Contact Lens Pocket Guide.* Irvine, CA, Allergan Optical, 1987.

Weisbarth RE, Ghormley NR: Hydrogel lens care regimens and patient education. In Bennett ES, Weissman BA (eds): *Clinical Contact Lens Practice.* Philadelphia, JB Lippincott, 1991.

McKenney CD, Ajello M: Comparative case contamination: three disinfection systems. *Int Contact Lens Clin* 1991;18:14–19.

Contact Lens Modifications

NEIL R. HODUR

The modification of rigid contact lenses is an art as well as a science. Modification allows the contact lens practitioner to add that "certain something" that will improve the physiology and/or comfort of a contact lens. Enhancing the physiology and the comfort of contact lenses will increase patient satisfaction.

The modification of rigid contact lenses is not difficult but does demand patience and practice. This chapter outlines the materials necessary to modify rigid contact lenses and describes the procedures for successful modification.

MATERIALS AND SUPPLIES

The equipment necessary does not demand a tremendous monetary expense and can be obtained from many contact lens–finishing laboratories. The following sections comprise a list of necessary materials.

Contact Lens Modification Unit

There are many different contact lens modification units available. There are two general types, of which there are many variations. These are the Jacob's chuck spindle and the Contour spindle. The Jacob's chuck spindle utilizes a jaw locking device similar to commercially available power drills; a locking key is used to tighten the tools to the chuck. The tool is inserted into the spindle and tightened with the key, and the unit is ready for the modification to be performed. The Contour spindle utilizes a spindle that is ready to receive a tool; the tool is simply pressed onto the spindle. Once the tool is placed on the spindle, the unit is ready for use.

Both Jacob's chuck and Contour units should have variable speed motors that have a rheostat, which allows the practitioner to select the proper speed of rotation. As will be noted, different rigid lens materials require different speeds of rotation for optimal modification. The unit should have an on-off switch, with some form of variable speed. The normal speeds of rotation produced in commercially available units is between 900 and 1500 rpm.

The unit should also contain a splash guard to protect the practitioner from the splash of modification compounds. This guard should be removable for easy cleaning. The spindle should be well protected where it inserts into the unit to prevent the overflow of modification compounds into the motor (Fig. A3–1).

Some units are available with multiple spindles, which allow several modifications without having to replace tools. These units allow for rapid modification and reduce the mess that can sometimes accompany removing and placing tools. The modification unit should be compact and made of an aesthetically

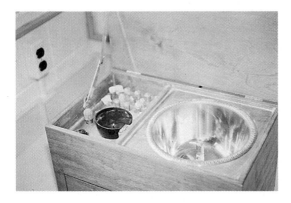

Figure A3–1. A typical lens modification unit. (Courtesy of Dr. Edward S. Bennett.)

appealing material. Formica-covered units are generally well accepted because they are pleasing to look at and easy to clean. The modification tools necessary for complete modification are listed in Table A3–1. These tools are usually provided with the purchase of a modification unit. The type and number of tools will vary among manufacturers but are generally in the range listed. Some tools are made of molded plastic. These usually provide the same modification ability as those made from brass but may have a limited life-span and have a tendency to overheat.

Holding Devices

A device to support the contact lens during modification is necessary and should be part of the contact lens practitioner's total armament of modification devices. There are many different types of holding devices; the most common is

Table A3–1. **Brass Modification Laps in the Following Radii (mm): Components of the Modification Kit**

7.87
8.00
8.25
8.50
8.75
9.00
9.25
9.50
9.75
10.00
10.50
11.00
11.50
12.50
13.00
Edge modification drum, usually $2\frac{1}{2}$ inch, with sponge
Cut-down stone, usually 90 degree
Sponge tree-cone polisher

the strong-hold suction-cup, sometimes called a "greenie." This suction-cup is a green or white two-piece rubber device that contains a bulb and support. The bulb provides suction, and the support actually holds the contact lens. One end of the support is concave in topography and will hold the convex side of a contact lens for modification of the concave (inside) surface. The other end of the support is a flat surface to hold the concave side of a contact lens for modification of the convex (outside) surface. The support has a hole drilled through its length to provide a means of directing the suction from the bulb. The suction-cup is arranged with the proper end support exposed, and the other end is placed into the bulb. The suction-cup is then placed into water, and some water is drawn into the bulb. This increases the holding capability because of the adhesive ability of water combined with suction. The contact lens is then placed on the support, and the bulb is squeezed to provide suction. Thus, the lens adheres to the suction-cup.

The suction device can be placed into a spinner tool, which is a cylinder of plastic or aluminum that has a central shaft supported by ball bearings (Fig. A3–2). This tool allows the suction device to spin freely, which can aid in the modification of the edge of a contact lens or dioptric power adjustments. Fitting curve, peripheral curve, and surface polishing should not be performed with a spinner unless it is not allowed to spin. If a spinning lens is placed on a spinning tool, no modification will be performed.

Other types of holding devices for the modification of contact lenses include a lucite or metallic rod, 7.5 to 10 cm in length, that is convex on one end and concave on the other. A contact lens is placed on the rod with the aid of double-sided tape or wax. It should be noted that the wax is the same as that used to seal boxes for shipment and is called, simply, boxing wax. A small piece of boxing wax is placed on one end of the modification rod, and a cross is made in the wax with the fingernail to allow space for displacement of wax when it is placed into contact with the lens. This device is especially useful when working with lenses less than 8.00 mm in overall diameter. Because the end of the suction cup usually is 8.00 mm, adherence of lenses less than 8.00 mm in overall diameter is difficult if not impossible.

In all instances, it is important to ensure that the contact lens is centered on the holding device and is well adhered. This will ensure that modifications are performed smoothly and accurately.

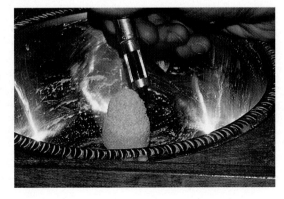

Figure A3–2. Use of a spinning tool to modify rigid contact lenses. (Courtesy of Dr. Edward S. Bennett.)

Lubricating, Polishing, and Cutting Materials

There are many different types of materials used in the modification of contact lenses. These materials are used for lubricating, polishing, and cutting a contact lens. Some of these materials are applied to the tool as a liquid and other materials are placed on a tool by an adhesive. The materials that are applied to a modification tool to create the actual modification are usually placed on the tool with some form of adhesive. The most common material applied to a modification tool, be it brass or plastic, is Demicel tape (Johnson and Johnson). A piece of tape is applied to the surface of a cutting tool to provide a cutting surface. Polished brass or plastic is not a good abrasive surface for the modification of contact lenses. A small piece of tape is applied to the center of the tool and smoothed out evenly in all directions until it forms a smooth surface continuous with the tool. The tape will add thickness to the surface of the tool, making the surface of the tape slightly flatter than that of the tool. The amount of flattening is approximately .05 mm. By placing more than one piece of tape on a tool, virtually any radius of curve can be formed on the tool. The nap of new tape must be broken in or else it will cause drag during modification; this is sometimes seen as a swirl pattern on the lens surface after a modification has been performed. The nap of the tape can be softened by using a fingernail on the taped tool after water has been applied to the tape. The tool is placed on the modification unit and allowed to spin at approximately 1000 rpm, and fingernail pressure is placed on the tape to soften the surface.

Other cutting materials can be used as well. Some of the more common materials are Telfa pads and silk pads. These may be purchased from contact lens laboratories, pre-cut to the diameter of the modification tools.

The previously described materials are used to cut a curve on the inside of a contact lens. Other materials are available to polish existing curves. These materials are:

1. Baby blanket (i.e., receiving blanket)
2. Velveteen
3. Flannel

These materials are not abrasive and are used to polish an existing curve or to blend the junction zone between two existing curves.

The polishing materials can be placed directly over a taped tool with the use of a neoprene O-ring. A piece of material, approximately 2.5 cm square, is cut from the material. The square is draped over the tool that has the proper curve, and the material is held in place with the O-ring (Fig. A3–3). A rubber band can be used in place of the O-ring.

If a self-adhesive polishing material is used, any tape on the tool must be removed, the tool must be cleaned of any foreign glue substance, and the polishing material is placed on the tool in a manner similar to placing tape on the tool. It is important to remove any residual glue, because it will cause a bulge in the new polishing surface. Some practitioners prefer to have two sets of tools, one for cutting curves with tape and another that has polishing surfaces for blending and polishing. This is very practical for those individuals who perform a great number of modifications or for those who prefer to finish their own contact lenses.

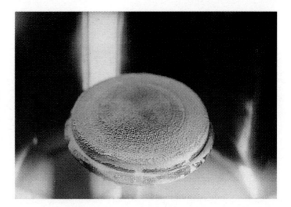

Figure A3–3. Velveteen is held in place with an O-ring. (Courtesy of Dr. Edward S. Bennett.)

Polishing and modification solutions are many. Water is the lubricant of choice for cutting a contact lens down in overall diameter and for truncation. Water does not have enough polishing ability to use as a compound for finishing a contact lens.

The most familiar modification compound is Silvo silver polish. This compound was used on polymethyl methacrylate (PMMA) lenses for many years. Silvo contains ammonia, an organic solvent, which can be placed in water. This compound works moderately well, but any residual ammonia may cause damage to rigid gas permeable contact lenses. There are many polishing compounds available through contact lens laboratories. The most common are X-Pal and Boston Polishing Compound. X-Pal is available as a powder and is mixed into solution with water. The Boston Polishing Compound is pre-mixed. Both work well with rigid gas permeable materials.

It is recommended in all cases that only polishing compounds designed to work with contact lenses be used. Compounds such as toothpaste can damage the surface of a contact lens, especially the current generation of rigid gas permeable lenses.

Comparator

A piece of equipment that is absolutely necessary is a $7\times$ or $10\times$ measuring magnifier, or comparator. The comparator allows the practitioner to measure the width of the optic zone, the width of fitting and peripheral curves, the overall diameter, and the front-surface optic zone. The edge characteristics can be visualized by reversing the comparator and viewing. Without the comparator, many modifications could not be measured, let alone evaluated. The comparator may also be used to evaluate the surface integrity of a contact lens, because scratches in either the front or posterior surface can be seen. A comparator has a measuring reticule on the face so that easy measurement of linear curve dimensions can be made. At first, it may take some practice to become proficient with the comparator. Practicing with known curve dimensions is the best way to become proficient.

MODIFICATION TECHNIQUES

Modification of contact lenses can be broken into two categories; those that are common and those that are not. The common in-office modifications are:

1. Front-surface polish
2. Posterior-surface polish
3. Blending of curves
4. Front-surface power modification
5. Re-edging

The uncommon modifications are:

1. Changing the radius of a fitting or peripheral curve
2. Changing the width of a fitting or peripheral curve
3. Reducing the overall diameter
4. Placing a truncation on a contact lens

The common modifications are routinely applied to rigid contact lenses in a practitioner's office. These modifications allow the practitioner to tailor a contact lens to an individual patient. This also allows the practitioner to place his or her own "signature" on a contact lens—that little extra that makes a particular practitioner special. Many practitioners routinely apply blends and edges to a lens to match the individual patient's corneal needs and topography.

FRONT SURFACE POLISH

Patient Symptoms

The symptoms a patient exhibits when the inside surface of a contact lens is in need of polishing are similar to that of front-surface symptoms. The patient will complain of recently decreased wear time and blurred vision, especially at the end of the day.

A front-surface polish of a contact lens is applied to a contact lens on a yearly basis. This re-forms a smooth front surface of a contact lens, ensuring the best possible wettability. Lenses that have not been polished in over 1 year usually have telltale poor wetting characteristics, and the patient may complain of a foreign-body sensation or a dry, scratchy feeling. A front-surface polish, when properly applied, can do wonders for a contact lens. Over time, tiny front-surface scratches accumulate, even on the most careful patient's lens. These scratches in the surface will reduce the adhesive ability of the lens and the pre-corneal tear layer. A front-surface polish will help seal the front surface and bring back normal surface wettability. This modification can be performed easily in the office.

Equipment

1. Comparator
2. Modification unit
3. Edge modification drum
4. Contact lens holding device
5. Polishing compound

The set-up is as follows. The modification unit is set up with the edge modification drum. The speed is set for the type of contact lens plastic that is being polished. Suggested speeds are:

PMMA: 1500 rpm
Silicone acrylate: 1300 rpm
Fluorosilicone acrylate: 1100 rpm

The lens is inspected with the comparator. The front-surface integrity is examined. Debris and scratches on the lens surface are evaluated. If debris or scratches are seen, the lens is placed on a strong-hold suction-cup with the convex surface exposed. A modification sponge is placed into the edge modification drum and is wetted with water before the instrument is turned on. The water is worked into the sponge with finger pressure to ensure that the sponge surface is not dry and scratchy. The unit is turned on and adjusted to the proper speed. A few drops of polishing compound are placed onto the center of the rotating sponge. The modification compound is allowed to disperse via centrifugal force. The lens is brought down into the sponge so that the front surface is completely immersed into the sponge perpendicular to the rotating surface. The contact time of the lens and sponge is 1 second; the lens is then retracted from the sponge. This is repeated five times. This should be sufficient to polish the front surface of the contact lens. The idea is not to polish out scratches, but to polish over the scratch. Debris will be removed from the lens during this procedure as well. The lens is then removed from the suction-cup, cleaned, and soaked in a soaking solution before it is returned to the patient. The lens should be allowed to soak for 15 minutes before it is worn.

It is imperative that the operator understand that scratches should not be removed from the contact lens surface. Scratches are in the surface of the lens. If the scratches are removed, plastic is removed from the surface of the lens, and it is very likely that the power of the front surface will be altered. The front surface of a rigid contact lens is the power surface, and any change in the radius will alter the power of the lens. The procedure is to polish over the surface of the lens, therefore polishing over the scratches on the surface. This will seal the surface and allow the normal wetting characteristics of the lens to return.

When a contact lens is received from a laboratory, a fine haze may be seen on the surface. This may interfere with the wetting of a new contact lens once it is placed on an eye. Even though the contact lens is cleaned, this haze may persist. This is the result of manufacturing residue, which is difficult to polish off the surface of the lens. This material should be removed with one of the commercially available laboratory lens cleaners. Polishing the debris on the surface of the contact lens will generally just rearrange this manufacturing residue. This has frustrated many practitioners. All new lenses should be cleaned with a laboratory cleaner to ensure that the lens surface will demonstrate normal wetting characteristics when new.

INSIDE POLISH

Polishing the inside surface of a rigid contact lens is sometimes necessary. Debris from metabolic byproducts (e.g., mucus) can sometimes lodge on the inside surface of a contact lens and cause discomfort. Minor scratches can sometimes form on the inside of a contact lens as well. Debris buildup is common on the fitting and peripheral curves as well. This is removed in a manner different from polishing the inside, central posterior curve. To polish the inside curve of a rigid contact lens, the following materials are necessary:

Equipment

1. Comparator
2. Contact lens modification unit
3. Tree-cone modification sponge
4. Polishing compound

The contact lens should be inspected with the comparator. If the inside surface has buildup and/or scratches, polishing of the inside surface of the lens is necessary to improve comfort and wettability.

The tree-cone sponge is placed on the modification unit, and the speed is adjusted for the type of plastic to be modified. The cone is wetted with water to ensure that the sponge is soft and pliable. The lens is placed on the holding device so that the concave surface is exposed for modification. The unit is turned on, and the lens is brought to the sponge perpendicularly. The inside of the lens is touched to the sponge so that the lens surface is completely covered by the sponge. The contact time is approximately 1 second. This is repeated five times. Surface scratches are polished over, not removed. If the scratches are removed, surface plastic from the inside of the contact lens may be removed, changing the surface radius and therefore altering the curvature of the inside of the contact lens. Debris and metabolic byproducts are removed from the inside surface of the contact lens with this procedure. If the buildup is on the fitting or peripheral curve, the material may not be removed with the cone sponge. This material can be removed in a manner that is similar to placing a curve on the back surface of a contact lens.

BLENDING THE JUNCTION ZONE BETWEEN TWO CURVES ON THE INSIDE OF A RIGID CONTACT LENS

Patient Symptoms

Patients in need of a blend will generally complain of a scratchy feeling of the lens. This feeling is present as soon as the patient places the lens on the eye and generally becomes more bothersome the longer the lens is worn. This is especially true of new lenses. If the patient has been wearing contact lenses for longer than 5 hours during the day, a complaint of heat or reduced wearing time may indicate that a blend, or an increase in the existing blends, is necessary to increase tear flow under the contact lens.

A blend is a polish applied to the inside of a contact lens to bridge the junction zone between two curves. Each curve junction zone may need a blend to decrease the radical change in radius between two curves. When a contact lens is manufactured, the back surface is manufactured from steepest curve to flattest curve. The base curve is the steepest curve on the inside surface of a contact lens. The fitting curve or curves are applied to the inside of the contact lens next. The fitting curves are flatter than the base curve but steeper than the peripheral curve. The peripheral curve is the last curve to be applied to the inside surface of the contact lens. Each curve junction zone should be blended. The are four categories of blend:

1. Touch
2. Light (#1)
3. Medium (#2)
4. Heavy (#3)

The blend classification is arbitrary, and varies from one practitioner to another. A general rule for classifying blends is to examine the junction zone between two curves. If the junction zone can be seen clearly, there is either no blend or a touch blend. If the junction zone has a hazy appearance but the curves can still be seen, a light blend has been applied. The hazy area between the two curves appears to be approximately 0.05 mm wide and extends into each curve width equally. If the hazy area between the two curves appears to be 0.1 mm wide, the blend is considered to be a medium blend. In a medium blend, the junction zone between the two curves is very difficult to see. If the hazy area between the two curves is greater than 0.1 mm wide and the junction zone between the two curves is obliterated, then a heavy blend has been applied.

Equipment

1. Comparator
2. Contact lens modification unit
3. Blending tool
4. Blending material to cover the blending tool
5. Contact lens holding device
6. Contact lens polish

The contact lens is inspected for a blend. If a blend is to be applied, the selection of the proper radius tool is necessary. The proper tool is one that has a radius halfway between the radii of the two curves that are to be blended. For example, the base curve of a contact lens is 7.50 mm, the fitting curve is 9.50 mm and the peripheral curve is 11.50 mm. A blend is to be placed on each junction zone between two curves. The first blend tool between the base curve and the fitting curve, would have a radius of 8.50 mm, halfway between the radius of the base curve and the fitting curve. The second blend tool would have a radius of 10.50 mm, halfway between the fitting curve and the peripheral curve radii.

The next decision in blending is to determine the degree of blend. This is done by observation of the contact lens on the eye with the use of sodium fluorescein. Bearing of a curve, or decreased tear circulation within a curve, dictates the amount of blend necessary. This is an individual choice. In any event, if the amount of blend necessary is not certain, always place less blend on the lens than might be necessary. The lens can always be re-blended, or additional blend can be placed on the lens. Once a lens has been blended too far, going back to the original curves is impossible.

The contact lens is evaluated for blend with the use of a slit lamp biomicroscope. The inside surface of the lens is evaluated with the comparator. The proper tool is selected for the blend. The lens is placed on the holding device with the concave surface of the lens facing out. The tool is prepared with the proper polishing material placed on the surface. This can be a Telfa pad, velveteen, or flannel. The tool is immersed in water to soften the polishing surface. The tool is placed on the modification unit, and the speed is adjusted for the contact lens material. The unit is turned on, and polishing compound is applied to the rotating tool. The lens on the holding device is placed in contact with the rotating tool approximately 1.00 mm off-center.

Two techniques can be used for the actual modification. Both are used for all modifications that involve the alteration of inside curves on a contact lens.

1. The lens is placed slightly off-center on the rotating tool, and the lens is slowly spun in the opposite direction as the rotating tool. Complete contact of the lens to the tool is very important to avoid applying blends or curves in an unequal manner. The lens is removed from the rotating tool, and the technique is applied once again. This is repeated until the desired modification is complete. Removing the lens from the holding device and viewing the lens with the comparator is necessary from time to time, to monitor the progress of the modification (Fig. A3–4).
2. The lens is placed slightly off-center on the rotating tool, and a series of small, deliberate figure-of-eight patterns are made over the center of the rotating tool. Care must be taken to ensure that equal pressure and equal lens contact to the tool are made. This will avoid unequal amounts of modification. The lens is removed from the holding device and inspected with the comparator to monitor the progress of the modification.

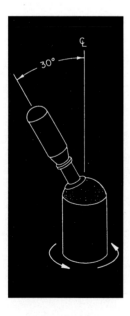

Figure A3–4. Modifying or blending peripheral curves. (Courtesy of Dr. Edward S. Bennett.)

FRONT-SURFACE POWER MODIFICATION

From time to time, power modification of a contact lens is necessary. The reasons for this modification vary, but in many instances, the patient has undergone a change in prescription. If the rigid contact lens is judged to be in good condition, a power modification can be made to the front surface of the contact lens to improve visual acuity. In most cases, this power modification is between +0.50 and −0.50 D. It should be remembered that only the front-surface topography is changed during power modification. No inside surface changes should be made to alter the power of a contact lens. To produce more divergent power, the front-surface center of the lens is flattened. To create more convergent power, the front-surface periphery is flattened, making the front-surface center more steeply curved.

Equipment

1. Lensometer
2. Edge modification drum
3. Water
4. Contact lens polish
5. Contact lens spinner (for convergent power only)
6. Modification unit
7. Strong-hold suction-cup

Procedure

Divergent Power

The contact lens should be inspected for surface defects. If the front surface of the contact lens is not clean or if there is defect, a substitute lens should be considered. If the front surface is debris-laden, clean the lens thoroughly and re-inspect. The power of the lens should be measured before modification and recorded.

To place divergent power on the front surface of a contact lens, there are two methods that have met with equal success.

Method 1. A piece of modification material, usually baby blanket, is placed on a hard, flat surface. Water is added to loosen the nap of the material. Polishing compound is placed on the center of the modification material. The lens is placed on the polish with the concave surface pointing upward. The second finger of the hand is placed on the lens at the junction of the first knuckle from the fingertip. The hand is positioned so that it is parallel to the modification material and the lens. A series of tight circles are made with the lens on the material and polish. It is important that only the center of the lens is pressed onto the material. A light amount of pressure is all that is necessary. It is equally important that the hand remain parallel to the modification material at all times. This is to insure that the lens is not rocked back-and-forth, creating a warp in the front surface. The amount of time spent modifying the lens varies. Practice is recommended before attempting this technique on a patient's lens. With a little practice, adding −0.50 D of power becomes very easy.

Method 2. This technique utilizes the modification unit and the edge modification drum. The lens is secured to the strong-hold suction-cup with the convex side out. The sponge is wetted with water to ensure that it is soft and pliable. The lens is placed on the holding device so that the convex surface is exposed for modification. The unit is turned on, and polishing compound is placed at the center of the sponge. The lens is brought to the sponge perpendicularly. It is important that polishing compound be added constantly while performing this procedure. Lens power should be checked several times during this process to avoid overcorrection; every 10 seconds of modification is a generally accepted maximum between lensometry readings (Fig. A3–5).

Placing convergent power on the front surface of the lens is more difficult than adding minus power. It is performed in a manner similar to that described for adding minus power with the modification unit; however, the lens is not brought to the sponge perpendicularly, but rather at an angle, so that material is removed from the periphery of the lens. The lens power and optics should be checked often during this procedure to ensure that no distortion is being introduced to the lens.

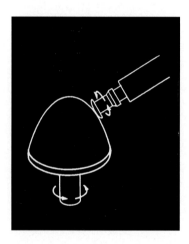

Figure A3–5. Adding minus power to the front of a rigid contact lens. (Courtesy of Dr. Edward S.

Contact Lens Complications

ARTHUR B. EPSTEIN

Nothing in life is without risk or completely problem-free. This is also true of contact lenses. Complications are an unfortunate and unavoidable part of contact lens wear. This appendix is about understanding and preventing contact lens complications.

Contact lens complications are the result of specific causative factors, many of which are identifiable and preventable. Every complication is caused by either an individual factor or specific combination of factors. Some causative factors are intrinsic to contact lens wear, whereas others may be secondary to less serious complications. The contact lens specialist must also be knowledgeable about non–contact lens–related ocular disorders, which may occur in a contact lens wearer. Contact lens wear can also modify the presentation of ocular diseases, making differential diagnosis difficult.

Thankfully, most contact lens complications are due to a limited number of potential causes. Often, a single underlying cause or a specific combination of causes can be found. The interaction of individual elements may make identification of specific factors difficult. However, uncovering the "why" of a complication is the only way to make sure that it will not happen again.

For many of the wrong reasons, too many doctors avoid any investigation or analysis when a patient has a complication. Imagine where the airline industry would be today if they unquestioningly accepted crashes as an inescapable consequence of flying. Although it may be true that flying is a requisite for most airplane crashes, flying is not the underlying cause of the crash, and contact lens complications are not the invariable result of wearing lenses. This is especially true of extended wear lenses. Extended wear may be a requisite for extended wear complications, but other, more specific factors are the real cause of the problems.

With some effort, it is possible to substantially reduce, if not eliminate, contact lens complications. Over the past few years, my patients have had far fewer problems than ever before. This reduction in complication rate was accomplished by intensively investigating and subsequently analyzing every patient complication. In most cases, the identification of likely causes and their systematic elimination helped reduce future complications to a negligible level. Every patient benefits when the causes of complications are identified.

Being able to recognize a complication is important, but this knowledge by itself does little to help the practitioner help his or her patients. This appendix first focuses on the possible causes of complications. You will find that many contact lens complications are, in turn, the causes of other contact lens complications. Every practice is different. What I present in this appendix is the result of many years of experience in a large, multi-office practice limited to contact lenses in a suburb of New York City. Depending on the nature and location of your practice, your experience may be somewhat different. However, understanding the basic causes of complications will permit you to develop a

251

strategy for isolating and hopefully eliminating complications among your own patients.

WHO IS TO BLAME FOR CONTACT LENS COMPLICATIONS?

Although it may be self-reassuring, blaming our patients and their bad habits for causing complications is unproductive. The first rule of preventing complications is to accept responsibility for them.

When patients forget to wash their hands before handling their lenses and end up with red eyes, is it their fault or yours? Perhaps both. Nearly every patient I've ever seen who had a problem did not really want to be in trouble. I've never met a patient who wanted to go blind or lose an eye. Nearly every patient will follow directions he or she understands. More importantly, patients must understand the consequences of not following instructions.

I firmly believe that non-compliant patients truly do not want to be non-compliant; they just fail to understand what is expected of them. If you, as a doctor, accept responsibility for your patient's failure to follow directions, it will motivate you to insure that all patients know exactly what you expect of them and what they need to do to avoid problems.

After a patient experiences a complication, communication becomes even more important. In many offices, a patient with a contact lens complication immediately evokes a response of guilt and fear from the practitioner. Instead of carefully interviewing the patient to help uncover the cause of the complication, many doctors treat the patient with kid gloves. The result is that most patients go unquestioned, and without answers, etiologies remain undiscovered, and important patterns go unrecognized.

Even patients with serious complications will not automatically blame you for their problem. Although extensive questioning might seem inflammatory, my experience suggests that most patients view this as professional and caring. They understand that seeking the cause will help make sure that this won't happen to them again.

Communication is essential if you want to eliminate complications in your practice. Investigate every complication with the same thoroughness and attention to detail that the National Transportation Safety Board gives to a plane crash. In time, you will discover patterns and potential causes. Do this unfailingly, and I promise your complication rate will fall.

WORKING WITH PATIENTS TO PREVENT CONTACT LENS COMPLICATIONS

Contact lens complications do not happen by accident. They are caused by recognizable and often predictable factors. It follows that complications should be preventable. If the causes of a contact lens complication can be identified, they probably can be eliminated. Even under the worst conditions, contact lens complications are rare. The precise factors causing them may remain elusive despite the most diligent introspection and investigation. That should not deter you from trying to identify things that predispose your patients to problems. Even if you identify only one element in a multi-factorial array, eliminating that single factor may be sufficient to eliminate the complication completely.

BASIC CORNEAL COMPLICATIONS— DISRUPTIONS TO NORMAL CORNEAL BARRIERS

Even under the best of conditions, the cornea is a delicate tissue in an environment that can easily turn hostile. Wearing a contact lens places many unique stresses and demands on corneal physiology and integrity. A serious contact lens complication that affects the cornea must first breach its formidable barriers and safeguards. There are many ways that contact lenses disrupt normal corneal integrity. The most obvious disturbance to normal corneal integrity is by mechanical disruption. Contact lens abrasions occur through the removal of corneal tissue by the lens, through a foreign body trapped beneath the lens, or through patient error. Rarely, a traumatic abrasion can be caused by a projectile or other object hitting the eye of a lens wearer; often, contact lenses have a protective function in these situations.

Abrasions are common with all types of contact lenses. Rigid lenses commonly cause insertion abrasions, edge abrasions, and foreign-body track abrasions (Fig. A4–1). Abrasions caused by rigid lenses can be severe. Massive, full-thickness epithelial abrasions can occur from poor lens insertion technique.

Despite the frequency and severity of rigid lens abrasions, they rarely are associated with secondary complications such as infection. Rigid lenses are poor hosts for pathogenic bacteria, thus minimizing the likelihood of superinfection.

Damaged soft contact lenses can cause significant epithelial abrasions. Interestingly, many patients will present complaining of intermittent discomfort. Logically, a ripped lens should constantly be uncomfortable. However, the edges of a tear can go in and out of apposition with routine lens handling. When the edges are separated, the lens is uncomfortable, but when they are together, lens comfort is almost indistinguishable from that of an intact lens.

Soft lenses also act as bandages, mitigating some of the patient's discomfort and delaying his or her immediate motivation to attend to the problem. Lens tears produce two basic types of abrasions. The typical abrasion is superficial

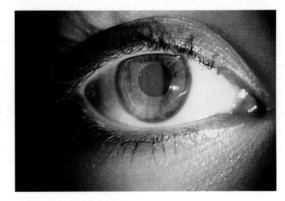

Figure A4–1. Unusual foreign body track beneath a rigid lens. Note the branching, almost dendritic appearance.

with irregular borders corresponding to the area the lens travels over the corneal surface. The abrasion is shallow, with an irregular, "ground-glass" appearance.

In cases in which the lens defect is more pronounced, full-thickness epithelial abrasions can occur. In these cases, lens movement is limited by the abrasion itself, placing all of the bearing and excavating forces on a smaller area, thus causing a deeper abrasion. As with all corneal defects, an abrasion caused by a damaged lens increases the potential for superinfection and corneal ulceration.

Although patching of corneal abrasions is routine, it is absolutely contraindicated in contact lens–related abrasions. Several reports of minor contact lens abrasions developing into severe microbial infections after patching have appeared in the literature. The normal ocular environment is altered by contact lens wear; the warm, moist conditions present in a patched eye increase the risk of infection by virulent organisms.

SUPERFICIAL PUNCTATE KERATOPATHY

The most commonly observed slit lamp finding and the leading cause of epithelial barrier disruption in contact lens wearers is superficial punctate keratopathy (SPK). SPK is easily revealed using fluorescein stain. With careful observation, SPK may be apparent in white light as well. The causes of SPK are so diverse that a full chapter could be devoted to this finding alone.

Although SPK is a contact lens complication, it is more often the result of other factors in addition to lens wear. As is true of many other corneal complications, the associated breakdown in the epithelial barrier represents the greatest danger to corneal health. Because SPK is almost always the result of a combination of factors, it is discussed in greater detail with each potential cause.

CONTACT LENS–INDUCED EPITHELIAL EDEMA

Epithelial edema is another common, disruptive, contact lens–induced corneal finding. Contact lens–induced edema is typically transient and is often so subtle that it may be difficult to observe clinically. Because of its ephemeral nature, edema is the most insidious of all lens-induced problems. The best way to visualize lens-induced edema is with fluorescein stain. Mild epithelial edema often appears as a surface mottling or waffling (Fig. A4–2). As the edema becomes more severe, SPK is found (Fig. A4–3).

Contact lens–induced edema is dependent on lens thickness, material permeability, and to some extent, mechanical (bearing) impingement on the corneal surface (Fig. A4–4). The thicker and less permeable the lens, the less oxygen is transmitted through it. Clinical experience also suggests that when the lens binds so tightly that the lens–cornea tear film is minimal, oxygen transmission is reduced, and epithelial edema is more likely to occur (Fig. A4–5).

Soft lenses produce epithelial edema; rigid lenses are more likely to cause stromal edema. Pronounced cases of stromal edema are seen as central corneal clouding, especially when older, less permeable materials are used. Because most modern rigid gas permeable (RGP) lenses are sufficiently permeable, the

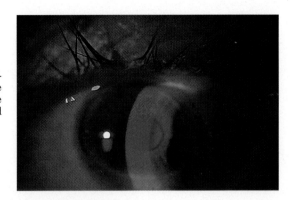

Figure A4-2. Epithelial waffling caused by edema. Note the fine superficial punctate keratopathy often associated with this finding.

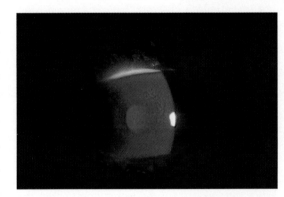

Figure A4-3. Epithelial edema and superficial punctate keratopathy in the central cornea.

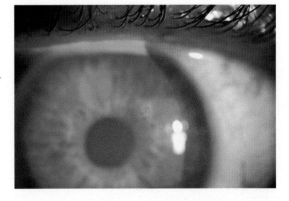

Figure A4-4. Pinpoint area of edema caused by microtrauma from a defective soft contact lens.

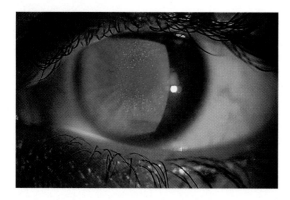

Figure A4-5. Diffuse epithelial edema with superficial punctate keratopathy caused by acute hypoxia in a hybrid (Softperm) lens wearer.

lenses are thinner and less reactive, and bearing areas are more limited, epithelial edema is rare with rigid lenses (Fig. A4-6).

The different structural and fitting characteristics of various types of contact lenses help explain the variability in pathology observed between myopic and hyperopic lens wearers. The greater amount of peripheral pathology in myopic soft lens wearers is caused by increased bearing and edema caused by peripheral lens thickness. This is more marked inferiorly in patients wearing toric lenses. In hyperopic patients wearing lenses with thicker centers, there is a greater tendency for central corneal problems.

The disruption of the epithelial barrier from edema has been well documented. Most hydrophilic lenses do not supply sufficient oxygen to meet corneal requirements, even during daily wear. Because the resultant edema is transitory and difficult to visualize, it is likely to be far more common than most clinicians realize. This disruption of the epithelial barrier combined with its ubiquitous nature virtually insures its role in the genesis of more serious pathology.[1]

Epithelial edema aids in the penetration of toxins, sensitizing agents, and pathogens. Edema is also a factor in corneal surface roughening and enhanced adherence of gram-negative bacteria such as the especially virulent *Pseudomonas aeruginosa*. Several recent studies have found a strong link between epithelial edema and the development of microbial keratitis in contact lens wearers.[2-4]

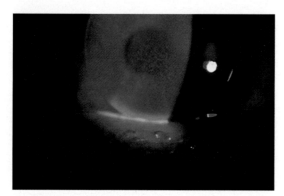

Figure A4-6. Diffuse hypoxic edema in a thick, low-Dk, rigid gas permeable lens wearer.

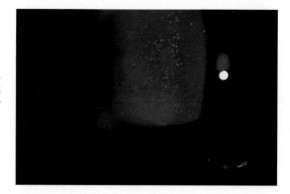

Figure A4–7. Epithelial microcysts in clusters, stained with fluorescein (see Fig. A4–8).

EPITHELIAL MICROCYSTS

Epithelial microcysts are another relatively common soft contact lens complication that can breach the intact corneal surface. Microcysts are present in the deeper epithelial layers, but they are best observed when they reach the corneal surface and fill with fluorescein stain (Fig. A4–7). Nests of microcysts may also be observed in retro-illumination (Fig. A4–8).

Although the cause of microcysts is not completely understood, corneal hypoxia is believed to be an essential precursor. Microcysts are much more commonly seen with extended wear. There is also some evidence that thin lenses that are tightly adherent to the corneal surface are more likely to produce microcysts. An explanation for this is that thin, floppy lenses drape so tightly that they virtually exclude the tear film from the cornea–lens interface and thus impede the outflow of waste products. As waste products build up, they become encapsulated within cyst-like intra-epithelial blebs that are seen as microcysts.

Although microcysts were initially described as taking many weeks to months both to occur and to resolve, several authors have reported microcysts occurring in just days with disposable lenses. My own experience suggests that microcysts are an infrequent complication of daily soft lens wear. They are a rare occurrence even in extended wear when the lenses are properly fitted

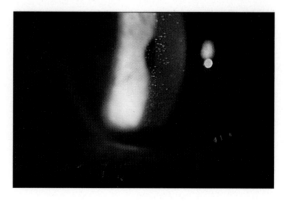

Figure A4–8. Epithelial microcysts in clusters, without fluorescein (see Fig. A4–7).

with adequate movement and tear film exchange. Microcysts are much more commonly observed with some brands of disposable lenses, probably because of their thin, draping design.

PROBLEMS RELATED TO LENS FIT

Although contact lens complications are frequently blamed on poorly fitted lenses, such direct cause and effect is rare. However, marginally fitted lenses are a decided risk factor in the genesis of more serious complications.

In some cases, the link between contact lens and complication is clinically significant. The association between disposable lenses and epithelial microcysts has been discussed previously. This does not mean that every patient who wears disposable lenses will develop microcysts. It does mean that the contact lens practitioner must be aware of the potential for this complication and should act accordingly through adequate follow-up.

A major frustration for contact lens fitters is the inability to relate lens parameters to corneal topography. This is especially true with soft contact lenses, in which the complete parameters of the lenses are not readily available. Even if this information was available, and the relations understood, devices providing detailed corneal topographic information are financially out of reach for all but a small number of contact lens practitioners.

Analysis of fitting relationships must therefore be accomplished after the fact. Fluorescein staining patterns offer important information about abnormal lens–cornea bearing relationships. Bearing typically appears as frank SPK or a change in normal epithelial appearance (Figs. A4–9 and A4–10). Punctate response can range from faint with light bearing to dense and coalesced when bearing is heavy.

In the absence of technological assistance, experience remains the best guide for dealing with lens fitting problems. Exacting trial and error fitting combined with careful follow-up may be necessary to achieve a successful, problem-free fit. It also adds to the fitter's experience and understanding of lens–cornea relations. Fluorescein staining should also be a routine part of every contact lens examination.

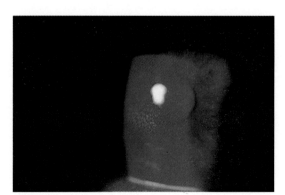

Figure A4–9. Focal area of traumatic edema in a keratoconic soft lens wearer.

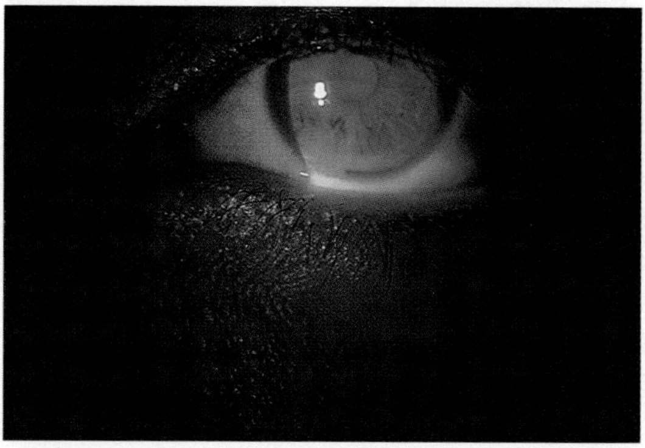

Figure A4–10. Wetting disturbance superimposed on epithelial edema. Note the underlying
mosaic caused by elevated
areas of epithelial basement
membrane.

ACCESSORIES TO THE CRIME: LIDS
AND EXTERNAL ACCESSORY STRUCTURES

Ocular health is extremely dependent upon the function of the eyelids and the
integrity of the tear film. This is especially true in the contact lens wearer.
Many contact lens complications have their genesis in dysfunction of the lids
and the external accessory structures. Lid disease should be viewed as both an
independent complication and an important risk factor for additional problems
in contact lens wearers.

MEIBOMITIS

Meibomitis (Fig. A4–11), and to a lesser extent its close relative blepharitis,
are ubiquitous problems. Nearly every adult patient has one or both of these
conditions. Meibomian gland dysfunction can be especially problematic for the
contact lens wearer. Under normal conditions, meibum is an unsaturated lipid
that is liquid at body temperatures. In many patients, for reasons that are not
completely clear, the meibomian gland orifices become blocked with thick,
waxy secretions (Fig. A4–12). Manual expression of inspissated glands pro-

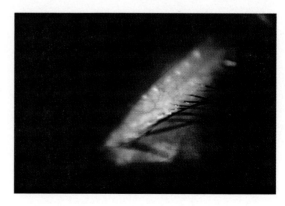

Figure A4–11. Inspissated
meibomian glands.

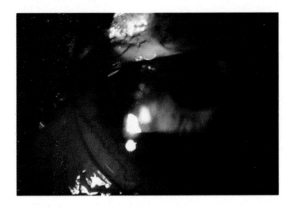

Figure A4–12. Large, blocked meibomian gland filled with meibum *(arrow).*

duces a formed column of congealed meibum that looks much like toothpaste being squeezed from a tube.

The stagnant meibum becomes increasingly saturated and laden with free fatty acids (Fig. A4–13). This causes inflammation when the meibum comes in contact with the lid skin and ocular surface. *Staphylococcus* bacteria also have a fondness for meibomian gland secretions. Bacterial lipase activity causes further lipid saturation, and when the *Staphylococcus* bacteria enter the ocular environment, normal ocular defense systems stimulate the release of exotoxin.

Staphylococcal exotoxin has a role in the genesis of infiltrative keratitis, including focal, diffuse, and ring infiltrates and, most classically, marginal keratitis. Phlyctenular keratoconjunctivitis is also thought to be caused by staphylococcal exotoxin. Because toxins pool in the tear film, they most commonly affect the inferior cornea and conjunctiva adjacent to the lower lid. However, any concurrent disturbance to normal epithelial barriers such as a corneal abrasion or edema can increase the penetration of toxins and modify the clinical picture. The ocular signs of lid disease include thickened and vascularized lid margins, blocked meibomian gland orifices, and frothing at the lower lid margins caused by saponification (soap-making) of the abnormal meibum. Patients often complain of dryness, burning, and occasionally itching. Physical signs include conjunctival and corneal fluorescein punctate staining,

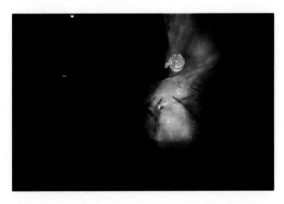

Figure A4–13. Severe meibomitis accompanied by a large lipid deposit at the lower lid margin. Meibomitis causes increased tear film concentration of free fatty acids as well as a diminished tear film volume that contributes to soft contact lens deposits.

especially around the lid margins. Intra-palpebral rose bengal staining is another frequent finding.

Sensitivity to staphylococcal exotoxin is variable. Some patients present with lids that are thickened, vascularized, and severely inflamed, yet they have no other signs or symptoms of lid disease. Other patients barely have a trace of visible lid disease yet have severe ocular surface disease. Because meibum acts to prevent surface evaporation of the tear film, decreased meibum will decrease tear volume. Diminished tear volume concentrates toxins and contaminants. The synergistic effects of decreased tear volume and increased exotoxin concentration can severely affect the contact lens wearer.

Effective treatment requires regular daily use of hot compresses applied to the closed lids. After raising the temperature of the lids past the melting point of the congealed meibum, simple massage helps to express the glandular contents. This procedure may be necessary two or more times a day. Patients should be warned to use care to avoid burning the sensitive skin surrounding the lids. In more severe manifestations of lid disease, topical antibiotic ointment and for some patients, treatment with oral tetracycline may be required. It is also important to explain the chronic nature of this condition to patients. Meibomitis is never cured—only managed.

BLEPHARITIS

Blepharitis, a condition that involves the eyelashes, is closely related to meibomitis and usually co-exists in the same patient (Fig. A4–14). There are two commonly recognized forms: seborrheic blepharitis and staphylococcal blepharitis. These two conditions are more likely opposite ends of a continuous spectrum, because most cases of blepharitis involve both bacterial and seborrheic elements. Classical seborrheic blepharitis appears as scaling and crusting around the lid margins, which are thickened and inflamed. Dandruff-like waxy flakes called scurf are seen on the eyelashes. Scurf and lid-borne bacteria may fall onto the ocular surface. Like meibomitis, blepharitis can have a significant effect on contact lens wear.

Treatment is similar to that for meibomitis. Additionally, lid scrubs using a mild detergent such as dilute baby shampoo or commercially available lid cleansers are helpful in controlling blepharitis. In cases in which bacteria play

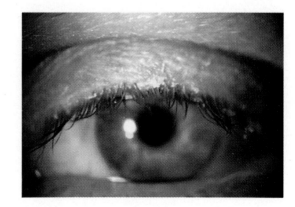

Figure A4–14. Blepharitis.

a significant role, treatment with antibiotic ointments is appropriate. The mere presence of blepharitis or meibomitis is not an absolute contraindication to contact lens wear. However, because these conditions are associated with increased risk of more serious complications, caution is advised.

THE LIDS—PTOSIS AND COMPLICATIONS FOLLOWING BLEPHAROPLASTY

Healthy eyelids are an important element in maintaining a functional environment for contact lens wear. Ptosis, whatever its etiology, can have a significant effect on contact lens wear. Paradoxically, this condition can also be caused by contact lens wear. In rigid lens wearers, sufficient evidence exists to link commonly used lens removal maneuvers and dehiscence of the insertion of the levator muscle. Although more common in rigid lens wearers, ptosis has also been reported in soft contact lens wearers. One report of contralateral ptosis in unilateral soft contact lens wearers was especially provocative. Although the etiology in this case was not readily apparent, it appears likely that it was mechanical in origin.[4a]

A ptosis may also cause contact lens complications. There are significant differences in oxygen availability beneath the upper lid and the exposed cornea. Depending on the peripheral thickness and the inherent permeability of the contact lens, the area beneath the upper lid may become hypoxic and edematous. The resultant disruption in corneal barrier function may be sufficient to stimulate vascularization and other complications affecting the superior cornea.

Contact lens–related superior limbic keratoconjunctivitis (CLSLK; Fig. A4–15) is also likely to be related to focal edema beneath the upper lid area. In one interesting case I encountered, a patient developed unilateral CLSLK. After careful investigation, the CLSLK was found to be challenge-positive to the preservative Polyquad. The involved eye had a unilateral ptosis and demonstrable epithelial edema in the affected area.

I have also observed superior corneal microcysts in a small number of patients with low, tight lids. They appear as a cluster of microcysts in an arcuate

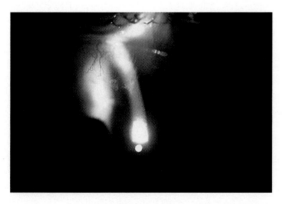

Figure A4–15. Contact lens superior limbic keratoconjunctivitis. Classically described hazy wedge pannus with lipid deposits is present at the leading edge of the sheath of invading vessels.

pattern around the superior limbus. The remainder of the cornea is clear and free of microcysts. In these cases, the tight superior fit reduces the tear film and, secondarily, causes focal hypoxia.

POST-BLEPHAROPLASTY EXPOSURE KERATITIS

Although generally rare, contact lens wearers may encounter difficulty after undergoing blepharoplasty. When cosmetic eye surgery is performed over-zealously, significant lagophthalmos may occur. Exposure keratitis occurs as a result of the gap between the upper and lower lids when the patient sleeps. Affected patients complain of significant ocular discomfort and redness when they rise, and in severe cases, they may be awakened by pain. Slit lamp examination shows a dense inferior staining pattern where the ocular surface is exposed during sleep. This condition can be so severe as to effectively preclude contact lens wear.

Treatment consists of prophylactic ointments before sleep and liberal use of wetting agents during the day. However, the best cure is prevention. Patients contemplating lid surgery should be directed to ophthalmic plastic surgeons or ophthalmologists who have significant experience performing lid surgery. If the patient insists on a plastic surgeon, it is important to insure that the Bell's reflex is intact; a majority of patients who experience post-surgical problems have a deficient Bell's phenomenon. Testing for this reflex is simple: have patients attempt to forcibly close their eyes while you hold their upper lids open. Attempts at forced eyelid closure against resistance will normally cause both eyes to roll upward and outward.

DRY EYES AND CONTACT LENS WEAR

True Dry Eye

True dry eye occurs with or without lens wear. Because dry eye is rare in the prime contact lens–wearing population, few normal contact lens patients actually have a significant dry eye problem. Surprisingly, many patients with clinically dry eyes actually do better wearing contact lenses than not wearing them. In my experience, dry eye, even when significant, is reason for caution but certainly not an absolute contraindication for contact lens wear. Dry eye can occur from aqueous deficiency, mucin deficiency, and subsequent wetting disturbance. As previously discussed in the section on meibomitis, inadequate meibomian gland secretion can cause excessive tear film evaporation.

Most tests for dry eye are woefully inaccurate as a predictor of success or failure for the contact lens wearer. This is especially true of Schirmer strip testing. In a 6-month (unpublished) study conducted in my office, Schirmer test results bore no correlation to initial comfort or ultimate success in our patient population. The reliable diagnosis of dry eye relies more on symptoms than on test results. Patients who consistently report dry eye symptoms without wearing lenses probably have true dry eyes. In such cases, decreased Schirmer testing suggests, but does not confirm, aqueous deficiency. A small or non-existent lacrimal lake at the inferior lid margin, most easily visualized with fluorescein, also suggests lacrimal insufficiency. Intra-palpebral rose bengal staining is also commonly observed in severe dry eye.

Mucin deficiency dry eye is heralded by rapid tear film break-up times. Strands of stringy mucus are often present in the tear film of these patients. This condition is due to goblet cell dysfunction and may be related to existing ocular surface disease. Dry spots may appear that cause discomfort and lead, paradoxically, to reflex tearing. The excess tears can wash away more mucin, thus exacerbating the problem. Soft contact lenses are frequently effective in maintaining surface hydration in these patients. Frothing at the inferior lid margin, meibomian gland inspissation, and inferior corneal or conjunctival rose bengal staining pattern suggest diminished meibum and evaporation-related dry eyes.

CONTACT LENS–INDUCED DRY EYE

Most contact lens wearers with the diagnosis of "dry eye" do not actually have dry eyes. If the patient's dry eye ends when the lenses are removed, they most likely have contact lens–induced pseudo–dry eye rather than true dry eye. In some cases, patients with marginal dry eye problems become symptomatic while wearing contact lenses. These patients can often be treated palliatively with wetting agents to increase tear volume, warm compresses to increase meibomian gland function, and vitamin A drops when mucin deficiency is suspected.

Chronic dry eye symptoms in many patients really represent an adverse physiologic response to a marginally fitted contact lens. Under normal conditions, many wearers walk a fine line between acceptable physiology and hypoxic failure. Eventually, some patients cross that line. Reasons include a lens that does not provide sufficient oxygen flux, decreased oxygen availability (high altitudes or airplane travel), low humidity, or metabolic stress induced by exogenous toxins. As corneal metabolism shifts toward increased anaerobic metabolism, increased levels of lactic acid are produced and secreted into the pre-corneal tear film. A soft lens acts like a sponge in this situation, and it quickly soaks up the lactic acid to maintain osmotic equilibrium. As the lens becomes increasingly acidic, it also dehydrates. The more dehydrated the lens becomes, the tighter it fits and the less its oxygen flux potential. As this condition progresses, patients become increasingly aware of their lens and less comfortable as the desiccation continues. Their eyes become red, and eventually they are forced to remove the lenses. Upon questioning, most patients report that the lens was dry and rubbery upon removal. If they continue to wear a lens under these conditions, there is a risk of spiraling metabolic distress, eventually resulting in "tight lens syndrome," an unpleasant complication that is covered in the next section (see Environmental Factors).

Management of patients with soft lens–induced dry eye requires refitting. Although it seems illogical, lower-water-content lenses are usually best in these cases, because these lenses are less subject to parameter change in the face of environmental stress. Because low-water-content lenses dehydrate less than high-water-content lenses, they are less likely to start a dry eye crisis.

Dry eye conditions, both true and contact lens–related, generate additional risk for more serious complications. Decreased tear volume increases the concentration of tear-borne toxins. Shifts in tonicity can be disruptive to corneal barrier functions. Vigorous attention to dry eye conditions reduces the potential for more serious problems.

ENVIRONMENTAL FACTORS

Lens Contamination

Lens contamination may be a significant problem by itself but commonly serves as a convenient but erroneous catch-all for a variety of contact lens problems. True contamination does exist but should be a diagnosis of exclusion. Most lens spoilage due to contamination involves soft lenses. Occasionally, the source of lens contamination is readily apparent. A patient who has eaten hot peppers may discover the unpleasant consequences of failing to completely wash his or her hands before handling the lenses. Certain dyes produce obvious and lasting effects when soft lenses come into inadvertent contact with them. Other contaminants such as hairspray have a specific appearance on either rigid or soft lenses. The most diagnostically challenging contaminants are those that do not produce visible changes in the lens. When an otherwise healthy and well-adapted lens wearer reports a sudden onset of contact lens–related irritation or intolerance, contamination must be suspected. Symptoms and signs vary depending on the solubility and toxicity of the contaminant. Signs range from mild conjunctival injection to keratitis and even anterior chamber reaction. Symptoms may vary from increased lens awareness to discomfort severe enough to preclude lens wear.

Some soft lens contaminants are water soluble. These may be leached from the lenses by burying them in a concentrated salt slush made from crushed salt tablets or reagent grade sodium chloride and non-preserved saline or distilled water. Irreversible contamination requires replacement of the lenses and, to be safe, the lens case. RGP lenses can also be contaminated, sometimes by common household products. Silicone acrylate lenses suffer surface contamination when exposed to certain hand creams. Makeup and hairspray are common contaminants of both rigid and soft lenses. Contamination is almost always accidental; however prevention through education is easily achievable for most patients.

Lipid Deposits

The presence of large lipid deposits, or jelly bumps (Fig. A4–16) as they are sometimes called, on a soft contact lens makes a dramatic picture. They may

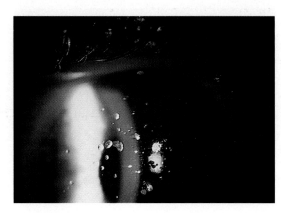

Figure A4–16. Multiple jelly-bump lipid deposits scattered on a soft contact lens.

also be a significant risk factor for microbial keratitis. These jelly bumps occur preferentially, in fact almost exclusively, on lenses worn under relatively hypoxic extended wear conditions. The relation between hypoxia and lipid deposits is so strong that I consider it to be virtually inviolate. Question patients with daily wear soft lenses having jelly bumps and more often than not they will admit to at least occasional extended wear. One theory suggests that these deposits are due to focal drying.[5] This fails to explain the basic observation that these deposits almost never form on lenses removed nightly, whereas the same lens worn on extended wear schedules is encrusted with heavy deposits. A more plausible explanation for jelly bumps is that under extended wear conditions, the osmotic flow across the gradient caused by relative hypoxia on the corneal side carries with it large-chain fatty acids. As these large molecules travel through the pore structure of the lens, some become trapped, creating a binding site for additional lipid molecules.

An important study found that the irregular surfaces present on these deposits make excellent binding sites for *Pseudomonas* bacteria.[6] The authors suggested that this may be the bacterial source in serious corneal infections. Large lipid deposits can cause significant corneal surface disturbance; I have observed multiple corneal depressions surrounded by a rim of edematous epithelium corresponding to an area compressed by large lipid deposits. With fluorescein staining, these depressions have the appearance of octopus suction cups (Figs. A4–17 and A4–18). The back-surface depressions in the lens mate with the corresponding corneal depressions, thereby fixing the lens in place. Although not conclusive, the presence of *Pseudomonas* organisms overlying a corneal surface disruption makes a compelling explanation for corneal infection.

The Air, Humidity, and Elevation

We sometimes forget that contact lens wearers depend on the vagaries of their environment for maintaining comfort and ocular health. An extreme example of environmental risk might be a farmer wearing soft contact lenses. The conditions prevalent in this type of work increase the risk of *Acanthamoeba* keratitis. The *Acanthamoeba* organism exists in soil and standing water, both of which are intrinsic to the farm environment. It would be prudent to educate such a patient about the risks of *Acanthamoeba* contamination. Altitude and

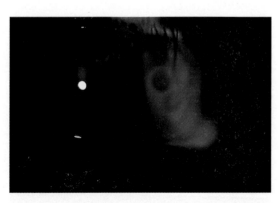

Figure A4–17. "Octopus" suction-cup depression caused by overlying lipid spots (see Fig. A4–18).

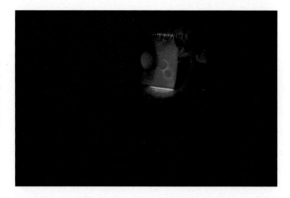

Figure A4–18. Suction-cup impressions caused by overlying large lipid deposits in a soft lens wearer. The rim of the depression is elevated by focal edema caused by compression trauma (see Fig. A4–17).

humidity are two elements that play a great role in contact lens comfort and possible complications. Practitioners in high altitude or very dry environments are familiar with the problems caused by the greater physiologic stress in these environments. Decreasing PO_2 and lower humidity diminish the amount of oxygen available to the cornea. Although there has been little investigation of physiologic corneal adaptation to sudden environmental shifts, it is well recognized that other body systems undergo rapid adaptation to such changes. For contact lens wearers, sudden changes in environment increase the risk of problems. A vacation at high altitude or in an overly dry environment will sometimes cause a contact lens complication. Often, the problem begins during or shortly after a prolonged airplane flight, because airplane cabins are dry and have reduced atmospheric pressure. Exposure to a different spectrum of pathogens can also increase the risk of contact lens–related complications. Suggest that patients wear glasses on long flights. If they prefer to wear lenses, urge them to use wetting drops frequently and remove the lenses at the first sign of trouble.

Environmental Toxins

Environmental toxins are an important concern. Toxins can be airborne or hand-borne (Fig. A4–19). Bacteria often enter the ocular environment through

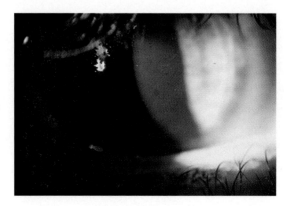

Figure A4–19. Hair spray coating on a soft lens.

contaminated lens cases or dirty hands. Patients working with insecticides or other toxins sometimes pollute their lenses. When faced with bizarre complications, a good history is critical. In one case, I discovered that a contact lens–wearing patient with a unilateral fixed and dilated pupil had used flea powder on her pet dog before inserting her contact lens. We found that the flea powder contained insecticides that had long-acting parasympatholytic effects.

TIGHT LENS SYNDROME

Tight lens syndrome is an unfortunate and confusing name for a contact lens complication. Although the name is descriptive, lens tightening is the result and not the cause of tight lens syndrome. Unfortunately, many doctors mistake cause and effect and blame the patient's problem on a too-tightly-fitted lens, which is not the case. It has been difficult to pinpoint an exact etiology for this condition. Patients with tight lens syndrome are nearly always overnight wearers. The condition is most commonly seen in aphakic patients on extended wear schedules. Slit lamp examination shows a diffusely injected eye (Fig. A4–20). The injection may have a violaceous appearance because of its intensity. There may be a watery discharge and significant lid edema. The cornea is typically edematous with possible diffuse white cell infiltration of the epithelium. The tears often contain cells, and anterior chamber reaction can occur. In severe cases, shut-down of the endothelial pump can produce massive edema. Although a significant reduction in acuity can occur, severe ocular discomfort and photophobia are what cause the patient to visit the practitioner.

Normally, corneal cellular metabolism can be thought of as a miniature nuclear reactor. The damaging products of energy production, free radicals, are balanced by anti-oxidant chemicals, which are present in finite quantities and specifically produced by corneal metabolism. Like the carbon rods in a nuclear reactor, anti-oxidant chemicals absorb damaging free radicals and thereby keep physiologic reactions in check, preventing damage to local tissues.

Like the pseudo–dry eye seen in soft lens wearers, tight lens syndrome involves a sudden shift toward increased anaerobic metabolism. However, tight lens syndrome differs because the failure of normal metabolic pathways is compounded by concurrent deterioration of anti-oxidant reserves and produc-

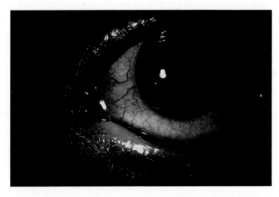

Figure A4–20. Acute red eye, also called tight lens syndrome, because the contact lens is often immobile.

tion. Cyanide inhibits the cytochrome system, which is essential for aerobic adenosine triphosphate (ATP) production and function of the hexose-mono-phosphate shunt, which produces the anti-oxidant nicotinamide-adenine dinucleotide phosphate (NADPH).

Eventually, the build-up of toxic by-products such as lactic acid becomes so overwhelming that the epithelium becomes damaged and a localized inflammatory response is initiated. Polymorphonuclear leukocytes and other inflammatory cells rush in to mop up local damage by releasing hydrolases and other oxidants. In most tissues, these highly reactive and toxic chemicals are actively balanced by anti-oxidants. However, the lack of direct blood supply to the cornea limits the influx of additional anti-oxidants. With much of the normally present anti-oxidant supply depleted and no additional supplies being manufactured in the absence of normal corneal metabolism, inflammatory cell activity causes significant damage to the epithelium, especially to the more metabolically active and vulnerable basal cell layer. The high concentration of lactic acid diffusing into the tear film is absorbed by the contact lens. This causes a progressive decrease in water content and steepening of lens parameters—hence the "tight" in tight lens syndrome.

Management of this condition is complicated by a protracted course, probably because of basal layer damage. It can take up to 2 weeks for the basal layer to regenerate and for complete resolution to take place. Severe cases can affect every layer of the cornea and produce a significant anterior chamber reaction. If the endothelium is affected, there may be significant corneal edema. Most cases are milder and resolve quickly. Treatment with topical steroids or antibiotic–steroid combinations can be helpful.

ACUTE TOXIC REACTIONS— CORNEAL POISONING—TOXIC OCCLUSION SYNDROME

Several years ago I encountered a bizarre complication that affected several patients in rapid succession. All were new soft lens wearers and all reported nearly identical symptoms. Shortly after lens insertion, halos surrounding lights developed. This rapidly progressed into a steam bath–like fog so dense it was visually disruptive. Severe photophobia and intense ocular pain with blepharospasm developed rapidly. After careful investigation, this complication was traced to a single batch of lens disinfectant. The manufacturer's analysis reported no problems with the product but suggested spoilage might be a factor. I suspect that improper formulation was more likely.

Interestingly, a similar complication was reported several years later by C. Edward Williams, O.D. He called it "soft contact lens toxic occlusion phenomenon" because of the occlusive nature of the soft lens fit.[7] The most severely affected of his patients described the same fogging and intractable pain and photophobia found among my patients. Slit lamp examination revealed epithelial sloughing. In his cases, no single causal factor was identified, although the preservative benzalkonium chloride (BAK) was implicated.

The intensity and severity of this complication suggest acute corneal poisoning. All patients reported a sudden and profound fogging effect. Severe corneal edema was evident. The only thing that could account for these findings is a complete shutdown of the cornea's physiologic pump mechanism. Although the shutdown was long-lasting, it was not irreversible, and in all cases the patients recovered.

Exogenous contaminants, whether passively or actively introduced into the ocular environment, can have profound effects on corneal function and integrity. It is impossible to completely eliminate environmentally induced complications. However, awareness of the environment's contribution to contact lens problems will help prevent them.

IMMUNE RESPONSE IN CONTACT LENS WEARERS

The cornea and, to a lesser extent, the entire ocular surface represent a unique immunologic area. The eye will react to a variety of endogenous and exogenous sensitizing stimuli. Infiltrative keratitis is a common immune-mediated response in contact lens wearers, although many cases of infiltrative keratitis are not contact lens–related.

Infiltrates have many causes, but nearly all are immune in character. They can vary tremendously in appearance, ranging from flat and flocculent to raised with well-defined borders. Infiltrates are often accompanied by an acute red eye response (ARE).

CONTACT LENS–RELATED STERILE CORNEAL INFILTRATES

Corneal infiltrates are a commonly encountered complication of contact lens wear. A corneal infiltrate represents an accumulation of immunologically active cells. Most infiltrates are epithelial or subepithelial. Hypersensitivity to staphylococcal exotoxin is a likely cause of most corneal infiltrates and infiltrative keratitis in contact lens wearers because of the ubiquitous nature of these bacteria on the lid margins and surrounding ocular skin surfaces (Fig. A4–21). In a majority of cases, routine contact lens manipulation is the source of contamination. Normal ocular defense systems promote the release of exotoxin. Compromise of the corneal epithelial barrier in a contact lens wearer, either from lens-induced edema or mechanical disruption of the epithelial sur-

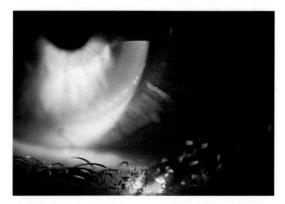

Figure A4–21. A classic example of marginal *Staphylococcus* infiltrates.

face, enables exotoxin penetration. Hypoxia also produces infiltrates, but they are more proximately due to disruption of corneal barriers by focal edema. Mechanical compromise or well-localized edema typically produces circumscribed, dense infiltrates. When the compromise is more diffuse, the response is a more diffuse infiltrative keratitis.

Infiltrates can also be associated with serious microbial keratitis. Some infiltrates are infectious, whereas others are sterile and represent a focal immune response. Several common causes of infiltrates must be considered and are discussed later in this appendix (see Microbial Keratitis).

Sterile infiltrates are typically small (<1 mm), raised, well-circumscribed, and covered by intact epithelium, and they do not stain with fluorescein (Fig. A4–22). Pain may be significant but not overwhelming. Sterile infiltrates are self-limiting and usually require no treatment. Infectious infiltrates are larger, more irregular, more invasive, and more painful. True ulcers usually stain with fluorescein.

Although it may be tempting to differentiate sterile from non-sterile infiltrates based on clinical observation, this is a dangerous approach, because judgment errors can be catastrophic. For this reason, aggressive antibiotic treatment of corneal infiltrates is indicated. Steroid use should be initially avoided, although in cases in which the visual axis is involved and vision is threatened, treatment with topical steroids may be indicated after any possibility of infection has been eliminated.

Differential Diagnosis, Prevention, and Treatment of Corneal Infiltrates

Although contact lenses are a frequent cause, there are many other causes of corneal infiltrates in the contact lens wearer. Adenoviral infection (e.g., epidemic keratoconjunctivitis and pharyngoconjunctival fever), idiopathic causes (e.g., Thygesson's SPK), herpes simplex and zoster infections, *Acanthamoeba* infection, Epstein-Barr virus, and *Chlamydia* infections can all present with corneal infiltrates. These infections are discussed in more detail in the section on microbial keratitis.

Initial treatment for any contact lens–associated infiltrative keratitis is cessation of contact lens wear. In most cases, non-infectious infiltrative keratitis resolves rapidly and spontaneously. Because infiltrates are often part of an

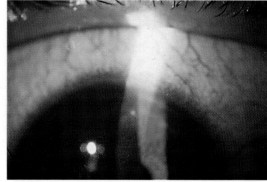

Figure A4–22. Typical contact lens–related sterile peripheral infiltrate.

infectious process, they must be approached with great suspicion and caution. When proven sterile infiltrates involve the visual axis, cautious use of topical steroids or antibiotic–steroid combinations may speed resolution and result in a more favorable visual outcome.

Treatment of infiltrates in contact lens wearers must always take into account the possibility that corneal integrity may be compromised, even in sterile infiltrates. Superinfection with virulent organisms can occur. Because sterile infiltrates in contact lens wearers are often related to lid disease, both prevention and treatment require attention to the condition of the lids. Regular lid hygiene, including massage after application of warm compresses, is advisable in any contact lens patient with lid disease.

The differential diagnosis of infiltrative keratitis in the soft contact lens wearer can be extremely challenging. Rapid resolution with cessation of lens wear strongly suggests a contact lens–related etiology. Lens wear in a patient with viral infiltrative keratitis will have little or no effect on the course of the disease, although because it is a potential source of irritation, it is not advised. In Thygesson's SPK, contact lenses are often an effective therapy. Discontinuing contact lens wear can actually cause the condition to worsen. Thygesson's SPK is a persistent condition, whereas both viral and contact lens–related infiltrative keratitis are self-limiting. Other infectious agents, such as herpes virus, *Chlamydia* organisms, and Epstein-Barr virus, must also be considered.

GIANT PAPILLARY CONJUNCTIVITIS

Giant papillary conjunctivitis (GPC), a common immune response, was among the first complications of soft contact lens wear to be recognized. GPC may also occur with rigid lens wear and even focally in response to exposed sutures. Despite the frequency of GPC in contact lens wearers, its precise etiology remains obscure. GPC is most likely the result of a combination of immunologic and mechanical factors. The immune response to antigen-rich protein deposits on the contact lens surface is the most prominent feature in soft lens wearers. Like many immune-mediated conditions, GPC often flares during times of heightened immunologic activity, such as during the spring allergy season.

Affected patients typically present complaining of itching, increased lens awareness, and moderate to severe lens coating (Fig. A4–23). Often, the affected lens, covered by an adhesive-like mucous coating, will ride up and stick beneath the upper lid (Fig. A4–24). Slit lamp examination shows giant papillae on the tarsal conjunctival surfaces of the upper lid. The papillae may be inflamed, and a significant amount of mucus may be present (Fig. A4–25).

Initially, lens replacement alone is sufficient to quiet the condition. Invariably, GPC will recur, each time with a shorter latency then before. Ultimately, lenses become irreversibly spoiled only hours after initial insertion. Effective treatment requires an understanding of the basic mechanisms of GPC. Normal proteins deposit on the lens surface and become antigenic through a combination with contaminants or toxins present in the ocular environment. Surface antigens stimulate an immune response in the upper lid, where lid–lens contact is greatest. Vast quantities of tear-borne antibodies are produced, which then attack and coat the lens surface. Through a poorly understood "black-box" mechanism, these proteins are themselves converted into antigen. The more antigen present, the greater the ocular response. The cycle rapidly spirals out of control.

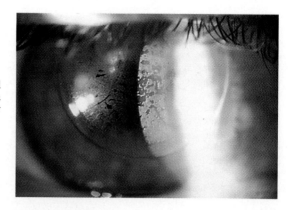

Figure A4–23. Heavily coated rigid gas permeable lens in a patient with giant papillary conjunctivitis.

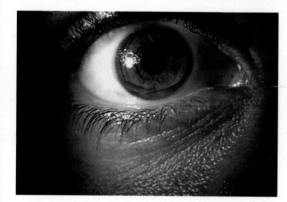

Figure A4–24. A classic finding seen with giant papillary conjunctivitis: well-coated soft contact lens riding high beneath the upper lid.

Figure A4–25. Giant papillary conjunctivitis beneath the upper lid.

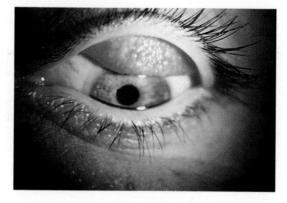

The most direct way to treat GPC is to eliminate, or at least reduce, the antigenic load on the lens surface by choosing a contact lens that minimizes protein build up. Among conventional lenses, the CSI (Crofilcon) soft lens excels in reducing surface protein. The CSI-T is best because of its thin edge design. Extended wear may be problematic but is not contraindicated. A very effective way to reduce surface antigen is through frequent lens replacement. Daily wear disposable lenses are excellent for this purpose. During GPC flare-ups, the frequency of lens replacement can be increased. In severe cases of soft lens–related GPC, a switch to RGP lenses may be helpful. Surprisingly, switching RGP wearers with GPC to soft lenses is frequently helpful in controlling the condition.

Keeping the lens surface clean is critically important, especially with conventional daily wear lenses. The most effective method is to use an alcohol-based surfactant cleaner, which helps solubilize surface proteins, allowing the surfactant component to more effectively remove them. Peroxide disinfection can also be useful by helping lyse protein. Preserved solutions should be avoided, because preservatives can combine with surface proteins to increase antigenicity. Peroxide-activated subtilisin-A–based enzyme cleaners are helpful in severe GPC. As an adjunctive measure, topical vitamin-A drops reduce symptoms and decrease upper lid inflammatory response.

Studies have linked meibomian gland dysfunction and GPC. This suggests that attention to lid condition may be important in patients with GPC. The reasons for this relation may involve the antigenic contribution of staphylococcal exotoxin or the role of meibum as an immunologic barrier preventing contact between the lens and upper lid surfaces.

Although a conservative approach to managing GPC usually works well, medical treatment with topical mast cell stabilizers may be necessary in recalcitrant cases. Steroids are generally not useful. Because medical treatment is palliative, not curative, management of GPC through conventional means is best. Medical treatment should be reserved as a last resort when lens wear is necessary and all other measures fail.

THE LIMBAL AREA

Staphylococcal Marginal Disease

Staphylococcus is a ubiquitous bacterium. In non–contact lens–wearing patients, *Staphylococcus* bacteria can cause a large variety of findings. Circumlimbal corneal injection and sterile peripheral corneal infiltrates are common. Phlyctenules are raised nodules at or near the limbus accompanied by a vascular ingrowth. Marginal infiltrates in the lower cornea in the presence of lid disease are due to the pooling effect of antigen in the tear film. This reaction is a type IV delayed hypersensitivity.

In contact lens wearers, the picture changes dramatically. Contact lenses can increase the penetration of staphylococcal exotoxin, which can occur anywhere on the corneal surface. Of greater concern is that contact lenses may harbor numerous gram-negative bacteria, which can super-infect sterile infiltrates.

RING INFILTRATES—WESLEY RINGS

Ring-shaped infiltrates are an unusual and exceedingly rare contact lens complication. They may be either complete, running uninterrupted around the

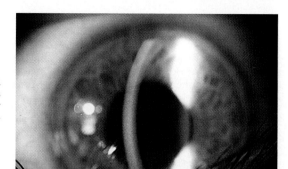

Figure A4–26. Rarely reported ring infiltrate in a soft lens wearer, presumably caused by *Staphylococcus* exotoxin hypersensitivity.

corneal circumference, or partial. The infiltrate is usually separated from the limbus by a small clear zone and may be flat or elevated.

In one case, a patient with extreme photophobia and ocular pain experienced a mild unilateral infiltrate followed several months later by more pronounced ring infiltrates in both corneas (Figs. A4–26 and A4–27).[8] Both infiltrates were raised with irregular but well-defined borders. Treatment with topical antibiotics and anti-inflammatory drops produced rapid resolution. A depression corresponding to the area of the infiltrate persisted. Careful investigation failed to produce any clear-cut causative factors. However, corneal ring infiltrates have been associated with staphylococcal hypersensitivity, *Acanthamoeba* keratitis, herpes virus, allergic reactions (often with a double ring), and immune disorders such as rheumatoid arthritis and Sjögren's syndrome. Because of the presence of severe lid disease, staphylococcal hypersensitivity appears to have been the most likely cause of this complication.

PROBLEMS WITH SOLUTIONS

Many contact lens complications are related to care products. The preservatives and disinfectants used in these products are naturally toxic. For most patients, this toxicity is mitigated by the relatively low concentrations used

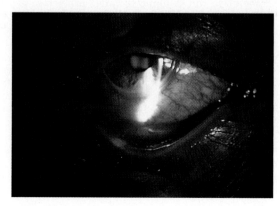

Figure A4–27. Acute stage of disease in patient in Figure A4–26.

and the specificity of the preservatives or disinfectants for pathogens compared with activity against normal ocular tissues. Even "modern" preservatives can produce allergic and toxic reactions. Residual hydrogen peroxide can cause a paracentral smile-shaped stain in susceptible patients. Polyquad and Dymed, both of which are generally non-reactive, have been associated with a variety of unusual complications such as infiltrative keratitis and punctate keratopathy.

Hypersensitivity

One of the first reported soft contact lens complications was allergy to thimerosal. Thimerosal, a methyl-mercury compound, is extremely sensitizing to a large percentage of the population. In this classic reaction, the patient presents with a bright red eye, often accompanied by a serous discharge and itching. This delayed hypersensitivity reaction frequently takes 2 weeks to occur after the offending solution is first used. Although sometimes dramatic in appearance, solution hypersensitivity is almost always self-limiting, easy to diagnose, and simple to resolve.

Occasionally, other factors play a role in hypersensitivity response. As an example, epithelial edema increases the permeability of the cornea to sensitizing chemicals, enhancing the chances for a reaction. Additionally, other allergies can help trigger a reaction. Occasionally, trauma or micro-trauma can mobilize the inflammatory cascade sufficiently to promote a hypersensitivity reaction.

Toxicity

Toxic reactions to chemical preservatives are commonly seen in soft contact lens wearers. Patients typically present with SPK that is greatest in the areas of lens bearing or tear pooling. Depending on the level and type of toxicity, the soft lens can act as a reservoir, allowing the tears to carry the toxic agent to the lower fornix, where the bulk of the response is observed. With more toxic elements, the entire cornea is involved, with the greatest response in areas of increased contact through bearing or associated edema. This can create unusual staining patterns, such as ring SPK associated with peripheral bearing in a soft lens wearer.

Occasionally, a combination of products or a specific lens material and a preservative can combine to cause problems. The CSI (Crofilcon) material has been linked to reactions with several solutions, including Allergan's Hydrocare and Alcon's OptiSoft. In the latter case, the product formulation caused concentration of the Polyquad preservative on the lens surface, resulting in an unusual diffuse punctate keratopathy (Figs. A4–28 and A4–29). Fluorinated silicone acrylate rigid lens materials may react with lens care products containing high concentrations of the preservative Dymed. Affected patients complain of decreased wearing time, increased lens awareness, and photophobia. The lenses appear glued to the cornea with a viscous, debris-filled tear layer. Dense SPK and imprinting of the cornea often occurs. This complication completely and rapidly resolves with a change in care products.

Misuse of both contact lens and non–contact lens ophthalmic solutions can also create problems for the contact lens wearer (Fig. A4–30). Many ophthalmic medications are preserved with compounds that are toxic to the cornea.

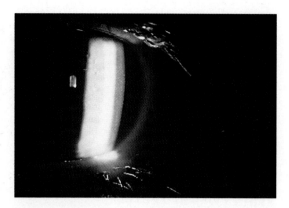

Figure A4–28. Diffuse atypical superficial punctate keratopathy caused by a rare toxic response in a patient using OptiSoft solution with a CSI lens. Note the unusual, dense, fine, white punctate lesions with a "crunchy" texture (see Fig. A4–29).

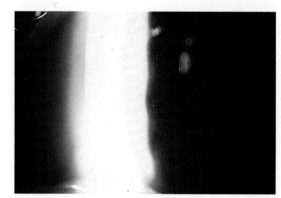

Figure A4–29. Higher magnification of Figure A4–28.

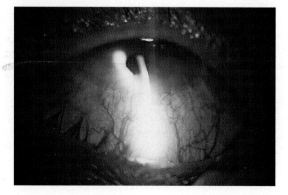

Figure A4–30. Toxic reaction to lens cleaner instilled directly in the eye. Patient was aphakic. Note the vascularization at the limbus and the infiltrate surrounding the vessels.

BAK, a quaternary ammonium preservative, is one example. When a product containing BAK is instilled with soft lenses in place, the lens absorbs the preservative and acts as a reservoir, increasing its effective concentration. Typical complications include burning, stinging, and diffuse SPK. Idiosyncratic reactions are possible with more severe findings such as a severe keratitis or iritis.

Solution toxicity has been implicated as a factor in other contact lens complications. Chlorhexidine, a bactericidal once commonly used in soft lens solutions, could bind to lens surface proteins and achieve toxic levels. Typical reactions included SPK, diffuse conjunctival injections, and rarely, limbal chemosis.[9,10] CLSLK has been associated with solution hypersensitivity. Although thimerosal is most frequently implicated, no specific factor has ever been conclusively identified.[11,12]

SOLUTIONS, INFILTRATES, AND CORNEAL ULCERS

There always seems to be some new controversy pitting the interests of contact lens manufacturers against the observations of clinicians. Most companies are honorable. However, some occasionally seem to forget that patients' needs are more important than profit.

Like the majority of contact lens complications, solution-related problems are exceedingly rare. This makes it all the more difficult for the individual practitioner to recognize that one or two complications are part of a larger pattern. A good example is the central corneal pigmentary disturbance associated with the preservative Dymed. This finding is an apparently benign rust-colored line that radiates horizontally across the corneal mid-line with a whorl-like central dip. It would not have been discovered had an astute practitioner not used large amounts of a Dymed-based care product and recognized this subtle presentation.

Because adverse reactions are so rare, most go undiscovered. For this reason, clinical trials are often ineffective in discovering potential contact lens complications. Rarely, a unique environment or special conditions increase the potential for penetration of specific complications. Individual practitioners may encounter a series of adverse reactions that the rest of the contact lens world somehow misses. Regardless, these complications are real.

The reasons manufacturers choose specific preservatives can be curious. During the early years of soft contact lenses, the high rate of adverse reactions to thimerosal prompted the U.S. Food and Drug Administration to approve sorbic acid as a non-sensitizing alternative. Although still in use, this preservative was admittedly a stop-gap solution with numerous problems. The initial use of sorbic acid also coincided with the approval of extended wear soft lenses. Sorbic acid is an unstable compound. Under the acidic conditions common to extended wear, it readily breaks down into an aldehyde. These aldehyde break-down products cause the lens discoloration associated with sorbic acid. More importantly, these products also have the potential for hardening and roughening corneal surface proteins. Under extended wear conditions, the corneal surface may be sufficiently compromised to permit the penetration of toxins or enhance the adherence of gram-negative bacteria. Shortly after the introduction of extended wear lenses and sorbic acid–based products, a dramatic increase in the incidence of corneal ulcers occurred. Although extended wear was blamed and did prove to be a significant risk factor, the role of sorbic acid in this complication has never been thoroughly investigated.

CONTACT LENS–RELATED CORNEAL COMPLICATIONS

Mechanical Problems

Contact lenses are, in the final analysis, mechanical devices. The fit of a lens, whether soft or rigid, is nothing more than aligning one non-spherical surface with another. Under ideal conditions, the lens virtually floats on a layer of tears, and the lens and cornea barely touch. Unfortunately, this is rarely the case.

Complications caused by a poor peripheral lens–cornea relation occur most often in soft lens wearers in whom the peripheral-to-central curve relations are fixed. In rigid lens wearers, these relations can be altered as part of the fitting process. Mechanical factors can affect the lens–cornea physiologic relation. Excessive lens bearing forces cause focal edema. Increased lens thickness reduces oxygen transmission and increases edema and the subsequent penetration of toxins. Normal physiologic barriers can be overcome. Routine epithelial cell turnover sloughing may be disturbed.

Peripheral Corneal Epithelial Hypertrophy

Peripheral corneal epithelial hypertrophy (PCEH) is an interesting and reasonably common soft lens complication.[13] Surprisingly, it has been infrequently described. The condition presents as a build-up of excess epithelial tissue in the peripheral cornea around, but slightly separated from, the limbus (Fig. A4–31). It is most easily visualized after instillation of fluorescein. The excess epithelial tissue has an irregular, heaped-up appearance. Initially, this tissue doesn't stain, but it is clearly highlighted by fluorescein pooling. After about 1 minute, the abnormal, more permeable tissue absorbs fluorescein and shows late staining.

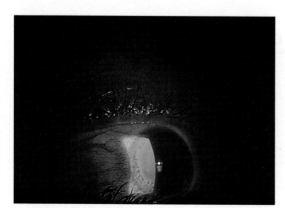

Figure A4–31. Peripheral corneal epithelial hypertrophy. Note the edematous peripheral cornea with areas of negative and contrasting positive fluorescein uptake.

PCEH is far more common in extended wear patients. Patients wearing high-minus or toric soft lenses are also often affected; this may be because of the thicker edge design of these lenses. In general, lens designs with tight peripheral fitting relations are more likely to produce this finding. Concurrent findings include peripheral furrow staining, localized edema with associated vascularization, and micro-geographic basement membrane changes.

Furrow Staining

Furrow staining often appears along with PCEH. In this condition, small, well-defined grooves appear in the peripheral cornea adjacent to the limbus (Fig. A4–32). The furrows are perpendicular to the limbus and may radiate circumlimbally for 360 degrees or appear in specific areas. Furrow staining is most visible immediately after instillation of fluorescein because of pooling in the depressed furrows. However, some later-stage staining does occur. Like PCEH, furrow staining is more commonly observed with extended wear and in patients wearing lenses with tight peripheral fitting relations.

Peripheral Epithelial Edema

Although some soft lens patients develop PCEH or furrow staining, others show only peripheral epithelial edema. Epithelial edema is best visualized immediately after the lenses are removed. After instillation of fluorescein, a zone of irregularly swollen epithelium becomes evident. There is often a characteristic waffled pattern. As the edematous epithelium loses its protective barrier functions, it is more easily penetrated by toxins. Bacterial adherence is thought to increase. Normal barriers to vascularization are disrupted, and there is an increased tendency for vascular invasion of the peripheral cornea.

Contact Lens–Related Flecked Arcus

Contact lens–related flecked arcus is a relatively common but easy to miss finding. It occurs in the peripheral cornea of soft contact lens wearers and is almost always found in the presence of PCEH. It resembles an incomplete

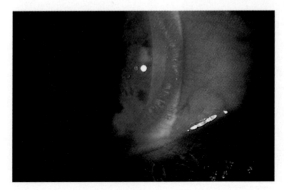

Figure A4–32. Furrow staining in a soft lens wearer.

arcus with multiple, irregularly shaped, white or gray fleck-like figures extending 360 degrees around the peripheral cornea (Fig. A4–33). This condition can be mistaken for an atypical arcus or limbal girdle of Vogt; however, unlike these two findings, flecked arcus resolves several weeks after temporary cessation of lens wear or after refitting with an appropriate contact lens.

Although the precise etiology remains uncertain, there are several possible explanations for this unusual finding. The most likely is that chronic edema causes basement membrane thickening and produces the irregular figures described. A second explanation is that local edema and epithelial disruption may allow increased penetration of exotoxin, resulting in deposition of an immune complex. The unusual shapes may correspond to areas of increased penetration and heightened antigen–antibody activity surrounding micro-capillaries. Finally, lipid leakage could also produce this clinical picture, but the condition would probably take longer to resolve than the several weeks it takes for flecked arcus to disappear.

This condition is self-limiting, and management consists of eliminating or reducing peripheral lens bearing. Refitting the patient with larger, flatter-fitting lenses appears to be highly successful. Although no secondary complications have been observed in conjunction with flecked arcus, the underlying cause is most likely disruption of the epithelial barrier.

Peripheral Corneal Vascularization

Contact lens–induced corneal vascularization is a common and dreaded complication, because it is difficult to manage and impossible to completely eliminate. There are many potential causative factors; hypoxia, immune mechanisms, and chemical hypersensitivity have been implicated but never proven. Experience suggests that mechanical factors, anatomic disruption from prior surgery, and secondary hypoxia are important elements in the development of peripheral corneal vascularization. An example of this is vascularization of radial keratotomy incisions in post-surgery soft lens wearers (Fig. A4–34).

There are two distinct forms of contact lens–related vascularization. Superficial vascularization occurs in or around the level of the corneal epithelium. Deep stromal vascularization typically occurs in the deepest one third of the stroma. The morbidity of these two variations differs greatly. Superficial vas-

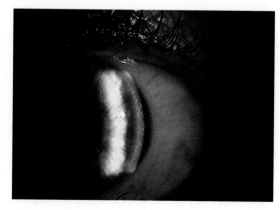

Figure A4–33. Flecked arcus is typically seen in conjunction with peripheral corneal epithelial hypertrophy.

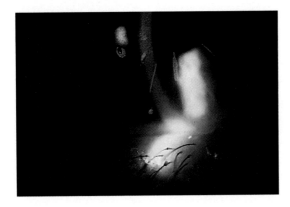

Figure A4–34. Vessel present in a radial keratotomy incision after soft lens wear.

cularization is almost always benign, with few complicating factors. Conversely, deep stromal vascularization is a more foreboding finding, because deeper vessels can leak large amounts of blood and lipid into the stroma. The result can be irreversible damage and severe visual loss.

Soft contact lens wearers are most commonly affected. Most vascularization occurs beneath the upper lid, radiating centrally from the superior limbus. Reduced oxygen tension beneath the upper lid may be the primary cause. Vascularization can also arise from other sites that are affected by chronic hypoxia.

After the process begins, it can progress rapidly if not carefully monitored. The degree of ingrowth varies from less than 1 mm to greater than one half of the corneal diameter. In advanced cases, the visual axis may be compromised. Most contact lens–related vascularization is superficial.

Patients with vascularization are often wearing thick or tight lenses. Some lenses appear to have steep peripheral-to-central curvature relations. Unfortunately, information on these important fitting characteristics is difficult if not impossible to obtain. High-minus lenses (Fig. A4–35) and prism ballasted lenses (Fig. A4–36) typically cause vascularization at their thickest points. Aphakic patients are at additional risk because of decreased oxygen transmission through the thick center of the lens and also because prior surgery ap-

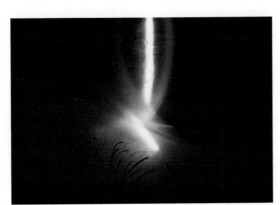

Figure A4–35. Isolated neovascular vessel in a patient wearing high-minus lenses.

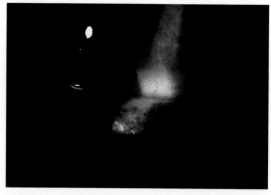

Figure A4-36. Deep stromal vascularization in the inferior cornea associated with long-term wear of a prism ballast toric soft lens.

pears to compromise the normal physiologic barriers to vascularization (Figs. A4–37 and A4–38). Low-riding and immobile rigid lenses can cause inferior vascularization.

Management of superficial vascularization requires increasing oxygen availability to the affected corneal area. Changes in lens designs and materials can be helpful. Corneal mapping devices offer insight into peripheral corneal topography and fitting relations. In more recalcitrant cases, reduction of wearing time and even cessation of lens wear may be indicated. RGP materials currently offer greater oxygen transmissibility than their soft lens counterparts. For that reason, and because rigid lenses usually rest away from the limbal area, they may provide a viable alternative to soft lenses in many cases.

The presence of deep stromal vascularization is far more ominous and must be treated with extreme caution. Aggressive steps to increase oxygen flux to the affected area are necessary. Frequent and careful monitoring is essential. In the absence of rapid improvement, cessation of all lens wear is prudent, at least until the vessels have significantly diminished in caliber.

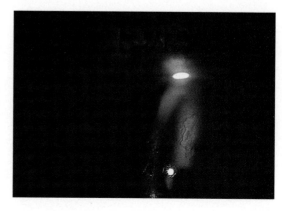

Figure A4-37. Extensive superior vascularization in an aphakic patient.

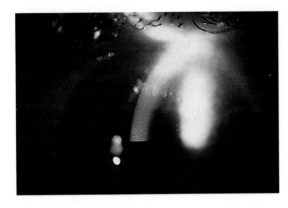

Figure A4–38. Pannus with lipid leakage at the vessel margins.

Intra-corneal Hemorrhage

Intra-corneal hemorrhage occurs almost exclusively in soft lens wearers. Several reports have appeared in the literature.[14–16] Like contact lens–related vascularization, hemorrhage can occur superficially or in the deeper corneal layers. Superficial corneal hemorrhage typically appears at the terminus of a corneal vessel (Fig. A4–39). It is self-limited and often light bulb–like in appearance. All reported cases have been of single hemorrhages, although multiple hemorrhages can occur (Figs. A4–40 and A4–41).

The cause of lens-related superficial hemorrhage is unknown. Several authors have suggested that it may be mechanical, with lens manipulation causing a rupture in the vessel wall. Others have suggested that vascular ingrowth produces fragile, less competent vessels that are more prone to leakage. Another possible explanation is that intra-corneal hemorrhage may be a form of immune-mediated vasculitis occurring in these new vessels.

Deep stromal hemorrhages in contact lens wearers are far less common but potentially more devastating. Whereas superficial hemorrhages are self-limiting, often resolving spontaneously within several days and leaving no residual effects, deep stromal hemorrhages cause significant blood staining of the

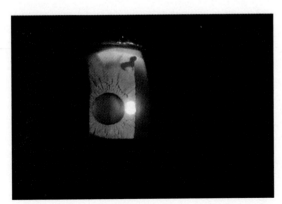

Figure A4–39. Single intracorneal hemorrhage showing the feeder vessel in an aphakic soft lens wearer.

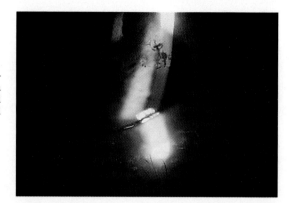

Figure A4-40. Unusual, centaur-shaped hemorrhage in a soft lens wearer who presented with multiple intracorneal hemorrhages (see Fig. A4-41).

stroma, concurrent leakage of lipids, and potentially, profound visual loss. The effects may be so severe that a penetrating keratoplasty becomes necessary to restore visual function. It is important to emphasize that the potential complications of stromal vascularization are devastating. For this reason, it is important to deal aggressively with this condition, even if it means discontinuing lens wear completely.

CONTACT LENS–ASSOCIATED SUPERIOR LIMBIC KERATOCONJUNCTIVITIS

SLK is a non–contact lens–related inflammatory condition first described by Theodore in 1954.[17] SLK often involves middle-aged women and is associated with thyroid disease. A condition with a similar clinical presentation but occurring exclusively in soft contact lens wearers was first reported by several authors in the early 1980s[11, 12, 18–20] CLSLK presents with intense injection of the superior bulbar conjunctiva, often accompanied by a localized SPK. A V-shaped wedge of corneal edema, infiltration, and vascularization progresses toward the central cornea (see Fig. A4–15). Discrete epithelial opacities often

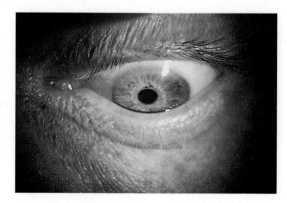

Figure A4-41. Multiple intracorneal hemorrhages in a soft lens wearer (see Fig. A4-40).

occur at its leading edge. The upper tarsal conjunctiva may show a fine papillary hypertrophy.

Patients are often uncomfortable, reporting burning, itching, and increased lens awareness. CLSLK can be sight-threatening if it progresses through the visual axis. Etiologic factors include preservative hypersensitivity and excessive lens movement. Treatment involves eliminating preserved care products, refitting when appropriate, and using topical anti-inflammatory drops in severe cases.

COMPLICATIONS ASSOCIATED WITH DESICCATION

Superior Limbal Epithelial Splitting

Epithelial splitting is a relatively rare but frequently reported soft contact lens complication. Perhaps this is because the appearance of a full-thickness rent in the corneal epithelium is quite dramatic. However, many patients remain asymptomatic, with the finding fortuitously observed during a routine examination. More typically, they present complaining of a foreign-body sensation.

The full-thickness lamellar crack usually occurs in the superior corneal epithelium (Fig. A4–42). The crack is thin, irregular, and often arcuate, following the limbal curvature. It absorbs fluorescein readily. Several investigators have failed to elucidate the cause of this unusual complication, although mechanical factors are likely contributory. Focal desiccation is another possible cause.

Epithelial splitting occurs with nearly every type of soft lens, including both large- and smaller-diameter lenses and high- and low-water-content materials. Management consists of refitting, although there is no rhyme or reason regarding why one lens causes the problem and another does not.

Full-Thickness Epithelial Cracking (Erosions)

Thin, high-water-content lenses desiccate more rapidly and more thoroughly than lower-water-content, thicker lens designs. Under some conditions, these lenses can desiccate the corneal surface so thoroughly that severe, full-thick-

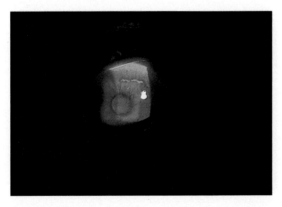

Figure A4–42. Epithelial splitting adjacent to the superior limbus.

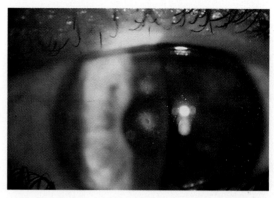

Figure A4–43. Central epithelial fractures from an ultra-thin high-water-content soft lens. Note the fractured appearance and the irregular margins.

ness erosions occur. These deep abrasions have a cracked appearance around their margins (Figs. A4–43 and A4-44). Large areas of epithelium extending to the basement membrane are removed. Although desiccation has been described as either the cause of or as associated with a good deal of epithelial staining, full-thickness desiccation abrasions are unique and unmistakable.

This type of damage typically occurs in the central cornea. The reason is that the thinnest part of a lens, the center of a minus lens, desiccates the most rapidly. Ultra-thin high-water-content lenses should be avoided, especially in myopic prescriptions, because the center portion of the lens will be exceedingly thin. Although these deep abrasions heal quickly, superinfection is possible. As with all contact lens–related abrasions, patching is contraindicated. Treatment with broad-spectrum topical antibiotic drops is advisable.

3-9 Staining

The 3- and 9-o'clock areas of the peripheral cornea are frequently involved in a variety of contact lens complications because this area is especially susceptible to drying and exposure in contact lens wearers. Most 3-9 staining is seen in rigid lens wearers. In rare cases in which small-diameter soft lenses fit eccentrically, chronically exposed peripheral corneal surfaces may show a variant of

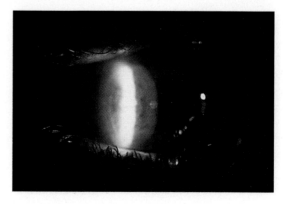

Figure A4–44. Central scarring of Bowman's layer in a long-term wearer of an ultra-thin high-water-content lens.

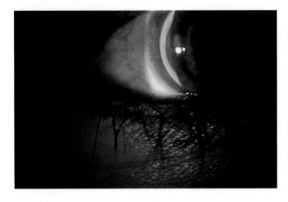

Figure A4–45. Typical 3-9 staining in a rigid gas permeable lens wearer.

3-9 staining. Clinically, 3-9 staining may vary from mild to severe, initially appearing as a localized punctate keratitis in the 3-9 position (Figs. A4–45 and A4–46). In severe and chronic cases, it can progress to form a desiccated and depressed area called a dell, a vascularized limbal mass, or a pseudo-pterygium.

Despite the ubiquitous nature of this finding, there remains considerable disagreement regarding the etiology and appropriate treatment of this condition. Classically, 3-9 staining is described as being caused by peripheral desiccation caused by interference with the wiping action of the lids because of the lens edge. Other clinicians believe the lens actually performs the wiping action, with the lids responsible for moving the lens around. In this scenario, 3-9 staining is caused by a problem with the lens fit. Diminished lateral movement secondary to a peripheral bind is what causes the drying effect.

Clinically, many patients with 3-9 staining also have problems with blinking. Effective treatment involves eliminating blink problems, lens-positioning problems, and movement problems, especially in lateral translation, and addressing underlying dry eye problems through lid hygiene and lubricants. Changes in lens diameter (using smaller and looser fitting lenses) often helps. In other patients, larger-diameter lenses provide better corneal coverage and improved tear film distribution. Sometimes, tremendous improvement can be achieved by a simple change in care products.

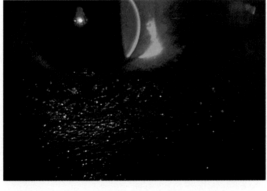

Figure A4–46. Coalesced 3-9 staining in a rigid gas permeable lens wearer.

Dellen

Corneal dellen are depressed areas that occur at the limbus. Most are small, saucer-shaped, relatively shallow, and do not stain unless actively inflamed or mechanically abraded by a lens edge. Dellen are thought to be caused by chronic and profound drying. An adjacent area of raised tissue is a common finding. The elevation may produce a disturbance in surface wetting that causes sufficient drying to give rise to the dellen (Fig. A4–47).

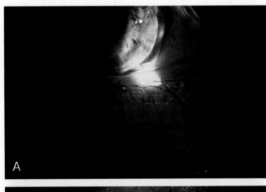

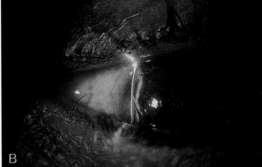

Figure A4–47. *(A)* Dellen at edge of a rigid lens. *(B)* Dellen in a rigid lens wearer. Note the thinned area highlighted by the slit lamp section. *(C)* Dellen in a rigid lens wearer.

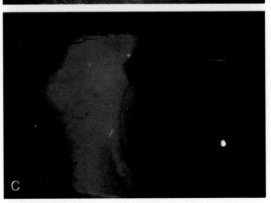

Clinically, dellen are usually preceded by long-standing 3-9 staining in rigid contact lens wearers. As the condition progresses, the area becomes progressively thinned, and local scarring may result. Dellen generally have little effect on vision, but the fragile epithelium overlying the dellen is easily disrupted and can increase the possibility of infection and ulceration.

Management of dellen include the same basic elements of managing 3-9 staining. In addition, cessation of lens wear until the area rehydrates and returns to normal may be necessary.

Although nearly all dellen occur in rigid lens wearers, transient, dellen-like depressions can occur at the edge of a thick soft lens. The edge of the lens is often surrounded by edematous conjunctiva, which may contribute to surface drying. Soft lens dellen resolve quickly with no lasting effects. They usually respond to changes in lens edge design or temporary cessation of lens wear when necessary.

Vascularized Limbal Keratopathy

Vascularized limbal keratopathy (VLK) is a rare limbal inflammation occurring in rigid lens wearers. Described as progressive and locally invasive, it is heralded by the ingrowth of a raised, vascularized mass of epithelial tissue at the limbus. VLK appears to share many of the same causative factors that stimulate other conditions such as 3-9 staining and dellen. However, unlike dellen and most cases of 3-9 staining, VLK often responds well to frequent ocular lubrication and the use of topical decongestants.

Pterygium and Pseudo-pterygium

A pterygium is a hyperplastic fibrovascular overgrowth of conjunctival tissue onto the cornea surface. Pterygia are usually the result of chronic exposure and most frequently occur in patients who are exposed to the elements, such as farmers and seamen. Some authorities believe contact lenses may inflame the pterygia and are thus contraindicated. I have not encountered significant problems with soft lens wear in these patients. In several cases, the lesions actually regressed slightly after soft lens fitting, suggesting a beneficial bandage effect. Unfortunately, these changes did not appear to be therapeutic or overly significant.

A pseudo-pterygium is yet another complication of long-standing 3-9 staining. In this condition, an invasive inflammatory frond of tissue extends centrally and is adherent to the underlying corneal epithelium. Sub-epithelial scarring occurs, and unlike VLK, the changes may be irreversible.

EDEMA-RELATED CONTACT LENS FINDINGS

Edematous Corneal Formations and Central Corneal Clouding

Edematous corneal formations (ECF; Figs. A4–48 and A4–49) and central corneal clouding (CCC) are two complications which are rapidly becoming extinct. They are of greater historical than practical interest, because both complications occur almost exclusively with polymethyl methacrylate (PMMA)

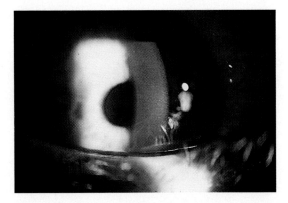

Figure A4–48. Edematous corneal formation in a PMMA rigid lens wearer seen without fluorescein (see Fig. A4–49).

lenses. ECF describes a pseudo-dendritic formation in the corneal epithelium. It occurs in PMMA wearers suffering from chronic, long-term edema. ECF takes weeks or longer to resolve.

Central corneal clouding describes an epithelial haze that is visible using sclerotic scatter. It represents dense epithelial edema caused by acute hypoxia in the central cornea beneath impermeable PMMA lenses. It resolves rapidly after the eye is exposed to oxygen. Treatment for both conditions consists of refitting with more permeable materials.

Deep Stromal Striae

Deep stromal striae are most commonly seen in patients wearing thick, extended wear, aphakic contact lenses. Thin striae occur in the deeper layers of the stroma as a clinically observable consequence of greater than 6% corneal edema. The number of striae observed may correlate with the degree of edematous swelling.

Management ideally requires refitting with more permeable lenses. In practice, this may not be possible given the current state of contact lens technology. This is especially problematic in aphakic patients for whom more perme-

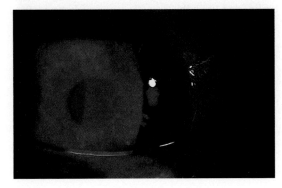

Figure A4–49. Pseudo-dendrite. Edematous corneal formation in a PMMA rigid lens wearer is highlighted by fluorescein (see Fig. A4–48).

able lenses may not be available yet extended lens wear is essential because of handling problems. I have monitored patients with significant striae without additional sequelae for a period of several years.

Epithelial Wrinkling

Epithelial wrinkling is an uncommon complication of soft lens wear. The folds are usually numerous, running parallel to each other in the central cornea (Fig. A4–50). Although a specific etiology has not been conclusively demonstrated, epithelial edema probably is a contributing factor.

The most likely explanation for this condition is that epithelial swelling pushes the cornea up against the lens, causing it to fold back on itself. The resultant ripples are most easily visualized with fluorescein, which pools in the furrows. Epithelial folds rapidly disappear after the lenses are removed.

FULL-THICKNESS FOLDS

Full-thickness corneal folds are an extremely dramatic and very rare complication of soft lens wear.[21] I have encountered only two cases, and both were unilateral. Both patients initiated the examination because of reduced acuity in the affected eye. On slit lamp examination, the lens had a rippled appearance, with deep furrows running obliquely through the entire lens. It looked very much like a rippled potato chip. At first it appeared that only the lens was wrinkled. However, after the lens was removed, the same rippling effect was present on the cornea (Figs. A4–51 through A4–53). Close inspection revealed that the entire cornea was affected and the ripples were full-thickness. One patient was wearing a conventional injection-molded–design soft lens and the other a lathe-cut Crofilcon lens. In both cases, the cornea returned to normal within approximately 1 hour. Both patients were refitted and had no recurrence or lasting consequences. Because of the depth of the folds, it seems likely that this condition is due to more than just mechanical forces. The cause is more likely to be a combination of mechanical and osmotic pressures that combine to produce both suction and molding forces.

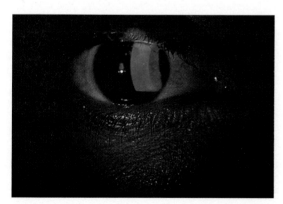

Figure   A4–50.   Epithelial wrinkling caused by chronic edema in a soft lens wearer.

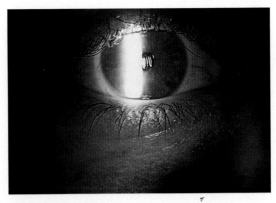

Figure A4–51. Full-thickness corneal folds seen without fluorescein (see Figs. A4–52 and A4–53).

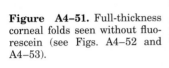

Figure A4–52. Full-thickness corneal folds in a soft lens wearer seen at low magnification with fluorescein (see Figs. A4–51 and A4–53).

Figure A4–53. High magnification of Figure A4–52 (see Fig. A4–51).

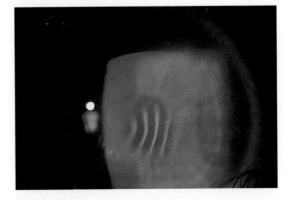

SOFT CONTACT LENS–RELATED ENDOTHELIOPATHY

An interesting and exceedingly rare finding in soft lens wearers is a condition that looks very much like Fuchs' dystrophy. Endothelial thickening and disturbance of the normal endothelial cellular architecture become apparent. A dusting of gutta-like excrescences may be evident. Unlike Fuchs' dystrophy, soft contact lens–related endotheliopathy does not appear to be progressive. Specular microscopy shows a slight reduction in cell count compared to normal. This exceedingly rare condition is associated with prolonged extended wear of soft lenses. Although discontinuation of extended wear is prudent, contact lens wear can be continued if the patient is carefully monitored.

SPECIFIC CORNEAL STAINING PATTERNS

Smile Staining

Corneal smile staining occurs in an arcuate pattern in the inferior paracentral cornea of soft lens wearers. This area seems to have a predilection for coalesced punctate staining. There are several possible reasons for smile staining. The area has a tendency for drying because of blink dynamics and tear distribution. The drying effect is both mechanically irritating and also tends to concentrate toxins in this area. The combination of mechanical disruption and increased absorption of toxins, individually or together, may be responsible for this characteristic finding. Toxicity from residual hydrogen presents with an inferior paracentral staining pattern (Fig. A4–54).

Eliminating contact lens–induced corneal staining is usually challenging and often frustrating. The first step to resolution is finding the cause of the staining. Isolating a specific cause is not an easy task nor is it always possible. In general, toxic reactions to preservatives or other solution components are the most common cause. Rarely, interaction between lens materials and solution components can produce epithelial damage and staining. Because bacterial

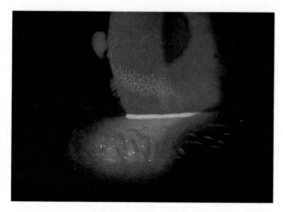

Figure A4–54. Coalesced arcuate staining pattern in a patient with sensitivity to residual hydrogen peroxide.

exotoxins and free fatty acids associated with lid disease are other common causes of staining, instituting a lid hygiene regimen is frequently productive. Because dry eye conditions diminish tear volume and concentrate toxins in the tear film, adjunctive treatment for dry eye and tear film deficiencies may be helpful. Vitamin A drops and lubricants are often useful.

Another potential cause of staining is the interaction between lens design and corneal topography. Increasing lens diameter or using a thinner lens will more evenly distribute bearing forces and will help to eliminate mechanically caused staining.

Doughnut Staining

Doughnut-pattern punctate staining is usually due to mechanical factors, specifically excessive peripheral curve bearing (Fig. A4–55). This occurs when the central curvature of a lens is in alignment but the peripheral curvature is tight. The lens is often small in relation to the overall corneal diameter. Sensitivity to care products or preservatives exacerbate the condition through increased penetration in the annular pattern. Hypoxia worsened by excessive lens–cornea contact may also be a factor. Treatment is the same as that for smile staining.

Toxic Staining

Soft contact lenses are much like sponges. They absorb almost everything in their immediate environment and slowly diffuse it back out. Some of these substances are toxic to the epithelium. The clinical picture of mild toxicity is usually painted by concurrent edema or mechanical factors that increase absorption in the affected areas. With moderate toxicity, the mere presence of the toxic substance is sufficient to damage the epithelial surface. Because the entire cornea is directly involved, the staining pattern is diffuse. The sponge-like properties of the soft lens even the pattern out, although inferior tear pooling may increase the effect locally. Severe toxicity causes a more profound response affecting the conjunctiva as well as the corneal surface.

Occasionally, binding of an otherwise innocuous preservative increases the

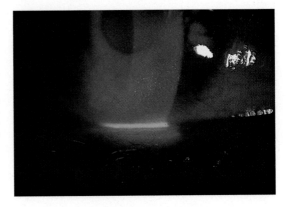

Figure A4–55. Well-circumscribed area of diffuse superficial punctate keratopathy overlying an area of epithelial edema, caused by toxic reaction to a preservative. The doughnut-shaped stain corresponds to an area of soft lens bearing.

concentration to toxic levels. This has occurred with several preservatives, including BAK. In rare cases, combinations of care product components combine or interact to reach toxic levels. Treatment is the same as that for smile staining.

MICROBIAL KERATITIS

Awareness of infectious keratitis is vitally important for the contact lens practitioner. Bacterial infections are of concern both because of the causal relation with contact lens wear and the potential for serious visual loss. Infections, even when not related to contact lens wear, can cause serious ocular damage. In either case, differentiating an infectious process from a less serious contact lens–related inflammation may be difficult. The differential diagnosis may be made even more difficult by the modifying effects of lens wear on the ocular inflammatory response.

INFECTIOUS CORNEAL ULCERS

Although serious contact lens complications are rare, the possibility of their occurrence is frightening, especially to the lay person. The single most feared complication and the one responsible for generating tremendous adverse publicity is the infectious corneal ulcer (Fig. A4–56). Although they are rare, infectious corneal ulcers are potentially disastrous. The precise etiology of infectious ulcers remains obscure; however, logic points to two distinct pathogenic elements. First, contamination of the lens or care products is a prerequisite, especially when infection is from pathogens exclusive to the normal ocular environment. Second, a breach must occur in the normal corneal barriers for any infection to occur. Few species of bacteria are capable of invading and infecting an intact cornea.

Understanding the actual mechanism of infection requires piecing together elements from many different studies. Most microbial keratitis in contact lens wearers is due to gram-negative organisms such as *Pseudomonas aeruginosa*. These bacteria flourish in the bio-film that coats contaminated contact lens cases.

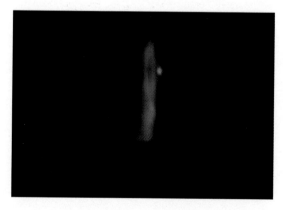

Figure A4–56. Early but rapidly progressing *Pseudomonas* ulcer in a soft lens wearer. Note the fluffy border and density of the lesion.

On contact lenses, *Pseudomonas* adheres to roughened surfaces like jelly bump lipid deposits. A recent study demonstrated the relation between oxygen permeability and binding of *Pseudomonas* to corneal epithelium, suggesting that epithelial edema is a significant and essential part of the development of this condition.[4]

Overnight wear, especially of soft contact lenses, has been described as the primary risk factor for developing bacterial infections of the cornea.[22] Extended wear is an important factor but only in that it serves as an umbrella for many different, more specific, and more approachable risk factors. Corneal edema, contact lens deposits, and surface disruption secondary to mechanical factors or solution interactions are all more proximate causes of infection. As suggested previously, many of these factors can be identified and eliminated.

The clinical presentation of bacterial keratitis depends on the pathogen involved and the stage of the infection. Bacteria such as the dreaded *Pseudomonas* organism are so virulent that patients often present with a frightening clinical picture. A large portion of the corneal surface can be involved, with significant destruction of normal corneal architecture. The cornea ulcerates with excavation into the stroma. *Pseudomonas* produces a thick, adherent mucous bio-film with a white or yellowish white appearance. Visual loss from scarring can be substantial after healing is complete.

Fortunately, most corneal ulcers in contact lens wearers are not severe. In fact, it is usually more difficult to decide whether an ulcer is a true ulcer or a non-infectious infiltrate. Peripheral corneal lesions, especially when small, are often sterile. Central lesions must always be viewed with more suspicion, because the threat to vision is greater, as is the likelihood of an infectious etiology. Differentiating between sterile and infectious corneal lesions can be difficult but is clinically important. General guidelines must be used with extreme caution but can be helpful. Small lesions, raised lesions, and lesions in the corneal periphery are generally sterile. Severe ocular pain is an important indicator of possible pathogenicity. However, all of these clues aside, the only way to know that a lesion is sterile is if the patient presents with a lesion that is resolving. Even then, if there is an epithelial defect, superinfection is still possible.

Discussion of the many possible bacterial pathogens that cause corneal infection in contact lens wearers is beyond the scope of this appendix. Treatment strategy depends on the location and size of the lesion. Small peripheral ulcers should be treated with broad-spectrum antibiotics and monitored closely. Lesions that are unusual in appearance and those associated with great pain, regardless of location, should be treated aggressively. Larger lesions, especially when central, must be cultured and treated aggressively usually with fortified antibiotics given every hour around the clock. Hospitalization to insure compliance may be advisable. The use of topical steroid drops should be avoided until the infection is clearly under control and then should be used only when the visual axis is threatened.

It is important to emphasize the cooperative role of the corneal specialist in the management of potentially serious corneal ulcers. Do not take chances: if in doubt, refer it out. Corneal ulcers rapidly can turn into disasters. The referral should be made as soon as possible after a suspicious lesion is discovered. If the patient will be seen in a short time, medication should be avoided, because this will preclude productive culture. If significant time will elapse before the patient is seen by the specialist, it may be advisable to begin a course of fortified antibiotics in consultation with the specialist.

VIRAL KERATITIS

Many viruses can cause conjunctivitis and keratitis. Although viral keratitis is not related to contact lens wear, contact lens wearers do develop viral infections. Most viruses run their course without serious or long-lasting impact on the eye. Because there is no treatment for these infections, cessation of contact lens wear is usually all that is necessary until the infection passes. Several viruses are capable of causing profound and permanent damage to the cornea. It is important for the contact lens fitter to be familiar with the viral keratopathies. Prompt treatment may be necessary to limit potential damage from the infection. Viral infections can present a confusing clinical picture, especially in the contact lens wearer. The differential diagnosis is sometimes difficult but nonetheless is important.

Herpes Simplex Keratitis

Herpes simplex keratitis is one of the leading causes of blindness in the United States. It is fairly common and can occur in contact lens wearers. The initial presentation is variable, often beginning with a follicular conjunctivitis and non-specific punctate keratopathy. The infection may or may not be bilateral and is more likely to occur in patients who are immune-compromised. Patients frequently complain of foreign-body sensation, tearing, and photophobia. Vesicles may appear on the eyelids and ulcerative blepharitis may occur. Preauricular lymphadenopathy is also common. Corneal hypoesthesia is an important sign that is typical of, but not exclusive to, herpes simplex virus (HSV) infection.

Epithelial dendritic lesions are pathognomonic for HSV (Fig. A4–57). These dendrites are linear branching lesions with characteristic true end bulbs. They last for approximately 10 days, leave no scar, and can stain with both fluorescein and rose bengal. HSV infection can progress to stromal keratitis and is often recurrent.

Unfortunately, HSV keratitis can have tremendous variability in presentation. In a sense, HSV is the great pretender, and the corneal findings can paint a confusing clinical picture, especially in the contact lens wearer. In such

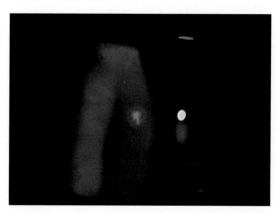

Figure A4–57. Herpes simplex dendrite masquerading as a contact lens–related infiltrate in a immune-compromised soft lens wearer. Fluorescein reveals the dendrite.

cases, laboratory testing is helpful in establishing a diagnosis. Topical anti-viral treatment is usually beneficial.

Epstein-Barr Keratitis

Epstein-Barr virus (EBV) is a member of the herpesvirus family. It can cause a keratitis including epithelial dendrites and stromal involvement. Various types of infiltrates have been reported with EBV infection, ranging from wispy, subepithelial infiltrates to dense, full-thickness infiltrates. Follicular conjunctivitis may also occur with EBV infection. Treatment is typically palliative because the condition is usually self-limiting. When the patient is extremely symptomatic or stromal keratitis is significant, topical corticosteroids may be used.

Pseudo-dendritic Keratitis

Pseudo-dendrites occur in several conditions. They have been reported with use of the preservative thimerosal, in *Acanthamoeba* keratitis, with EBV infections, and with herpes zoster infections. ECF also has a dendritic appearance but occurs in the deeper corneal layers (see Fig. A4–48).

Pseudo-dendrites are usually easy to differentiate from the true HSV dendrite. Pseudo-dendrites are characteristically elevated, lack true end bulbs, and typically do not stain with fluorescein but will stain with rose bengal.

THYGESSON'S SUPERFICIAL PUNCTATE KERATOPATHY

Thygesson's SPK is a relatively rare corneal surface disease. It is characterized by numerous coarse epithelial lesions distributed throughout the cornea. The individual lesions are irregular, round to oval, and often slightly elevated, with a characteristic popcorn-like appearance.

Patients may complain of a persistent foreign-body sensation; however, symptoms are variable and not related to the severity of surface disease. The conjunctiva is typically white, and the eyes appear normal. Photophobia and tearing may be significant. Thygesson's SPK responds rapidly to topical corticosteroid drops; however, recurrence is common after the drops are discontinued. Contact lenses are often effective in ameliorating symptoms. Although a viral etiology has been suspected, it has never been proven.

EPIDEMIC KERATOCONJUNCTIVITIS AND PHARYNGOCONJUNCTIVAL FEVER

Epidemic keratoconjunctivitis (EKC) and pharyngoconjunctival fever (PCF) are common adenoviral infections. Both are highly contagious, lasting from 1 to 3 weeks. Both are unrelated to contact lens wear. Patients typically present with acute keratoconjunctivitis, intense injection, a watery discharge, and chemosis. Although not always present, the corneal findings of multiple subepithelial infiltrates can predominate the clinical picture. These infiltrates typically occur within 2 weeks after the start of the infection.

Because of the similarity to contact lens–associated infiltrative keratitis, EKC and PCF can also present a confusing clinical picture in the contact lens wearer. Keys to making the differential diagnosis are preauricular lymphadenopathy, a mixed papillo-follicular conjunctivitis, membrane formation (in EKC), and conjunctival petechial hemorrhages, all of which are characteristic of adenoviral infection. In PCF, upper respiratory symptoms are common.

Treatment is usually not required. In severe cases, especially when infiltrates in the visual axis are dense and could compromise sight, treatment with topical steroid drops can be helpful in reducing inflammation and scarring.

ACANTHAMOEBA KERATITIS

Acanthamoeba is a ubiquitous protozoan organism present in fresh water and soil. Although the organism rarely infects the intact cornea, trauma and especially contact lens wear are significant risk factors for infection. The organism exists in two states: the trophozoite and a well-protected dormant cystic form. Acanthamoeba cysts are extremely resistant to nearly all forms of therapy, making treatment of infection extremely difficult. In contact lens wearers, exposure to contaminated water usually precedes infection. Use of non-sterile water to make saline and exposure to swimming pool or hot tub water are thought to be risk factors.

The clinical presentation is extremely variable, especially in the early stages of infection. Initially, the presentation may resemble non-specific contact lens–associated red eye with sub-epithelial opacities, infiltrates, and diffuse conjunctival injection. Discomfort may be minor, with tearing and diffuse injection the predominant features. As the disease progresses, pain becomes more common, often reaching intense levels. Acanthamoeba infection commonly mimics herpes infections, which are also quite variable in presentation. A surprising number of Acanthamoeba infections are initially diagnosed and treated as herpes keratitis. Dendritic lesions and lessened corneal sensitivity have been reported. Ring infiltrates have also been found accompanying Acanthamoeba infection.

Diagnosis requires laboratory confirmation of infection. Although treatment is difficult, the infection will inexorably progress when untreated. Referral to a corneal specialist is strongly advised. Although this infection is exceedingly rare, the results are often devastating. Minimizing risk requires educating patients about risk factors: use of non-sterile water to prepare saline should be avoided. Rinsing lenses, including RGP lenses, with tap water is also a potential source of infection. Swimming while wearing lenses may be a vector for infection. Heat disinfection, although otherwise virtually obsolete, may be advisable for patients exposed to conditions favorable to Acanthamoeba infection. The use of alcohol-based cleaning solutions is effective at killing both trophozoite and cystic forms of Acanthamoeba.

CHLAMYDIAL KERATITIS

Chlamydiosis is a common sexually transmitted disease. In the eye, chlamydial infection may be difficult to distinguish clinically. There is often a mixed papillo-follicular conjunctivitis, a mucus-laden ocular discharge, and possible urinary tract involvement. The cornea may show a diffuse punctate keratopathy with sub-epithelial infiltrates, especially superiorly. The conjunctival findings in chlamydial infection may be confused with GPC. In addition, the corneal findings may be difficult to differentiate from contact lens–related keratopathy. Systemic treatment using tetracycline or erythromycin is indicated in chlamydial infections because concurrent urinary tract infection is often present.

ANTERIOR SEGMENT DISEASE AND CONTACT LENSES

Contact lenses can cause anterior segment disease, and they can be helpful in treating it. This section presents many of the conditions that benefit from contact lens treatment. Some of the more common conditions that the contact lens practitioner needs to be aware of are also discussed.

Vogt's Striae

Vogt's striae are fine white lines at the level of Descemet's membrane. They are typically oriented vertically, although horizontal orientations have been seen. These striae are believed to be caused by stress, thinning, and protrusion of the cornea in thinning disorders such as keratoconus. Light digital pressure on the globe makes Vogt's striae disappear, confirming the diagnosis.

Fleischer's Ring

This is the most recognizable finding in keratoconus. Fleischer's ring is formed of hemosiderin deposited around the base of the cone in the deeper epithelial layers. A faint, white, fibrillar line can also circle the cornea at the base of the cone (Fig. A4–58). The cause of Fleischer's ring probably is related to tear film disturbance. In that sense, it is also related to the Hudson-Stähli line seen in normal patients. It is present in at least 50% of all keratoconus cases and becomes increasingly well defined with progression of the disease.

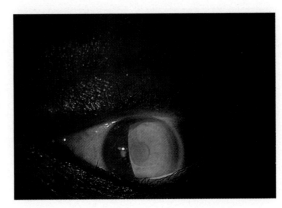

Figure A4–58. Fibrillar line around the cone in a keratoconic patient.

KERATOCONUS

Keratoconus is a non-inflammatory, variably progressive, thinning disorder of the central cornea. Axial thinning results in a cone-like protrusion that causes irregular astigmatism, increased corneal curvature, and ultimately increased optical distortion. The condition is usually bilateral but is typically asymmetric in both its presentation and severity.

Although the cause is unknown, keratoconus appears to have a hereditary basis in approximately 8% of cases. It is associated with several ocular and systemic disorders including atopy, Marfan's syndrome, Ehlers-Danlos syndrome, osteogenesis imperfecta, and Down's syndrome. Keratoconus is also associated with retinitis pigmentosa, retrolental fibroplasia, posterior polymorphous dystrophy of the cornea, and, as noted most recently, floppy eyelid syndrome.

Localized mechanical factors seem to play an important role in the genesis of keratoconus. Proponents of a mechanical etiology point to atopy and eye rubbing as strong contributing factors. Mechanical trauma caused by rigid contact lens wear has also been implicated as a possible contributing factor. Down's syndrome and floppy eyelid syndrome, conditions in which eye rubbing is a prominent finding, have both been associated with keratoconus.

In mild cases, the diagnosis of keratoconus may be difficult to reach, especially in contact lens wearers. An unexplained increase in corneal cylinder, especially with a history of atopy and eye-rubbing, is suggestive.

Corneal modeling devices have been extremely helpful in the diagnoses of marginal cases. However, care must be exercised when examining all contact lens–wearing patients. Transient corneal distortion can mimic keratoconus and present a confusing picture. In advanced cases, several findings are characteristic of the disease and aid in reaching the diagnosis.

CORNEAL SCARRING IN KERATOCONUS

Scarring is a frequent concomitant of keratoconus (Fig. A4–59). Some scarring seems to be part of the natural progression of the disease, and some patients present with scarring in the absence of prior contact lens wear. This "natural"

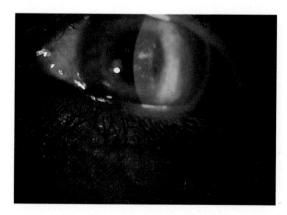

Figure A4–59. Apical scarring at Bowman's layer in keratoconus.

scarring characteristically occurs around Bowman's membrane and appears to be intrinsic to the overall degenerative process. In severe cases, scarring of the deeper cornea may be seen. Contact lens wear may also cause superficial scarring (Fig. A4–60). In many cases, this scarring diminishes or completely resolves after the patient is refitted. When a contact lens–wearing patient presents with superficial scarring, especially when it is associated with localized punctate keratopathy, a contact lens with reduced bearing in the affected area should be fitted. Resolution of the scarring can be rapid or can take several months to well over a year and can be partial or complete. Another explanation for the reduction of scarring in keratoconus patients is that the supportive qualities of a properly fitted rigid lens can reduce stress and subsequent scarring.

CORNEAL HYDROPS

Corneal hydrops, also known as acute keratoconus, is caused by a break in Descemet's membrane. The break permits a rapid inrush of aqueous humor. The resultant edema can produce significant visual loss and accompanying inflammation. This condition is transient, with the edema resolving over several weeks to months. Subsequent scarring can interfere with vision or, conversely, can reduce corneal curvature to more normal levels from secondary contraction. In some cases, the inflammatory component may be substantial, with anterior segment cell and flare. Reports of corneal perforation in acute hydrops make careful monitoring of potential infection prudent.

HURRICANE KERATOPATHY

Hurricane keratopathy, also known as swirl staining, occurs as a consequence of excessive lens–cornea bearing. The affected area develops a characteristic punctate keratitis that appears in a swirl pattern, mimicking the hurricane pattern of weather maps. Like most punctate keratopathy associated with rigid lens wear, super-infection is rare. If the condition persists, apical scarring will usually result. Treatment requires refitting the patient with a lens with diminished apical bearing.

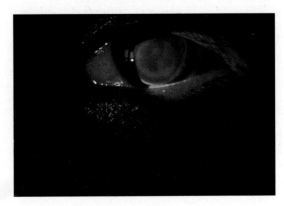

Figure A4–60. Central bearing with abrasion in a keratoconic rigid gas permeable lens wearer.

PELLUCID MARGINAL DEGENERATION

Pellucid marginal degeneration is a variant of keratoconus affecting the inferior cornea. There is a narrow zone of corneal thinning, 1 to 2 mm wide, parallel to the inferior limbus. The inferior thinning produces protrusion of the cornea above the thinned area and marked against-the-rule astigmatism and surface irregularity. The condition is usually bilateral and is difficult to distinguish from keratoconus in some patients. The condition is difficult to correct surgically. The area of greatest thinning is in the far periphery, making penetrating keratoplasty extremely complicated. A large donor button is needed, and suturing must be done in an area of very thin cornea. Alternately, an initial tectonic lamellar corneal graft can provide the stroma necessary for a subsequent conventional penetrating keratoplasty. Unfortunately, this technique requires two separate surgeries and a visual rehabilitation period of at least 1.5 years.

In advanced cases, pellucid marginal degeneration presents one the greatest fitting challenges. Custom-designed soft toric lenses and SoftPerm hybrid lenses have been used with good results.

KERATOGLOBUS

This rare, bilateral condition involves thinning of the entire cornea, especially in the periphery. The cornea is usually normal in diameter and, other than thinning, there are few distinctive signs. Keratoglobus may be present from birth or may be acquired in adulthood. It is rarely progressive.

Contact lens correction of this condition is required when distortion and irregularity become visually disabling. However, there is a marked propensity for corneal rupture or perforation secondary to even minor trauma. For this reason, protective eyewear is advisable, even when contact lenses are worn. Fitting large custom soft lenses is preferred when possible. Fitting keratoglobus patients with rigid lenses is similar to fitting post-penetrating keratoplasty patients; however, the irregular topography of the cornea often requires the use of soft/rigid piggyback systems.

PSEUDO-KERATOCONUS AND CORNEAL WARPAGE SPECTACLE BLUR

Warpage of the corneal surface caused by contact lens wear is a long-recognized complication of contact lens wear. This problem had been frequently encountered with PMMA lenses, and the literature contains many reports associated with corneal distortion and PMMA lens wear.

Spectacle blur is a minor and transient form of corneal warpage. Rigid lens–molding effects alter corneal topography sufficiently to evoke a noticeable change in prescription. Patients report blur immediately after removing their lenses, with the effect lasting a variable amount of time. With PMMA lenses, the primary cause is corneal edema. With modern materials, spectacle blur is most frequently associated with tightly fitted aspheric lenses. The molding effect can be minimized by refitting with a lens with a flatter base curve. PMMA wearers should routinely be refitted with more permeable materials.

CORNEAL WARPAGE

Warpage of the corneal surface occurs with both rigid and soft lenses. Almost all reports of corneal distortion in the literature involve rigid contact lenses, although it probably occurs as frequently in soft lens wearers.[23] Contact lens warpage can take several weeks or even months to resolve. When resolution fails to occur, keratoconus or other corneal pathology should be suspected as the cause of the topographic disturbance.

RIGID LENS WARPAGE

Rigid lens wearers, especially those wearing PMMA lenses, often have visual disturbance as a consequence of contact lens wear. Although it is agreed that they require refitting, there is much controversy regarding how to go about rehabilitating their distorted corneas.

Some practitioners suggest that patients discontinue rigid lens wear for several days before examination and refitting. This makes little sense. In PMMA wearers, Rengstorff demonstrated that at least 2 weeks without wearing lenses are needed before the cornea returns to a reasonably normal state.[24, 25] In RGP wearers, the lessened physiologic and mechanical effects of the lens should make cessation before refitting unnecessary.

When a patient has significant corneal distortion, it may take many months before the cornea stabilizes. Because eyeglasses are of little value, forcing the patient to do without adequate correction is at best cruel and often unacceptable. I have found that in cases in which the cornea is physically intact, immediate refitting usually makes the most sense. It also is least disruptive to the patient's routine. It may be necessary to refine the fit several times as the cornea returns to normalcy. However, with warranties and fit guarantees, this does not present the logistical problems it once did. Immediate refitting also seems to minimize the recovery time because the cornea is exposed to increased oxygen more gradually and is physically braced by the presence of the new lens.

It is important to explain to patients that several visits and lens changes may be needed to complete the fit. They should also be warned that switching to more permeable materials will sometimes result in transiently increased lens awareness.

SOFT LENS WARPAGE

Many soft lens wearers experience transient episodes of corneal distortion. Most commonly, this occurs unilaterally. In most normal binocular patients, these visual changes go unnoticed because the patient continues to see well with the other eye.

Prior to the advent of computerized corneal topographic analysis, quantification of soft lens–associated corneal topographic distortion (SLATCD) was virtually impossible. Conventional keratometric instruments are essentially useless in identifying this condition because of their limited measurement ability. This explains why SLATCD has been so infrequently described in the literature.

In many respects, SLATCD resembles keratoconus. Affected patients have decreased vision in the involved eye. There is often an oil droplet retinoscopic reflex, increased astigmatism, and increased topographic irregularity. A refractive end point is difficult to find, and acuity may be dramatically reduced. Topographic analysis often suggests early keratoconus; however, unlike true keratoconus, the condition typically resolves within several days or weeks.

Refitting, even with exactly the same lens, appears to be an effective treatment. In cases in which resolution does not occur, fitting with thinner and flatter contact lenses may be necessary. In some cases, refitting with toric soft lenses may be necessary to deal with residual astigmatism. When patients remain unstable, discontinuing lens wear or refitting with high-Dk RGP lenses is indicated.

DIFFERENTIAL DIAGNOSIS OF INCREASED REFRACTIVE ERROR OR DECREASED ACUITY IN SOFT LENS WEARERS

It is important to determine whether increased refractive error or decreased acuity is truly contact lens–related. Significant increases in spherical correction are rarely pathologically related to contact lens wear. Myopic creep can cause small spherical increases, but significant shifts are rare. This condition seems more likely to be associated with chronic lens-related edema. Most often, refractive shifts are caused by changes in the crystalline lens or as a presentation of systemic disease (e.g., diabetes).

Increases in regular or irregular astigmatism are more difficult to diagnose. First, are the changes corneal? Comparison of initial and current keratometry readings will be helpful. It is also important to determine whether the changes are transient or stable. Transient increases in astigmatism are likely to be contact lens–related. In most cases, lens replacement or refitting will hasten the return to normal. In cases in which large increases of astigmatism occur, underlying pathology must be ruled out.

Keratoconus is the most common condition associated with acute refractive change. Contact lens wear appears to be a risk factor for the development of keratoconus. A confirmed diagnosis can be difficult to establish in the early stages. Pellucid marginal degeneration can also produce significant increases in against-the-rule corneal astigmatism, even in its otherwise difficult to identify early stages. Other corneal conditions capable of effecting refractive change typically are accompanied or preceded by significant pathology.

In some patients, increases in corneal astigmatism appears to be permanent. Whether these changes are an early presentation of corneal disease or a naturally occurring refractive change can be equivocal. It is important to remember that no known disease causing only refractive change without other signs or symptoms causes irreversible corneal damage without warning. Patients should be reassured and followed expectantly. In most cases, changes in the patient's correction are all that is necessary.

EPITHELIAL BASEMENT MEMBRANE DISEASE

This condition describes a spectrum of diseases that are common but so variable in presentation that the contact lens clinician may be confronted with a potentially confusing clinical picture. In this condition, redundant or reduplicated basement membrane creates raised areas of corneal epithelium. The

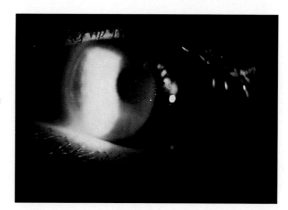

Figure A4–61. Geographic basement membrane dystrophy.

affected areas can arise spontaneously or secondary to trauma, especially from an organic object. Many cases are benign and produce no symptoms; however, diminished epithelial adhesion can cause spontaneous and recurrent corneal epithelial erosions. Typically, the patient is awakened by a sharp, intense pain in the affected eye. The pain persists and is accompanied by copious tearing and photophobia.

The appearance of these lesions is variable. Raised geographic areas–dots, microcysts, and fingerprint-like figures–can occur individually or together (Figs. A4–61 and A4–62) Fluorescein pooling around the raised areas usually enhances visibility and can draw the examiner's attention to the otherwise barely visible condition. Treatment includes patching, hypertonic salt solutions, lubricating ointments applied before sleep, and bandage contact lenses. In more severe or recalcitrant cases, anterior stromal puncture, epithelial debridement, and most recently, excimer laser ablation may be helpful.

LIMBAL GIRDLE

Although not related to contact lens wear, the limbal girdle of Vogt is a common finding, especially among the elderly population. It is worthy of men-

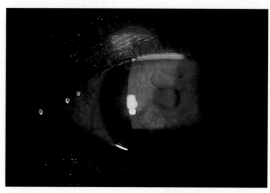

Figure A4–62. Geographic figures in epithelial basement membrane disease.

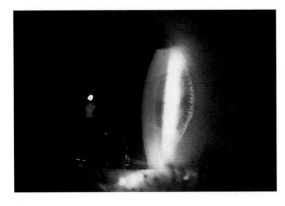

Figure A4–63. Limbal girdle of Vogt.

tion simply because it is so common. In many cases, the presentation is dramatic and at first notice, its circumlimbal location may suggest a contact lens–related complication. However, it is a normal degenerative process that is neither affected by nor affecting contact lens wear.

There are two types of limbal girdle classically described. Type I is thought to be an early presentation of calcific bond keratopathy. Type II is more common and consists of an irregular, white arcuate deposit separated from the limbus by a clear zone (Fig. A4–63). Finger-like projections radiate toward the corneal apex.

PINGUECULA

A pinguecula is a degenerative lesion of the bulbar conjunctiva. Typically yellow-white in appearance, pingueculae are found adjacent to the limbus, most commonly on the nasal side. Although differentiation from other more serious lesions is important, especially the similar-appearing Bowen's carcinoma in situ, pingueculae are usually of little concern.

In soft lens wearers, the edge of the lens may inflame the pinguecula and complicate fitting. Management requires refitting with a lens of a different diameter or thinner edge profile. In severe cases, excision of the inflamed pinguecula may be necessary.

TERRIEN'S MARGINAL DEGENERATION

Terrien's degeneration is a non-inflammatory peripheral corneal thinning disorder of unknown etiology. Lipid is deposited at the central leading edge of the thinned area. In its early stages, mild visual disruption from increased astigmatism and a vascularized arcus-like haze can suggest contact lens–related pathology.

Terrien's degeneration is usually bilateral, although it is asymmetrical in presentation. Some cases remain stable, whereas others can progress to produce significant corneal astigmatism and distortion. In advanced cases, perforation is possible. Contact lenses can be a useful adjunct in the visual management of affected patients.

SALZMANN'S DEGENERATION

Salzmann's degeneration is a whitish, raised, subepithelial area of opacification that occurs in adults. The nodules are often seen in the periphery, most commonly in an area that has previously been affected by disease. They may be vascularized. Awareness of Salzmann's nodules is necessary to distinguish them from neoplasms and other degenerative changes.

HUDSON-STÄHLI LINE

The Hudson-Stähli line is a rust-colored iron deposit in the epithelium that extends horizontally across the cornea where the upper and lower lids meet in closure. It is believed to be related to chronic irritation and tear film abnormalities. The line appears in an area of tear film concentration and stagnation, which increases the absorption of iron. Dry eye conditions that concentrate the tear film increase tear-borne iron and thus the Hudson-Stähli line.

Although the Hudson-Stähli line is a common finding in the normal population, its presence suggests tear film stagnation or an irritative process that may be of prognostic significance in contact lens wearers.[26] Because many contact lens complications occur in this area, the same anatomic peculiarities that cause the Hudson-Stähli line can increase the possibility of contact lens complications affecting the inferior para-central cornea.

SUBCONJUNCTIVAL HEMORRHAGE

Although a subconjunctival hemorrhage is a well-recognized and almost always benign entity, it seems no one bothered to tell the patients this. The subconjunctival hemorrhage is among the most frequent causes of emergency office visits.

The relation between subconjunctival hemorrhage and contact lens wear is not always clear; however, persistent or rough contact lens removal may be a precipitating factor. The edge of a soft lens sometimes blocks the spread of hemorrhage, leaving a clear zone around the limbus (Fig. A4–64). Doctors not

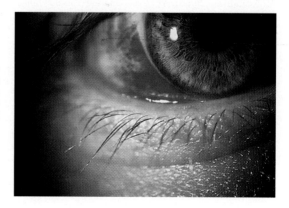

Figure A4–64. Subconjunctival hemorrhage in a patient wearing a soft lens. Note the delineation at the limbal border where the lens edge prevented extravasation of the blood.

familiar with contact lenses are sometimes confused by this, assuming incorrectly that the lens edge caused the hemorrhage.

When a patient presents with a subconjunctival hemorrhage, it is a good opportunity to show your staff what it looks like. I discovered the hard way that a spontaneous subconjunctival hemorrhage during insertion and removal training can be extremely frightening to an inexperienced contact lens technician.

BIBLIOGRAPHY

Abel R, Shovlin JP, DePaolis MD: A treatise on hydrophilic lens induced superior limbic keratoconjunctivitis. Int Contact Lens Clin 1985;12:116.

Aswad Ml, John T, Barza M, et al: Bacterial adherence to extended wear soft contact lenses. Ophthalmology 1990;97(3):296.

Bergmanson JP: Histopathological analysis of the corneal epithelium after contact lens wear. J Am Optom Assoc 1987;58(10):812.

Donnenfeld ED, Ingraham H, Perry HD, Imundo M, Goldberg LP: Contact Lens–related deep stromal intracorneal hemorrhage. Ophthalmology 1981;98:1793.

Epstein AB, Donnenfeld ED: Hudson Stahli line. Contact Lens Forum 1990;15(2):46.

Epstein AB, Donnenfeld ED: Immune ring infiltrates in a soft CL wearer. Contact Lens Forum 1988;13(10):45.

Epstein AB, Donnenfeld ED: Peripheral corneal epithelial hypertrophy. Contact Lens Forum 1989;14(11):54.

Fuerst DJ, Sugar J, Worobec S: Superior limbic keratoconjunctivitis associated with cosmetic soft contact lens wear. Arch Ophthalmol 1983;101:1214.

Hart DE, Tisdale RR, Sack RA: Origin and composition of lipid deposits on soft contact lenses. Ophthalmology 1986;93(4):495.

Imayasu M, Petroll WM, Jester JV, et al: The relation between contact lens oxygen transmissibility and binding of Pseudomonas aeruginosa to the cornea after overnight wear. Ophthalmology 1994;101(2):371.

Koch JM, Refojo MF, Hanninen LA, et al: Experimental Pseudomonas aeruginosa keratitis from extended wear of soft contact lenses. Arch Ophthalmol 1990;108(10):1453.

Laroche RR, Camobell RC: Intracorneal hemorrhaqe induced by chronic extended wear of a soft contact lens. CLAO J 1987;13:39.

Lawin-Brussel CA, Refojo MF, Leong FL, et al: Time course of experimental Pseudomonas aeruginosa keratitis in contact lens overwear. Arch Ophthalmol 1990;108(7):1012.

Lowe R, Brennan N: Corneal wrinkling caused by a thin medium water content lens. Int Contact Lens Clin 1987;14:403.

Maltzman B, Cinotti A: Extender-wear contact lenses. Contact Intraocular Lens Med J 1979;5(3):19.

Mutti DO, Seger RG: Eyelid asymmetry in unilateral hydrogel contact lens wear. ICLC 1988;15(8):252–255.

Paugh J, Caywood T, Peterson S: Toxic reactions associated with chemical disinfection of contact lenses. Int Contact Lens Clin 1984;11:680.

Refojo MF: Reversible binding of chlorhexidine gluconate to hydrogel contact lenses. Contact Intraocular Lens Med J 1976;2:47.

Rengstorff RH: Variations in myopia measurements: an aftereffect observed with habitual wearers of contact lenses. Am J Optom 1967;44:149.

Rengstorff RH: Variations in corneal curvature measurements: an aftereffect observed with habitual wearers of contact lenses. Am J Optom 1969;46:45.

Schein OD, Glynn RJ, Poggio EC, et al: The risk of ulcerative keratitis among users of daily-wear and extended-wear soft contact lenses: a case control study. N Engl J Med 1989;321:773.

Sendale DD, Kenyon KR, Mobilia F, et al: Superior limbic keratoconjunctivitis in contact lens wearers. Ophthalmology 1983;90(5):616.

Stenson SM: Superior limbic keratoconjunctivitis associated with soft contact lens wear. Arch Ophthalmol 1983;101:402.

Stenson SM: Soft lens related SLK. Contact Lens Forum 1986;11(12):22.

Theodore FH: Superior limbic keratoconjunctivitis. Ear Nose Throat J 1963;42:25.

Wallace W. Soft contact lens associated superior limbic keratoconjunctivitis. Int Eye Care 1985;1:427.

Williams CE: Soft contact lens toxic occlusion phenomenon. Contact Lens Spectrum 1986;1(11):14.

Wilson SE, Lin DT, Klyce SD, et al: Topographic changes in contact lens-induced corneal warpage. Ophthalmology 1990;97:734.

Questions and Answers About Legal Issues in a Contact Lens Practice

MARIAN C. WELLING

As a professional, the contact lens practitioner has a special relationship with his or her patients. As in any such relationship, there are legal implications and issues at stake. The law protects both doctor and patient, but it allocates risk in a way society feels is most fair. This means that the professional shoulders the main burden in a doctor–patient relationship. The following questions and answers are designed to help the contact lens practitioners understand some of the legal issues that affect contact lens practice.

CONTRACT LAW

Q. What is a contact lens fitting agreement?

A. A contact lens fitting agreement is a contract that you enter into with your patient. A contract is a promise or set of promises, the performance of which the law recognizes as a duty, and for breach of which the law gives a remedy. This means that a contract creates a legal duty on your part to perform the promises you made in the fitting agreement. Typical promises the doctor makes in this agreement are to evaluate eye health and vision status; to measure and fit the eye with contact lenses; to provide a pair of contact lenses, a care kit, and instructions on use; and to provide specified follow-up care.

In turn, the contract has created a legal duty on the part of the patient. The patient's promises normally consist of a promise to pay the fee and a promise to comply with the doctor's instructions. If either party fails to perform the promises, that party has breached the contract. When a contract has been breached, the law provides a remedy; this is most often damages. Damages are monies given to compensate the party who suffered the breach for their time, efforts, and any monetary loss.

Q. Does a contact lens fitting agreement protect the doctor from liability?

A. No. An agreement does not extinguish liability. A contract cannot do away with either a doctor's duty or a patient's right to sue. A doctor can be sued under many theories; lack of informed consent, product liability, and negligence are the most common. If a contract such as the fitting agreement exists, the doctor could also be sued for breach under contract theory.

Q. Should a doctor enter into a contract lens fitting agreement with a patient even though it doesn't offer protection from all liability?

A. Yes. The agreement should explain the fees and services to the patient and also emphasize the fact that the patient has promised to comply with instructions. It can also emphasize the fact that the fee is for both services and materials, so the patient understands why a refund of all his or her money is not made if the fitting is unsuccessful.

The contract is your evidence that a patient knows and understands the terms of your agreement from the outset.

Q. Is the contact lens fitting agreement legal even if it is not in writing?

A. Yes, either an oral or written agreement can be a contract and legally binding. Contracts are described as express or implied. An express contract is formed by language, either oral or written. An implied contract is formed by manifestations of assent other than oral or written language, such as by conduct.

Q. Is there an advantage to writing it down?

A. The advantage of a written contract is that there cannot be a dispute over the terms of the contract. The terms of the agreement should be discussed with the patient so that you are sure the patient understands what he or she is agreeing to. If the patient objectively manifests assent, he or she is bound by all contract terms that a reasonable person would have noted and understood. Blanket form recitals stating that the patient has read and understood every provision and agrees to be bound thereby will not prevent a court from applying the objective standard. The use of a written contract lessens the likelihood of disagreement or misunderstanding between the doctor and the patient.

Q. What is a contact lens service agreement?

A. Like the contact lens fitting agreement, a contact lens service agreement is a contract with the same legal implications therein. The main reason for the service contract is to provide the patient with prepaid services and materials for a specified time.

Q. Where do I get contact lens fitting agreements and service agreements.

A. It is best to hire an attorney to draft fitting and service agreements that have terms and conditions tailored to your specific requirements.

THE LAW OF INFORMED CONSENT

Q. How much must I tell a patient to satisfy the doctrine of informed consent?

A. In general, you must provide the patient with enough information so that he or she can make a reasonable decision. A doctor must consider disclosure of a variety of factors:
1. Diagnosis, including steps preceding diagnosis, tests and their alternatives, and disclosure of the risks of foregoing a diagnostic procedure.
2. The nature and purpose of the proposed treatment.
3. The risks of the treatment. Risks that are remote can be omitted. The threshold of disclosure varies with the product of the probability and the severity of the risk.

4. The probability of success in terms of the general population and the patient's specific probability of success.
5. Treatment alternatives that are generally acknowledged as feasible.

The doctrine of informed consent has developed out of a strong judicial deference toward individual autonomy, reflecting a belief that an individual has a right to be free from non-consensual interference with his or her person and a basic moral principle that it is wrong to force another to act against his or her will.

Q. What purpose does informed consent serve?
A. The doctrine of informed consent serves six salutary functions:
1. It protects individual autonomy.
2. It protects the patient's status as a human being.
3. It avoids fraud or duress.
4. It encourages doctors to carefully consider their decisions.
5. It fosters rational decision-making by the patient.
6. It involves the public in health care.

Q. How could I be sued for lack of informed consent?
A. There are two theories under which a patient can sue for a lack of informed consent. One is a battery theory, which is unconsented touching of another's person. The other is negligence, meaning the doctor failed to disclose enough information to the patient in order for the patient to make a reasonable decision.

The doctor has few defenses against battery. The patient does not have to prove through expert testimony what the standard of care was; the proof is only that the particular doctor failed to explain to the patient the nature and character of the particular procedure. Under battery theory, the patient need only show that an unconsented touching occurred. Under negligence theory, the patient must show that he or she would have declined a procedure if he or she had known all the details and risks. A doctor sued in a battery case has relatively little elbow room in which to establish a defense. A doctor sued for negligence in failing to disclose hazards has many possibilities on which to base a defense under the circumstances that existed.

Q. What is the standard of care concerning disclosure?
A. Although states are almost equally divided, a slight majority has adopted the professional disclosure standard, measuring the duty to disclose by the standard of the reasonable practitioner similarly situated. Expert testimony is required to establish the content of a reasonable disclosure.

Other states use the reasonable patient as the measure of the scope of disclosure. The effect of a patient-oriented disclosure standard is to ease the patient's burden of proof, because a jury could find that a doctor acted unreasonably in failing to disclose, despite unrebutted expert testimony to the contrary. This is because in these jurisdictions, the question of whether a doctor disclosed risks that a reasonable person would find material is for the jury to decide; technical expertise is not required because the standard is that of a reasonable person, not an expert of any sort.

PRODUCT LIABILITY LAW

Q. What is product liability?

A. Product liability is the generic phrase used to describe the liability of a supplier of a product to one injured by the product. There are five possible theories of liability available to someone suing for product liability: intent, negligence, strict liability, implied warranties of merchantability and fitness for a particular purpose, and express warranty and misrepresentation.

Q. Can a contact lens practitioner be sued under a product liability theory?

A. Yes. The most likely way the contact lens practitioner would be sued using a product liability claim would be under a strict liability theory, and the defect most likely to occur with contact lenses is inadequate warning. The law considers inadequate warning a product defect, which is why warnings are prominently displayed on many items you purchase.

The law says that a person in the business of selling a product, or a supplier of the product who makes money from the sale of the product, owes a duty to all foreseeable plaintiffs in the zone of foreseeable danger. This duty is breached if the product is defective when sold. Remember that inadequate warning about possible dangers of the product is considered a defect.

Misuse of the product by the patient is not a defense to a strict liability claim if the misuse is foreseeable. Over-wearing of contact lenses and misuse of or failure to use the correct contact lens solutions would be considered foreseeable misuse.

Q. How should contact lens practitioners protect themselves from a product liability suit?

A. The best way to protect yourself is to provide your patient with adequate warning about the dangers of contact lenses if the patient fails to carefully follow your instructions for wear, care, cleaning, disinfection, and handling. One test the court uses to determine if a product is unreasonably dangerous is if the product was dangerous beyond the expectation of the ordinary consumer. Another test is if there is a less dangerous alternative that was economically feasible. Make sure your patients understand wearing instructions and the importance of using the care products you prescribe. Warn against home remedies, even if they know someone else who uses them.

NEGLIGENCE

Q. How do contact lens practitioners protect themselves from a negligence suit?

A. Negligence is the tort that most doctors are referring to when they use the term malpractice, although there are many other legal theories a contact lens practitioner can be sued under and against which he or she should protect himself or herself.

There are four elements to the tort of negligence. The first is duty. You owe a duty of care to your patients. As a contact lens professional, your standard of care is that level of skill and learning commonly possessed by members in good standing of the same profession in the same or a similar community. If you call yourself a specialist, you will be held to a higher, national standard. There is controversy regarding whether there are specialists within the profession of optometry or whether optometry is a profession of generalists, and what standard should be used. Expert testimony is used to establish the standard of care.

The second element is breach of the duty of care. This is always a question of fact for the jury. Evidence that everyone in a profession is doing something is not conclusive proof that there is no breach. An entire profession can be negligent.

The next element is causation. The breach of duty must be the actual cause of the patient's injury. The patient must prove the injury would not have happened but for the breaching act of the doctor. The act must also be the legal cause of the injury, which in essence means that the injury was a foreseeable result of the breaching act.

The final element of the tort of negligence is damages. The patient must suffer actual damages. The extent of the injury does not have to be foreseeable. This means that any substandard act by the doctor that causes injury to the patient is compensable by law.

Q. How should a contact lens practitioner protect against a negligence suit?

A. The best defense is a good offense. Use due care in all interactions with your patients. Remember to evaluate whole eye health, and not just the contact lenses, on a regular basis. Document the results of tests, diagnosis, prognosis, and all interactions with your patients at the time they occur. This should include events such as a patient's failure to show up for an appointment and telephone follow-ups. Legible, consistent documentation is the best possible proof of due care.

Q. Is there anything else contact lens practitioners can do to protect themselves from lawsuits?

A. Yes. Studies have shown that a patient is much less likely to bring a lawsuit against a professional whom they like, even if they have been seriously injured by that practitioner's malpractice. This means that a professional who uses good communication skills, who takes the time to deal with the patient as a human being rather than a case, and perhaps shows some personal concern and compassion is much less likely to be sued under any circumstances. When patients see the practitioner as a caring human being, personally concerned with their eye health and visual performance, they will treat the practitioner with respect and understanding in return.

Q. Must a contact lens practitioner release a contact lens prescription to the patient?

A. Yes. The Federal Trade Commission (FTC), in its rulings called "Eyeglass I" and "Eyeglass II," say so. These administrative rulings have the force of law in all 50 states. The rules cover both eyeglasses and contact lenses. In writing a prescription for contact lenses, you do not need to include any measurements beyond those which you would have determined if the patient were to be fitted with eyeglasses. This means the prescription does not have to include keratometry readings, but you must include any specifications for contact lenses that state law requires to be included in the prescription. The FTC ruling requires you to prepare and release prescriptions. A prescription that you determine and write with due care that is valid for the time you specify serves to protect both you and the consumer.

BIBLIOGRAPHY

Calamari JD, Perillo JM. *Contracts; Black Letter Series,* 2nd ed. St. Paul, Minnesota, West Publishing Co., 1990.
Corbin AL. *Corbin on Contracts,* 18th ed. St. Paul, Minnesota, West Publishing Co., 1993.
Dobbs DB. *Handbook on the Law of Remedies: Damages, Equity, Restitution.* St. Paul, Minnesota, West Publishing Co., 1973.
Furrow BR, Johnson SH, et al. *Health Law: Cases, Materials,* 2nd ed. St. Paul, Minnesota, West Publishing Co., 1988.
McCormick CT. *Handbook on the Law of Damages.* St. Paul, Minnesota, West Publishing Co., 1935.
Prosser JM, Keeton WP. *Prosser and Keeton on the Law of Torts,* 5th ed. St. Paul, Minnesota, West Publishing Co., 1988.

Vertex Conversion Table and Diopter Conversion Table

VERTEX CONVERSION TABLE

Spectacle Lens Power	Plus Lenses — Vertex Distance/Millimeters								Minus Lenses — Vertex Distance/Millimeters							
	8	9	10	11	12	13	14	15	8	9	10	11	12	13	14	15
4.00	4.12	4.12	4.12	4.12	4.25	4.25	4.25	4.25	3.87	3.87	3.87	3.87	3.87	3.75	3.75	3.75
4.50	4.62	4.75	4.75	4.75	4.75	4.75	4.75	4.87	4.37	4.37	4.25	4.25	4.25	4.25	4.25	4.25
5.00	5.25	5.25	5.25	5.25	5.25	5.37	5.37	5.37	4.75	4.75	4.75	4.75	4.75	4.75	4.62	4.62
5.50	5.75	5.75	5.75	5.87	5.87	5.87	6.00	6.00	5.25	5.25	5.25	5.12	5.12	5.12	5.12	5.12
6.00	6.25	6.37	6.37	6.37	6.50	6.50	6.50	6.62	5.75	5.62	5.62	5.62	5.62	5.62	5.50	5.50
6.50	6.87	6.87	7.00	7.00	7.00	7.12	7.12	7.25	6.12	6.12	6.12	6.00	6.00	6.00	6.00	5.87
7.00	7.37	7.50	7.50	7.62	7.62	7.75	7.75	7.75	6.62	6.62	6.50	6.50	6.50	6.37	6.37	6.37
7.50	8.00	8.00	8.12	8.12	8.25	8.25	8.37	8.50	7.12	7.00	7.00	6.87	6.87	6.87	6.75	6.75
8.00	8.50	8.62	8.75	8.75	8.87	8.87	9.00	9.12	7.50	7.50	7.37	7.37	7.25	7.25	7.25	7.25
8.50	9.12	9.25	9.25	9.37	9.50	9.50	9.62	9.75	8.00	7.87	7.87	7.75	7.75	7.62	7.62	7.50
9.00	9.75	9.75	9.87	10.00	10.12	10.25	10.37	10.37	8.37	8.37	8.25	8.25	8.12	8.00	8.00	8.00
9.50	10.25	10.37	10.50	10.62	10.75	10.87	11.00	11.12	8.87	8.75	8.62	8.62	8.50	8.50	8.37	8.37
10.00	10.87	11.00	11.12	11.25	11.37	11.50	11.62	11.75	9.25	9.12	9.12	9.00	8.87	8.87	8.75	8.75
10.50	11.50	11.62	11.75	11.87	12.00	12.12	12.25	12.50	9.62	9.62	9.50	9.37	9.37	9.25	9.12	9.12
11.00	12.00	12.25	12.37	12.50	12.75	12.87	13.00	13.12	10.12	10.00	9.87	9.75	9.75	9.62	9.50	9.50
11.50	12.62	12.87	13.00	13.12	13.37	13.50	13.75	13.87	10.50	10.37	10.37	10.25	10.12	10.00	9.87	9.87
12.00	13.25	13.50	13.62	13.87	14.00	14.25	14.50	14.62	11.00	10.87	10.75	10.62	10.50	10.37	10.25	10.12
12.50	13.87	14.12	14.25	14.50	14.75	15.00	15.25	15.37	11.37	11.25	11.12	11.00	10.87	10.75	10.62	10.50
13.00	14.50	14.75	15.00	15.25	15.50	15.62	16.00	16.12	11.75	11.62	11.50	11.37	11.25	11.12	11.00	10.87
13.50	15.12	15.37	15.62	15.87	16.12	16.37	16.62	16.87	12.25	12.00	11.87	11.75	11.62	11.50	11.37	11.25
14.00	15.75	16.00	16.25	16.50	16.75	17.12	17.50	17.75	12.62	12.50	12.25	12.12	12.00	11.87	11.75	11.50
14.50	16.50	16.75	17.00	17.25	17.50	17.87	18.25	18.50	13.00	12.75	12.62	12.50	12.37	12.25	12.00	11.87
15.00	17.00	17.37	17.75	18.00	18.25	18.62	19.00	19.37	13.37	13.25	13.00	12.87	12.75	12.50	12.37	12.25
15.50	17.75	18.00	18.25	18.75	19.00	19.37	19.75	20.25	13.75	13.62	13.50	13.25	13.00	12.87	12.75	12.62
16.00	18.25	18.75	19.00	19.37	19.75	20.25	20.50	21.00	14.25	14.00	13.75	13.62	13.50	13.25	13.00	12.87
16.50	19.00	19.37	19.75	20.25	20.50	21.00	21.50	21.87	14.50	14.37	14.12	14.00	13.75	13.62	13.50	13.25
17.00	19.75	20.25	20.50	21.00	21.50	22.00	22.25	22.87	15.00	14.75	14.50	14.25	14.12	14.00	13.75	13.50
17.50	20.50	20.75	21.25	21.75	22.25	22.75	23.25	23.75	15.37	15.12	14.87	14.75	14.50	14.25	14.00	13.87
18.00	21.00	21.50	22.00	22.50	23.00	23.50	24.00	24.62	15.75	15.50	15.25	15.00	14.75	14.62	14.37	14.12
18.50	21.75	22.25	22.75	23.25	23.75	24.50	25.00	25.62	16.12	15.87	15.62	15.37	15.12	14.87	14.75	14.50
19.00	22.50	23.00	23.50	24.00	24.75	25.25	26.00	26.50	16.50	16.25	16.00	15.75	15.50	15.25	15.00	14.75

DIOPTER CONVERSION TABLE

Diopter	mm	Diopter	mm	Diopter	mm	Diopter	mm	Diopter	mm
36.00	9.37	40.12	8.41	44.25	7.63	48.37	6.98	52.50	6.43
36.12	9.34	40.25	8.38	44.37	7.61	48.50	6.96	52.62	6.41
36.25	9.31	40.37	8.36	44.50	7.58	48.62	6.94	52.75	6.40
36.37	9.27	40.50	8.33	44.62	7.56	48.75	6.92	52.87	6.38
36.50	9.24	40.62	8.30	44.75	7.54	48.87	6.91	53.00	6.36
36.62	9.21	40.75	8.28	44.87	7.52	49.00	6.89	53.12	6.35
36.75	9.18	40.87	8.25	45.00	7.50	49.12	6.87	53.25	6.34
36.87	9.15	41.00	8.23	45.12	7.48	49.25	6.85	53.37	6.32
37.00	9.12	41.12	8.20	45.25	7.46	49.37	6.84	53.50	6.31
37.12	9.09	41.25	8.18	45.37	7.44	49.50	6.82	53.62	6.29
37.25	9.06	41.37	8.16	45.50	7.42	49.62	6.80	53.75	6.28
37.37	9.03	41.50	8.13	45.62	7.40	49.75	6.78	53.87	6.26
37.50	9.00	41.62	8.10	45.75	7.38	49.87	6.77	54.00	6.25
37.62	8.97	41.75	8.08	45.87	7.36	50.00	6.75	54.12	6.23
37.75	8.94	41.87	8.06	46.00	7.34	50.12	6.73	54.25	6.22
37.87	8.91	42.00	8.03	46.12	7.32	50.25	6.72	54.37	6.21
38.00	8.88	42.12	8.01	46.25	7.30	50.37	6.70	54.50	6.19
38.12	8.85	42.25	7.99	46.37	7.28	50.50	6.68	54.62	6.18
38.25	8.82	42.37	7.96	46.50	7.26	50.62	6.67	54.75	6.16
38.37	8.79	42.50	7.94	46.62	7.24	50.75	6.65	54.87	6.15
38.50	8.76	42.62	7.92	46.75	7.22	50.87	6.63	55.00	6.13
38.62	8.73	42.75	7.89	46.87	7.20	51.00	6.62	55.12	6.12
38.75	8.70	42.87	7.87	47.00	7.18	51.12	6.60	55.25	6.10
38.87	8.68	43.00	7.85	47.12	7.16	51.25	6.58	55.37	6.09
39.00	8.65	43.12	7.82	47.25	7.14	51.37	6.57	55.50	6.08
39.12	8.62	43.25	7.80	47.37	7.12	51.50	6.55	55.62	6.07
39.25	8.59	43.37	7.78	47.50	7.10	51.62	6.54	55.75	6.05
39.37	8.57	43.50	7.76	47.62	7.08	51.75	6.52	55.87	6.04
39.50	8.54	43.62	7.74	47.75	7.06	51.87	6.50	56.00	6.03
39.62	8.51	43.75	7.71	47.87	7.05	52.00	6.49		
39.75	8.49	43.87	7.69	48.00	7.03	52.12	6.47		
39.87	8.46	44.00	7.67	48.12	7.01	52.25	6.46		
40.00	8.43	44.12	7.65	48.25	6.99	52.37	6.44		

Index

Note: Page numbers in *italics* indicate figures; those followed by a t indicate tables.

A

Abrasions, corneal, 116, 253–254
  keratoconus and, *303*
Acanthamoeba keratitis, 266–267, 275, 300
ACC Bivision lenses, 67–68, *68*
ACC translating design, 69–70, *72, 75, 76*
Acute red eye (ARE) response, 270
Acuvue lenses, 118, 121
Adaptation, to lenses, 64, 235–236, 236t
Adherence, lens, 115
Adventures in Color lenses, 192
Against-the-rule cornea, keratoconus and, 304
  prescribing for, 37–38
  toric soft lens for, 42, *44*
Age factors, 62, 87t
Agreement, lens-fitting, 312–313
Alden Optical Laboratories lenses, 192
Allergies, cleaning solutions and, 228, 276
  environmental, *265–267*, 265–268
  lenses and, disposable, 119–120
    extended wear, 104
    spherical, 219
  ring infiltrates from, *275*, 275
  toxic reactions and, 276–278, *277*
Anisometropia, after keratoplasty, 200
  from monovision lenses, 86
Anterior segment status, 80
Aphakia, adults with, 173–174
  children with, 134–136, *135*
  corneal vascularization and, *283*
  infants with, 165–173, 166t, 167t, *167–171*
  intra-corneal hemorrhage with, *285*
  lenses for, fluorosilicone acrylate, 172
    hydrogel, 172
    insertion of, 136–139, *137, 170,* 170–171, *171*
    rigid gas permeable, 172
  stromal striae and, 291–292
  tight lens syndrome and, 268
  unilateral, 140
Arcus, flecked, 280–281, *281*
ARE (acute red eye) response, 270
Arthritis, 275

Aspheric lenses, 66–67, *67, 68,* 73–74, 82–83
  keratoconus and, 149
  rigid gas permeable, 49–57, *50, 52, 53*
    corneal alignment of, *53*
    fitting of, 50–51
    flattening and, 51–56, *52, 53*
    problems with, 56–57, 57t
    uses of, 49
Asthenopia, 90t
Astigmatism, against-the-rule, 304
  corneal, 1, 39
    back-surface toric design for, 3t
    keratoplasty and, 199
    post-transplant, 213
  flowchart for, 60
  refractive, 10, 39
Athletic lenses, 125–131, 130t–131t
Axial edge lift approximation, 27t

B

Back-surface lenses, centration of, 34
  refractive correction of, *29*
  rigid gas permeable, 1–9
  vertex power of, 3–4
Balancing brightness test, 88
Base curve radius (BCR), aphakic lenses and, 167–168, *168*
  extended wear lenses and, 97, 109, 109t
  keratoconus and, 143, 143t
  orthokeratology and, 180
  Remba, 3t, 3–4
  Silsoft lenses and, *168*
  verification of, 8–9
Base curve–cornea relation, 21–23, *22*
Base–apex line, *12–14*
Basement membrane disease, 306–307, *307*
Bausch and Lomb Optima Toric lens, 43t
BCR. *See* Base curve radius (BCR).
Bifocal lenses, athletic, 129–131
  corneal measurement for, 60–62
  disposable, 122
  Fluoroperm ST, 70, 71t, *72*
  rigid gas permeable lenses and, 58–77, *67–76,* 71t, 73t